AMERICAN FOLK MEDICINE

PUBLISHED UNDER THE AUSPICES OF THE

CENTER FOR THE STUDY OF COMPARATIVE

FOLKLORE AND MYTHOLOGY, UNIVERSITY

OF CALIFORNIA, LOS ANGELES

American Folk Medicine
A Symposium

Edited, with an introduction, by WAYLAND D. HAND

UNIVERSITY OF CALIFORNIA PRESS

Berkeley   Los Angeles   London

*Publication of this book was supported in part
by NIH grant 1 R013 LM 02090-01 from the
National Library of Medicine*

University of California Press
Berkeley and Los Angeles, California

University of California Press, Ltd.
London, England

First Paperback Printing 1980
ISBN 0-520-04093-7
Library of Congress Catalog Card Number: 74-30522
Printed in the United States of America

1 2 3 4 5 6 7 8 9

Contents

Foreword

The UCLA Conference on American Folk Medicine, held December 13-15, 1973, was sponsored by the Center for the Study of Comparative Folklore and Mythology in cooperation with the Medical History Division of the UCLA School of Medicine and the Society for the History of Medical Science, Los Angeles. It was the first broadly interdisciplinary symposium of its kind ever to be held anywhere in the Americas. Twenty-five scholars representing many fields participarted in the conference. Professors John Q. Anderson and Bruce Jackson were unable to attend but sent papers. These are made a part of the proceedings of the conference. Professor Thelma G. James, an expert in the folklore of ethnic groups, was to have submitted a paper tentatively entitled "The Influence of Magic in Folk Medicine as Seen in the Collections Made in the Metropolitan Detroit Area," but she was taken ill before the conference and could not prepare the paper. With great aplomb Professor Thomas R. Forbes, Yale University, chaired the discussion sessions, "Summary and Prospect," at the end of the conference. Dr. Charles H. Talbot, Wellcome Institute of the History of Medicine, London, delivered the banquet address, "Classical Survivals in Folk Medicine," which appears as the lead article under the title "Folk Medicine and History."

The conference was planned by members of the Center for the Study of Comparative Folklore and Mythology and the Division of Medical History of the UCLA School of Medicine. Heading the four-man planning committee were Wayland D. Hand, Director of the Center (Program), and Robert G. Frank, Jr., Medical History (Local Arrangements). Michael O. Jones, History, and Donald J. Ward, Germanic Languages, rounded out the committee. In addition to its debt to the work of the committee, the conference owed its success to the efforts of Marjorie Griffin (Business Arrangements) and Elena Bradunas, who served as Liaison Officer.

All of us who were involved with the conference wish to express our particular thanks to Dean Sherman Mellinkoff of the UCLA School of Medicine and Martha Gnudi of the Society for the History of Medical Science, Los Angeles, for their help in the preliminary planning of the conference and Louise Darling, Librarian of the Bio-Medical Library, who made it possible for some of the sessions to be held in the library itself.

The conference was underwritten by the National Institutes of Health, and the publication of these proceedings was supported in part by NIH Grant 1 R013 LM 02090-01 from the National Library of Medicine.

In the name of the Center for the Study of Comparative Folklore and Mythology at UCLA, I wish to express gratitude to Wayland D. Hand for his efforts in directing the conference, to the National Institutes of Health, and to the other agencies and individuals who contributed to its success.

DONALD J. WARD

Introduction

WAYLAND D. HAND,
University of California, Los Angeles

The study of folk medicine in America, as elsewhere, has always been a common enterprise, claiming the attention, not only of people trained in the biological sciences, biochemistry, ethnobotany, ethnopsychology, ethnology, and so on, but also of travelers, cultural historians, anthropologists, and folklorists. First and foremost in this formidable array of scientists, of course, are medical doctors themselves and various practitioners in the expanding field of the health sciences. If this wide diversity of interest has brought multiple approaches to the assessment and study of the corpus of noninstitutionalized medicine, it has also brought specialization. In the case of many individual investigators, unfortunately, this specialization has resulted in too restricted a view of the whole ramifying field.

As one who has for many years worked primarily in only a single area of folk medicine, namely, folklore itself, I have come increasingly to feel the need for closer cooperation among all investigators concerned with medical care outside of professional medicine. The inveterate and pervasive appeal of folk medicine to large numbers of the sick and ailing in all cultures, including the most advanced countries in the world, must inevitably be faced. Long before Dr. D. C. Jarvis's *Folk Medicine* became a best-seller in the early 1960's— a book, after all, with little real merit as a treatment of American folk medicine—it was clear that millions of Americans were still clinging to old-fashioned medical recipes and were only reluctantly giving up time-tested home curative practices. Systematic efforts to debunk self-curing have been only partially successful. Not even the regular publicity given to sensational cases of fraud and death resulting from the unlicensed practice of medicine has diminished the natural proclivity to self-treatment that has continued to flourish from early times.

Sociologists and workers in the field of public health, cognizant of the persistence of folk medicine, have studied it as a part of the social process and have laid the groundwork, at last, for further studies in acculturation. Hospitals and other public institutions engaged in the delivery of health services have slowly tried to understand the many problems with which they are daily confronted by the reluctance of patients to put full trust in scientific medicine. Even medical schools, the last bastions of medical orthodoxy, are now increasingly taking ethnic, social, and cultural diversity into account as a necessary part of the training every doctor should receive. This is particularly the case if he is to practice medicine in rural areas or in the teeming inner city with its polyglot culture. Medical anthropologists and even faith healers are to be found in growing numbers in the modern medical establishment, if only in adjunct capacities. All of these developments have underscored the need for a broader view of the scope of folk medicine and the wit to deal with it in an enlightened medical policy.

As indicated above, I came to the study of folk medicine from the scholarly base of comparative folklore and mythology. As a by-product of my Dictionary of American Popular Beliefs and Superstitions, begun in the early 1940s, I have compiled a corpus of some three hundred thousand items of folk medicine, European as well as American, with token representation from elsewhere. Although this body of material was very rich in its purely folkloric component, until a few years ago it lacked the clinical depth and perspective that only a survey of medical writings could insure. This lack has now happily been repaired with timely assistance from the National Institutes of Health. At the present time efforts are being made to bring the holdings in Latin American and American Indian folk medicine up to a par with the Anglo-American corpus and the basic stocks from elsewhere in Europe against which American ethnomedicine is to be measured.

From my own research problems in connection with a systematic study of American folk medicine, manifest most often in inadequate coverage, incomplete data, wanting comparative treatment, and superficial analysis, there grew the conviction that scholars in various fields tributary to the study of folk medicine must somehow begin to work in concert. The founding of *Ethnomedizin: Zeitschrift für interdisziplinäre Forschung* in Hamburg in 1971, the readiness of medical historians to admit folk medicine to their scholarly concerns, and the increasing number of panel discussions of folk medicine in various learned societies led the director of the conference to the conclusion that the time was indeed ripe to convene the first general conference on folk medicine in the United States.

The proceedings of the conference tell their own story. Even though the ethnic treatment was not as wide-ranging as we had originally hoped and fewer disciplines and individual subject fields were covered than we had thought desirable at the time the program was planned, we nevertheless went ahead with the conference. We counted on a better representation in psychiatric medicine and medical psychology than we were able to schedule; but the one strong paper in this area, augmented by numerous references to psychological problems in other papers, helped, partially at least, to make up the deficiency. All in all, sufficient diversity of subject matter and viewpoint was developed during the three-day conference to give an adumbration of the general kinds of problems which workers in the field of American folk medicine are likely to encounter in their researches. The needs, and particularly the perspectives, came out more clearly in the discussions, of course, than in the papers themselves. Unfortunately these informal assessments could not be made a part of the published record, but it is heartening to know that participants in the conference, as well as the many auditors, have clear memories of what transpired and an even stronger sense of the positive effects and the accomplishments of the meetings.

It is not the director's purpose in this brief introduction to summarize any of the papers or even to rate the work or needs of given fields. Rather, he hopes to touch upon problems which all disciplines face and to suggest scholarly methods and approaches from which all fields stand to benefit. The need for systematic fieldwork, first of all, was echoed in several papers delivered at the conference, with the corollary desideratum of a strong data base to underlie theoretical formulations and working constructs. By common consent these needs are basic to successful work in folk medicine itself and all of its tributary fields. Directly related to field observation on a specific subject in a given area is the broader problem of geographical distribution and historical attachments. The misgivings of the banquet speaker, Dr. Charles H. Talbot, of the Wellcome Institute of the History of Medicine, London, about work in folk medicine largely in the modern geographical dimension, without thought to the possible time purchase, are in the main welltaken. To illustrate with a relevant matter from Latin American folk medicine and the theory of "hot" and "cold" diseases, "hot" and "cold" foods, "hot" and "cold" natural conditions, and so on: it is clear that the most careful fieldwork with informants exclusively in the modern setting would be notably enhanced if the investigator had knowledge of these "hot" and "cold" principles, which were enunciated in Galenic humoral pathology and then kept alive in the *Schulmedizin* of Europe for centuries until rudiments of the doctrine were carried to the New World with the early colonists.

Perhaps the best example of a modern work on folk medicine that takes into account folk beliefs and customs is Bakker's comparative work on the folk medicine of Waterland in the Netherlands.[1] A medical doctor in the town of Broek, near Amsterdam, Bakker collected folk medicine in connection with his daily practice throughout his career. Unsatisfied with a mere recording of modern Dutch folk medical beliefs and customs, Bakker copiously annotated his stout volume of over six hundred pages with comparative materials from writers on science and medicine from classical times forward. This excellent work of reference and others like it point up the need for more historical studies, particularly if the "learned" ancestry of many items of folk medicine is not to go unnoticed. To be understood in this connection is folk medicine, or common medical practice, which found its way into the accepted curing regimen and was then handed down in standard medical treatises century after century. In this way an item of scientific medicine in one generation might, in a sense, be discarded, only to be picked up and kept alive in an ongoing folk tradition, from which, in a free give-and-take, scientific medicine itself was occasionally enriched. It was in this general philosophical framework that three or four speakers at the conference suggested the connections between medicine and folk medicine and science and folklore at different periods of history. Cultural background of the kind adduced, of course, adds a whole new dimension of understanding and appreciation and affirms ongoing popular traditions that span not only centuries but whole continents as well.

In a generation brought up on the pragmatic approach to problems, workers in increasing numbers have come to insist on an analysis of function and meaning in folklore as it relates to modern life. Pursuant to these aims, several papers were addressed to the relationship of curer and patient and to the role of the folk medical practitioner in the community and society at large. The application of sociopsychological insights to the dynamic relationships existing among the healer, the patient, and the extended family group is a phenomenon that reaches its maximum potential, perhaps, in the study of shamanism. Yet the same element of trust and faith, as many of the conference papers show, is basic to almost any kind of folk curative procedure, not merely to one in which professionalism is as strong and its safeguards as well established as they are in the shamanic office. The same close rapport between doctor and patient, it may be observed, is essential at any level of medical practice, and one may therefore expect to find comparably close relationships between healer and patient in medical situations of all kinds, whether in very primitive societies or in more advanced cultures.

There is not much difficulty in tracing affinities between American folk medicine and medical beliefs and practices that derive from a common European past. The European counterparts are traced in Hovorka and Kronfeld's standard volumes on comparative folk medicine[2] and in various other compendious works dealing with the European scene. They are confirmed on this side of the Atlantic in annotated studies of all kinds that take European folk medicine into account. The same is true to some extent of American aboriginal medicine, particularly with regard to natural or botanic medicine, thanks to the efforts of numerous investigations, not the least of which is Virgil Vogel's standard work, *American Indian Medicine*.[3] It is generally assumed that in the exchange of cultural legacies at the folk level as they relate to the human body and its care, the Indian gave more than he received in the acculturative process. My own researches indicate, however, that the borrowing by Indians from the white tradition is considerably greater than is commonly supposed. Comparative research on individual matters will show the full extent of the borrowing of the North American Indian from the white man's repertories of natural and botanic medicine.

Magical medicine, of course, is an entirely different matter. Not enough has been done to show, even in a general way, how substantial an exchange of curative rituals and practices may have taken place since the time of contact. Passing the sick through clefts in trees and through other apertures is found sporadically in the Latin American tradition, as is "measuring," but my limited reading of American Indian medicine does not indicate that this old-world practice was known among the American Indians. Similar uncertainty holds true with regard to the magical transference of disease, including "plugging" and the magical implantation of a disease in a new host. In the interest of stimulating a search for some of these European divestment rituals in American Indian medicine, I am listing some of my studies on the subject that may serve as guidelines for a search of early American historical documents as well as for field investigations where some of these rituals may still be practiced.[4] Even if the existence of these curatives practices could be established, there would still remain the problem of determining whether they were native to the aboriginal peoples or whether they were introduced by the earliest colonists from Europe. In this task only historical research of the most exacting kind can bring to light the information that is needed.

These are a few of the interesting problems that may be looked into further as a direct result of the UCLA Conference on American Folk Medicine. Other such gatherings at proper intervals over the years will be able to reveal what progress has been made in dealing with the myriad problems of sickness and health, concerns that are as vital to human welfare as they are ancient and pervasive.

NOTES

1. C. Bakker, *Volksgeneeskunde in Waterland: Een Vergelijkende Studie met de Geneeskunde der Grieken en Romeinen* (Amsterdam: H. J. Paris, 1928).

2. Dr. O. v. Hovorka and Dr. A. Kronfeld, *Vergleichende Volksmedizin: Eine Darstellung volksmedizinischer Sitten und Gebräuche, Anschauungen und Heilfaktoren, des Aberglaubens und der Zaubermedizin*, 2 vols. (Stuttgart: Verlag von Strecker und Schröder, 1908-1909).

3. Vigil J. Vogel, *American Indian Medicine* (Norman: University of Oklahoma Press, 1970).

4. Wayland D. Hand, "'Passing Through': Folk Medical Magic and Symbolism," *Proceedings of the American Philosophical Society*, 112 (1968), 379-402; *idem.*, "'Measuring' with String, Thread, and Fibre: A Practice in Folk Medical Magic," in *Festschrift für Robert Wildhaber zum 70. Geburtstag am 3. August 1972*, ed. Walter Escher, Theo Gantner, und Hans Trümpy (Basel: Verlag G. Krebs AG., 1973), pp. 240-251; *idem.*, "'Measuring' and 'Plugging': The Magical Containment and Transfer of Disease," *Bulletin of the History of Medicine*, 48 (1974), 221-233; *idem.*, "Plugging, Nailing, Wedging, and Kindred Folk Medical Practices," in *Folklore and Society: Essays in Honor of Benj. A. Botkin*, ed. Bruce Jackson (Hatboro, Pa.: Folklore Associates, 1966), pp. 63-75. Related problems are to be found in my article "The Magical Transference of Disease," *North Carolina Folklore*, 13 (1965), 83-109. This volume of *North Carolina Folklore* appeared simultaneously under the title *Folklore Studies in Honor of Arthur Palmer Hudson*.

Folk Medicine and History

CHARLES H. TALBOT, *Wellcome Institute of the History of Medicine, London*

In this august assembly of scholars, experts in folklore, physicians, pharmacologists, and psychiatrists, I feel somewhat of an interloper, since I am merely a historian of medicine and particularly of medieval medicine. It is presumptuous of me even to think of passing any comments on all that has been said and done here during the past few days, but since I have been invited to do so, I will give you my reactions.

Let me say at once that I find it admirable that folklorists travel extensively and spend months, sometimes years, in collecting folklore details and recording them for posterity. I admire their devotion, their idealism, and their industry; and in my estimation they fulfill to perfection the command given in the Gospel: gather up the fragments lest they be lost.

But on the whole I find that folklorists are fascinated more by geography than history. They are more interested in showing the spatial extent of a belief or a custom than in plumbing its depths. Diffusion, rather than origin, seems to be their main concern. For this reason I would like to commend to them another scriptural text: by their fruits ye shall know them; or rather, if one may be permitted to modify the words in one small detail: by their roots ye shall know them.

If we know only the terminal belief or the present custom, we merely recognize the leaf. What we have to examine are the branches and the roots. These will give us a complete understanding of the widespread, organic growth of the tree that first emerged from a tiny seed and then developed over the centuries.

This is what folklorists ought to be interested in and ought to pursue.

Let me give you an example. In the books which record recent folk medical practices in the state of Pennsylvania, mention is made of the employment of the peony as a cure for epilepsy. The sources of this practice are traced back to books of the early eighteenth century, and it has been generally assumed that they go back no farther. During this conference, the date has been pushed back a little farther into the sixteenth century, and the use of the peony is now said to derive from a book by Romanus. The fact is that the peony was already being recommended as a cure for epilepsy in the twelfth century, when Bartholomaeus of Salerno mentioned it in *De aegritudinum curatione*. Where he picked up this remedy we do not know, but quite possibly he had read about it in Galen, who in the second century A.D. recorded that he had used it and found it efficacious. Since Galen was a Greek and was recording a folk medical practice of his day, it is likely that the use of the peony had a long history. Indeed, Pliny tells us in his *Natural History* that the plant took its name from Paion, who first discovered its medical properties. He appears in the *Iliad* as a healer, and consequently the belief in the efficacy of the peony goes back to at least 800 B.C., a long and illustrious tradition.

But this is by no means a unique example. All books dealing with folk medicine and providing lists of herbs that cure various diseases invariably include such plants as artemisia, centaury, achillea, chironia, and many others. Artemisia takes its name from the goddess Artemis; centaury derives from the centaur who was supposed to have discovered the medical properties of this plant and passed on the knowledge to Apollo and thence to Aesculapius; chironia also owes its name to Chiron the centaur; and achillea obviously stems from Achilles. These figures belong to the heroic age of Greece, and their connection with healing herbs that are in common use in folk medicine today indicates how ancient are the beliefs and practices we have inherited.

Most of the rituals for the gathering of herbs are also ancient. The prescriptions about the time of the year when medicinal herbs are to be gathered, about the observance of the phases of the moon, the days of the week, even the hours of the day, whether at sunrise, sunset, midnight, or midday, are survivals, not of the eighteenth century but of much earlier times. They can be traced back in almost unbroken line to the Middle Ages, to the Anglo-Saxon leech books of the ninth and tenth century, to Pseudo-Apuleius's herbal, to Marcellus of Bordeaux of the fourth century, to Pliny, and even beyond that. The propitiatory rites which are observed by the North American Indians when plucking a medicinal plant from the ground, the leaving of some little sacrifice, such as tobacco, to atone for having robbed Mother Earth of one of her creatures, also find an echo in such writers as Vergil and Pliny.

The so-called powwow charms, which occur so frequently in the folk medicine of Pennsylvania, are also much earlier than the eighteenth-century German sources from which they have been translated. I refer specifically to those charms which are concerned with the cure of toothache or with the arresting of nosebleed. The verses which were recited over the victim of toothache have been transmitted to us almost unchanged since they were first translated into the vernacular from Latin and incorporated into the *Lacnunga*, a collection comprising elements from the Byzantine liturgy and other Eastern texts. In fact, they derive from an apocryphal gospel and biography of Saint John the Evangelist which was circulating among the oriental churches from a very early date. The charms for nosebleed go back at least to the fourth century of our era, one of the earliest examples being found engraved on a Byzantine cup. In this particular case the saint invoked was Saint Zacharias, but other charms to stop bleeding call upon Longinus, the centurion who pierced Christ's side with a spear at the Crucifixion, or Saint Veronica, the pious woman who proferred a towel to wipe Christ's bleeding face as he carried the cross to Calvary. All these versions survive in one form or another in modern folk medicine.

Mention was made during the conference of the so-called Himmelsbrief, which appears in many forms and is attached to the names of various churches. This letter, which supposedly came from heaven, was concerned in its original form with the church at Jerusalem. Its diffusion in the West was due to the Irish missionaries, who were spreading the Gospel among the Germanic peoples. The Irish always had a penchant for teachings that were slightly unorthodox, and it was because of this proclivity that many pseudoreligious writings were disseminated among the half-pagan, half-Christian communities of the seventh and eighth centuries. Saint Boniface, the Anglo-Saxon missionary who was evangelizing the Germans, found his efforts at conversion put in jeopardy by this irresponsible conduct. The protagonist in encouraging belief in the Himmelsbrief was an Irish monk called Clement. So Boniface had him summoned before a synod, which, after protracted examination of the document, condemned Clement as a heretic and consigned the Himmelsbrief to the flames. Its persistence in folklore and folk medicine shows how deeply ingrained certain ideas may become. But what is really interesting is the long history that goes behind it, for it probably originated among the Syriac Christians and may have been centuries old before the Irish accepted it and propagated its teaching.

It would be wearisome to list the various beliefs that survive in folk medicine today and whose roots strike deep into civilizations that have long since died out. But one indubitable fact emerges: wherever we look in folk medicine we find the traditions, the customs, the remedies, the whole corpus of doctrine drawing substance and vigor from an almost timeless source, as if they belonged to the very nature of man himself.

The Madstone

THOMAS R. FORBES, *Yale University School of Medicine*

Lithotherapy, the use of stones or stonelike objects for the treatment of illness and injury, was a practice that extended back through the Middle Ages and into antiquity.[1] Some of the stones were precious or semiprecious gems such as diamonds or amethysts or topazes. Some, like coral and pearls, came from the sea. Others were actually or allegedly produced in the bodies of real or imagined creatures— the rooster, deer, dragon, and many others. Numerous so-called stones were in fact minerals. Some stones worked their cures when carried as amulets. Others were applied directly to a lesion or were ground to powder and became ingredients of supposedly healing mixtures. The virtues of stones were passed on verbally and from time to time were compiled into lapidary books by encyclopedists like Bishop Marbode of Rennes.[2]

Several kinds of stone were highly recommended for the cure of snakebite. The relative prominence of snake stones in European lapidary writings, incidentally, supplements other evidence that this superstition originated in warm countries of the East, where poisonous snakes constitute a far greater hazard to life than they do in Germany or France or England. Early travelers brought back many tales of snake stones from India. One variety of the stone was allegedly found in the head of a snake, particularly the cobra de capello. The stone was said to draw out the poison from the bites of all kinds of venomous creatures and even arrow poison. The technique was to apply the stone to the wound. The stone would adhere until it had drawn out all the venom and would then drop off, and the victim would be cured. Later the stone was soaked in milk, preferably human, whereupon the poison left the stone, passing into the milk and discoloring it. After this cleansing the stone could be used again.[3] Vincent of Beauvais mentions the snake stone in his *Speculum naturale*, compiled in the thirteenth century.[4] In Bengal it was believed that a snake stone could be found in the head of the adjutant bird,[5] a large stork which, incidentally, is protected by law in India because it kills many snakes.

Another kind of snake stone was the ophite, so called, according to Christopher Entzelt, a sixteenth-century lapidarist, "because it has the color of serpents."[6] Ophite, now a name applied to a kind of feldspar, or crystalline rock, seems originally to have been related to the famous *ovum anguinum*, or "snake's egg," described by Pliny. He tells a particularly unlikely tale about how the latter is produced by a coiled mass of snakes, then goes on to quote further details supplied, he says, by the Druids. Obviously much of this, including the belief that the true *ovum anguinum* will float upstream even when set in gold, is too much for Pliny's credulity. However, he does state that "for my part, I have seen this egg, about the bigness of a medium sized apple . . . , a badge of office among the Druids."[7] But Pliny says nothing about use of the stone to cure snakebite.

Anselm de Boodt, a lapidarist of the early seventeenth century, writes at length about both the "Snake stone famous among the Bohemians" and the *ovum anguinum*.[8] Glass amulets shaped like beads and known as adder beads or snake stones were observed in Wales and the Scottish Highlands at the end of the seventeenth century,[9] but King, an authority on gems, says that these were "nothing more than the central ornaments of Roman, British and Saxon necklaces."[10]

Best known of the stones alleged to remove or neutralize all kinds of poison was the bezoar. According to sixteenth-century lapidarists, it occurred in a variety of shapes, sizes, and colors. The name itself was derived from Arabic and Persian words meaning "antidote" or "protecting against poison." The bezoar was found in the digestive tracts of various animals, ruminants in particular. A stone from the white stag was greatly prized.[11] Concretions, sometimes around hair balls, do indeed occur in the stomach, intestines, and gall bladders of animals, including man; this much of the story is true.[12] Chemical analysis of one such stone from a deer showed it to be composed mostly of calcium phosphate. The stone was able to absorb water up to 5 percent of its weight.[13]

A famous test of the powers of the bezoar was performed by Ambroise Paré, the great sixteenth-century French surgeon. He wrote at some length about the concretion, found in sundrie shapes, but commonly it resembles an Acorne or Date-stone; it is sometimes of a sanguine color, and otherwhiles of a hony-like or yellowish colour, but most frequently of a blackish or darke greene, resembling the colour of mad Apples [the fruit of hawthorn], or else of a Civet Cat.

Paré was surgeon to Charles IX of France. One day the latter asked Paré about the efficacy of the bezoar. It must be remembered that lapidary superstitions were generally believed at the time. Paré replied cautiously and proposed that the stone be tested on a criminal sentenced to be hanged. The wretched man agreed gladly to take poison, obviously believing that if he then received a prep-aration of ground bezoar, his life would be saved and he would, as agreed, go free. He swallowed corrosive sublimate and then powdered bezoar and died in agony. Paré performed an autopsy and confirmed the cause of death. The great surgeon, a compas-sionate man, must have been horrified at the outcome of his experiment. It is to his credit that nonetheless he recorded the details for the enlightenment of his profession.[14]

The bezoar was often recommended for treatment of persons bitten by rabid dogs. Before any discussion of this remedy, it must be stated that in the centuries preceding Pasteur's discovery of an effective protection against rabies, a vast number of other treat-ments, none of them really successful, had accumulated. Some idea of their variety can be obtained from perusing simply the titles of the books and articles listed under the heading "Hydrophobia (*Treatment of*)" in the first series (1885) of the *Index–Catalogue of the Surgeon-General's Office*.[15] Procedures that were tried, sometimes repeatedly, included the following:

Amputation	Galvanic electricity
Application of ice to spine	Submersion
Cauterization	Sweating
Cold baths	Tracheotomy
	Venesection or cupping

Many drugs were recommended, some of them as "certain cure" or "infallible":

Alcohol	Atropine
Ammonia	Belladonna
Amyl nitrite	Cantharides
Anagallis	Chloral

Chloroform
Cinereus terrestris
Cinnabar
Cockchafer
Common salt
Curare
Dampier's powder
Datura stramonium
Ether
Euphorbia
Garlic
Gentian root
Guaco
Hairs of the rabid dog
Hashish
Hydrochloric Acid
Hydrocyanic acid
Iron subcarbonate
Laudanum

Lead acetate
Mercury
Morphine
Musk
Oil of Turpentine
Opium
Pilocarpine
Potassium bromide
Potassium cyanide
Potassium permanganate
Simaba cedron seeds
Scutellaria lateriflora (madweed)
Tincture of Calabar bean
   (physostigmine)
Tobacco smoke
Vinegar
Viper poison
Xanthium

In his struggle to find a cure for this terrible disease, an eighteenth-century Polish surgeon, called on to care for "eleven Persons bitten by a mad Wolf," administered six different treatment regimes to *five pairs of patients and to one individual.*[16] Fifty years later, a British surgeon, despairing of contemporary remedies, turned to the ancients:

> Every remedial measure recently tried for the prevention and cure of hydrophobia having confessedly proved ineffectual, I beg to call the attention of the profession to a method of treatment which is said to have proved eminently successful in ancient times. I allude particularly to the internal use of the Veratrum Album, or White Hellebore, to which, however, as an auxiliary, was commonly joined the external application of the actual cautery to the wound.[17]

About the middle of the nineteenth century, newspapers in Bexar County, Texas, were recommending "leaf tobacco, vinegar, calomel, sage, asparagus, ashroot tea, chloride of lime, caustic potash, excision of wound, mercury ointment, hot iron, lobelia, hydrochloric acid, spirits of hartshorn, etc."[18] for the treatment of hydrophobia. So it is small wonder that there should be a demand for a stone that seemed simply by its application to prevent ill effects from the bite of a rabid dog or other animal.

Madstone is a term that almost certainly originated in the United

States. The earliest use of the word cited in the *Oxford English Dictionary* is in 1864.[19] The history of madstone has been complicated by its application retroactively to stones dating from earlier centuries.[20] However, I have not encountered the word madstone in lapidaries or in other writings antedating the mid-nineteenth century. *Webster* and other authorities confirm that madstone is of United States origin; the fact that the word does not appear in the 1968 edition of *Webster's New World Dictionary* suggests that the term is disappearing from the American scene.[21]

As might be expected, several kinds of madstone were recognized. Some were truly stones or stonelike, described variously as "a brown, striated porous pebble,"[22] as "aluminous shale or other absorptive substance,"[23] as "a worn piece of white feldspar,"[24] a flattened pebble,[25] porous "calcareous rock such as halloysite,"[26] or as fine-grained, deep pink, and lighter than, but about as hard as, soapstone.[27] A second class included the various kinds of bezoar, frequently those from deer.[28] Finally, and perhaps uniquely, there was a polished seed from the Kentucky coffee tree, "offered to the Smithsonian Institution as a genuine madstone of proved efficacy for the sum of $1,000."[29] The term *madstone* was applied to other substances, including the ancient tabasheer, a vegetable material;[30] but as already indicated, such usage seems anachronistic.

Because of their porosity, most madstones were apparently quite absorbent. The stone was moistened before use and then, like the snake stone, applied to the wound, to which it either adhered or was bound with a bandage. The victim might then, it was said, experience a sucking sensation from the stone. It was supposed to cling until saturated with poison or until all of it had been extracted. The stone was then placed in warm milk. If bubbles (actually, air trapped in the interstices of the stone) appeared and if the milk turned greenish, the stone was ready for use again. Persons treated with it only many hours after being injured might become nauseated, vomit, and then sleep deeply.[31]

The madstone was credited with numerous cures. The reason for its apparent success, of course, was that most dogs that bite are not mad and most snakes that bite are not venomous.[32] In addition, the madstone could provide powerful psychological support at a time of great stress—for example, when no doctor was available. Let us examine some case histories of the madstone and its predecessors in this country.

Best known of them all was the Lee stone. In his introduction to *The Talisman*, first published in 1825, Sir Walter Scott speaks of a Sir Simon Lockhart of Lee and Cartland who helped to fight the

Saracens in the Holy Land late in the twelfth century. There as a ransom he obtained a pebble set into a coin. According to the story, water into which this talisman had been dipped would relieve fever, stop bleeding, and work other cures. Whatever may be said for this tale, the coin with its stone, known as the Lee penny, did exist early in the nineteenth century, by which time it was being used, according to Scott, mostly for the cure of persons bitten by mad dogs. He sensibly remarked that "as the illness in such cases frequently arises from imagination, there can be no reason for doubting that water which has been poured on the Lee penny furnishes a congenial cure." The stone was for a long time owned by the Lockharts of Lee, in Lanarkshire. It was described as small, roughly triangular, dark red, and set into a coin called a groat. The amulet was used by high and low in case of need; once in the reign of Charles I it was borrowed under a bond of £6,000 to combat an epidemic of plague in Newcastle.

The Reformed Protestant Church of Scotland, endeavoring in the seventeenth century to wipe out, or at least to diminish, superstition, considered the Lee penny. The Synod of the Presbyterian Church of Glasgow concluded that the amulet was used without

> any words such as Charmers and Sorcereirs use in their unlawfull practisess; and considering that in nature thair are many things seen to work strange effects, whereof no human wit can give a reason, it having pleast God to give stones and herbes a special virtue for the healing of many infirmities in man and beast, advises the Brethren to surcease thair process, as wherein they perceive no ground of Offence, and admonishes the said Laird of Lee, in the using of the said stone to take heid that it be usit hereafter with the least scandle that possibly maybe.[33]

The family of Joseph Fredd, of Loudoun County, Virginia, is said to have owned a famous stone for the cure of persons bitten by mad dogs,[34] and there is a report that this was actually the Lee penny brought to this country from Scotland in 1776,[35] but it seems very unlikely that the Lee penny became the Fredd stone, since early nineteenth-century reports about the latter do not mention a Scottish origin[36] and since Scott himself wrote in 1832 that the Lee penny was still in the possession of that family.[37]

In 1805, according to a justly indignant physician, "a Mr. Micow, of Virginia, announced to the public his being possessed of [a madstone], and proposed to the inhabitants of four or five adjacent counties to sell it for the moderate sum of 2000 dollars, in shares of 10 dollars each."[38]

The Reverend Mr. Lewis Chaustien of Frederick County, Virginia, cured a child bitten by a mad dog, according to the child's father. Pieces of a madstone were applied successively for twenty-four hours. The Reverend Chaustien "purged" the stone by putting it in hot water. Soon bubbles arose,

> and a small scum, like oil of a yellow colour, tinged with green, appeared on the top of the water, which Mr. Chaustien informed me was poison. After the stone had been some short time in water, it was taken out and put into warm ashes to dry. Mr. Chaustien showed me a certificate which accompanied the stone, and called it by the name of the *Chinese Snake Stone*, and which said that it came from Bombay in (I think) 1740.[39]

The word *madstone*, incidentally, does not appear in either of these accounts.

The *Dallas Weekly Herald* for May 22, 1875, carried a lengthy front-page account by a Mr. James of Fannin County, who on April 2 was bitten by a dog on the streets of Sherman, which was furious from the effects of hydrophobia. Passing down the street, he was approached by the dog, as he came snapping along, his mouth white with froth. Before Mr. James had time to offer any defence, the infuriated animal laid hold of one of his legs, and his teeth were sunk in the flesh! The dog ran on, but was soon overtaken and killd. Mr. James was induced to at once start out in search of a mad-stone, and on arriving at the residence of Mr. McKinney, in Collin Country, near Van Alstyne, the stone was found and applied to the wound, but refused to take hold. Three days from the time the wound was inflicted, a dull unnatural headache was felt, and the limb began to swell. The stone was again applied, and this time with the most satisfactory results. The stone at once commenced drawing, and so continued for thirty-one hours, becoming filled and dropping off four times, since which time Mr. James has felt not the slightest return of the symptoms of hydrophobia, and to the virtues of this stone he is, no doubt, indebted for his life.... The remarkable properties of this stone may in some degree be appreciated when it [is] stated that during the forty-seven years it has been in his [McKinney's] possession, it has been applied to four hundred different parties who have been bitten by rabid animals, and effected a permanent cure in every instance but two.... We do not know how the Esculapian fraternity of the day regard the madstone, but presume they consign it to the apron strings of "old women doctors." As for us, we cannot imagine a more striking proof of its efficacy than that adduced, which is strictly reliable.[40]

Four years later, another Texas madstone had its day in the papers. On May 3, 1879, the *Galveston Daily News* reported from Gainesville that "a man in town yesterday from the Pan Handle said he had been bitten by a mad dog and had ridden 350 miles in four days and nights, coming to a mad stone. The stone stuck nine times. This gentlemen says the Indians are on the war path. . . ."[41]

In 1877 it was reported that a Kentucky madstone had cured fifty-nine people in twenty-three years.[42] Good results in Nevada, Missouri, and Florida were reported in the press in 1888.[43] Several other alleged cures have been described in valuable reviews by Blanton, Cheshire, and Dobie.[44] But one watches in vain for contemporary mention of the madstone.

NOTES

This research was supported by NIH grant 5 RO1 LM 01538-02 from the National Library of Medicine.

1. See, for example, Joan Evans, *Magical Jewels of the Middle Ages and Renaissance* (Oxford: Clarendon Press, 1922), pp. 14–15; T. R. Forbes, "Chalcedony and Childbirth," in *The Midwife and the Witch* (New Haven, Conn.: Yale University Press, 1966), pp. 64–79; Forbes, "Lapis Bufonis: the Growth and Decline of a Medical Superstition," *Yale Journal of Biology and Medicine*, 45 (1972), 139–149.

2. Marbode, "Le Lapidaire," in *Poèmes* (Rennes: Verdier, n.d.), p. 147.

3. D. Hervey, "'Plotosus canius' and the 'Snake-stone,'" *Nature*, 62 (1900), 79; G. F. Kunz, "Madstones and Their Magic," *Science*, 18 (1891), 286–287; G. F. Kunz, *The Magic of Jewels and Charms* (Philadelphia: Lippincott, 1915), pp. 230–233.

4. Vincent de Beauvais, *Speculum naturale* (Nürnberg: Anton Koberger [ca. 1486], n.p.

5. Thomas Carson, *Ranching, Sport, and Travel* (London: Unwin, 1911), p. 33.

6. Christophorus Encelius, *De lapidibus & gemmis* (Francofurtus: Egenolphus, 1557), cap. 40.

7. M. E. Littré, trans., *Histoire naturelle de Pline* (Paris: Firmin Didot, 1865), liv. 29, cap. 12, pp. 305–306.

8. A. B. de Boodt, *Gemmarum et lapidum historia* (Hanovia: Wechelius, 1609), cap. 173, 174.

9. Kunz, *Magic*, pp. 226-227; J. Y. Simpson, "Notes on Some Scottish Magical Charm-stones, or Curing-Stones," *Proc. Soc. Antiquaries of Scotland*, 4 (1860-61), 211-224.

10. C. W. King, *Antique Gems* (London: Murray, 1860), p. 455.

11. *Le jardin de santé* (Paris: le Noir [1529]), n.p.; Andreas Baccius, *De gemmis et lapidibus pretiosis* (Francofurtus: Becker, 1603), pp. 182–187; Boodt, *op. cit.*, cap. 191–194; Encelius, *op. cit.*, cap. 49.

12. V. H. Cahalane, *Mammals of North America* (New York: Macmillan, 1947), p. 39.

13. H. C. White, "The Chemical and Physical Characters of the So-Called 'Mad-Stone,'" *Chemical News, London*, 88 (1903), p. 180.

14. Thomas Johnson, trans., *The Workes . . . of Ambrose Parey* (London: Cotes and Du-Gard, 1649), bk. 21, chap. 36, pp. 529–530.

15. (Washington, D.C., Government Printing Office, 1885), 6, pp. 594–599.

16. Wolf, "Account of Trials made with different Medicines, reckoned the most effectual in Cases of canine Madness, on eleven Persons bitten by a mad Wolf," *Gentlemen's Magazine*, 38 (1768), 260-261.

17. Frederick Adams, "Hydrophobia. Ancient Mode of Treating Persons Bitten by Mad Dogs," *London Medical and Physical J.*, 60 (1828), 1-5.

18. P. I. Nixon, *A Century of Medicine in San Antonio* (San Antonio, Texas; privately printed, 1936), p. 109.

19. J. A. H. Murray, ed., *A New English Dictionary on Historical Principles* (Oxford: Clarendon Press, 1908).

20. For example, Kunz, *Magic*, p. 225; White, *op. cit.*

21. The madstone must, incidentally, be distinguished from other stones once supposed to cure human madness.

22. Charles Whitebread, "The Magic, Psychic, Ancient Egyptian, Greek, and Roman Medical Collections of the Division of Medicine in the United States National Museum," *Proc. U.S. National Museum*, 65 (1924), 1-44.

23. Kunz, *Magic*, p. 235.

24. W. J. Hoffman, "Folk-Medicine of the Pennsylvania Germans," *Proc. Amer. Philosophical Soc.*, 26 (1889), 329-352.

25. W. J. Hoffman, "A Description of the 'Mad-Stone,'" *San Francisco Western Lancet*, 13 (1884), 4-5.

26. W. B. Blanton, "Madstones, with an Account of Several from Virginia," *Annals Med. History*, n.s. 7 (1935), 268-273; C. W. Dulles, "The Mad-Stone," *J. Amer. Med. Assoc.*, 34 (1900), 1208-1209; J. M. Flint, "What are Madstones?" *St. Nicholas*, 36 (1909), 271-272; Whitebread, *op. cit.*

27. J. B. Cheshire, *Nonnulla* (Chapel Hill: University of North Carolina Press, 1930), p. 204.

28. Blanton, *op. cit.*; A. M. Cleaveland, *No Life for a Lady* (Boston: Houghton Mifflin, 1941), p. 149; J. F. Dobie, "Madstones and Hydrophobia Skunks," in *Madstones and Twisters*, ed. M. C. Boatright, W. M. Hudson, and Allen Maxwell (Dallas, Texas: Southern Methodist University Press), p. 5; Dulles, *op. cit.*; Flint, *op. cit.*; Hoffman, "A Description"; Whitebread, *op. cit.*; W. G. Zeigler and B. S. Grosscup, *The Heart of the Alleghanies [sic]* (Cleveland: Brooks, 1883), pp. 157-158.

29. Flint, *op. cit.*; Whitebread, *op. cit.*

30. Kunz, *Magic*, p. 235.

31. Blanton, *op. cit.*; Cheshire, *op. cit.*, pp. 206-207; Dobie, *op. cit.*, p. 7; Hoffman, "A Description."

32. Blanton, *op. cit.*; James Mease, "On Snake Stones and Other Remedies for the Cure of Diseases Produced by the Bites of Snakes and Mad Dogs," *Philadelphia Med. Museum*, 5 (1808), 1-15.

33. Sir Walter Scott, *The Talisman*, Introduction and Note III.

34. W. H. Harding, "On the Chinese Snake-Stone, and Its Operation as an Antidote to Poison," *Med. Repository*, 10 (1807), 248-250; Mease, *op. cit.*

35. *Encyclopedia Americana*; "What Are Madstones?" *St Nicholas*, 35 (1909), 271-272.

36. Harding, *op. cit.*; Mease, *op. cit.*

37. Scott, *op. cit.*

38. Mease, *op. cit.*

39. Harding, *op. cit.*

40. "The Mad Stone," *"Dallas Weekly Herald*, May 22, 1875.

41. *Galveston Daily News*, May 3, 1879.

42. W. G. Black, *Folk Medicine* (London: Folk-Lore Society, 1883), pp. 144-146.

43. J. S. Farmer, ed., *Americanisms* (London: Poulter, 1889), p. 335; Murray, *op. cit.*

44. Blanton, *op. cit.*; Cheshire, *op. cit.*; Dobie, *op. cit.*

The Role of Animals in Infant Feeding

SAMUEL X. RADBILL, M.D., *Philadelphia*

Maternal nursing is an instinctive mammalian characteristic, even though it is shunned by some women for various reasons. When a replacement for the mother is used to suckle the child, the substitution is called wet-nursing. This is a practice commonly found in all times, places, and strata of society. It even occurs among animals. Often animals, instead of women, are employed to act as wet nurses, and the infants are placed directly at the animals' udders to suck. This was done in antiquity as it still is today. An ancient Egyptian representation shows a boy kneeling under a cow beside a newborn calf, both sucking at the udder;[1] and there is an ancient Mesopotamian wall relief also showing children nursing directly from the cows' teats.[2]

Cow's milk was relished from dim antiquity, and the cow was deified as a symbol of joy and love. Through her milk, the physical, moral, and intellectual qualities of the gods could be acquired by children. The Romans, however, although they may have admired the ferocity of the bull, were not so enamored of the docile traits of the cow and insisted that mothers nurse their own children. Children nursed by other animals appear in mythology, art, and literature as well as in common folk practice. Romulus and Remus are a familiar example. They are figured on coins, statuary, paintings, mirrors, helmets, and gravestones and appear frequently in Roman literature. Suckled by a wolf, the twin offspring of the war god Mars and earth mother Rhea symbolize Roman survival and prowess. Ovid also described the woodpecker's officiating at the nursing of the infants. Sacred to Mars, this bird apparently endowed them with brute strength by bringing them additional food.

The belief that mental, emotional, and physical characteristics, as well as disease, can be transmitted through milk was universally accepted until quite recently.[3] In the nineteenth century Brouzet in France even went so far as to recommend a law to prevent disreputable mothers from nursing even their own children, lest they communicate immorality as well as disease to them. Transference of animal qualities to humans could take place in other ways, too, such as ingestion, inunction, or even inhalation. Thus, chameleons' eyes fed to South American Indian boys make them sly; tails of jaguars, make them strong in battle; certain animal brains convey wisdom; and the heart of a fierce, feared animal in the diet gives strength and courage. In Finland little boys eat ants in the spring to make them grow strong. The flesh of a certain bird given by inoculation to young Carib warriors makes them brave and hardy, and Arabs in eastern Africa rub lion fat over the body to absorb boldness. Inhalation is practiced by the Kaffirs, who transmit desirable characteristics by burning things like leopards' whiskers, lions' claws, or other materials while the infant, wrapped in a blanket, is held over the burning substance to inhale the smoke.

Some food taboos are based on this belief. Although wet nurses are acceptable to Muslims, animal milk in a baby's diet is frowned upon by the Koran on the grounds that it communicates animal traits. Children suckling the same nurse are called milk sisters and milk brothers, and since milk is considered to be altered blood, they become blood relations and are not permitted to marry because of the antipathy to consanguineous marriage.[4]

The Israelites had few cows, so goats' milk and sheeps' milk were generally used.[5] A symbol for whiteness and purity, milk also denoted abundance. It was praised as a food in rabbinical literature, and the Hebrew sages suggested that if you want your daughter to be fair, feed her in her youth on milk and young birds. To the Jews any substance separated from the living body is taboo. Blood is in this category, and milk would be as well but for a *hiddush* which determined that milk is an exception from this general prohibition against eating anything cast off from the living body. The milk of a ritually unclean animal, or from an animal suffering from any disease that makes it unclean, or a ritually slaughtered animal that suffered from such a disease within three days of its death is taboo. The Hindu laws of Manu, like those of the Jews, interdict milk of one-hoofed animals, and the laws of Apastamba forbid, besides one-hoof animals, village pigs and cattle as food. There was an opinion among the Arabs that Jacob forbade eating the camel because he believed it caused sciatica;[6] and in the northwest Amazon region travelers reported that the bush-deer was tabooed as a food for married women because it supposedly would make their infants deformed, and no greater disgrace could befall a woman there than to be the mother of a deformed child.[7] There were many other food taboos for pregnant women intended to prevent various defects in the child. Indeed, the food taboos to protect the unborn child extended even to the father. While there have been logical hygienic grounds for these taboos, the spirit of totemism, a feeling of kinship with closely related animals, may also have been the underlying reason. Nevertheless, the Talmud rules that children are permitted to suck the teats of animals, even of those prohibited by ritual law, such as the ass or camel, if the child's welfare demands it.[8]

A large variety of animals served abandoned children as foster parents. The Persian Cyrus, raised by Cyno, a bitch, was thought to derive his name from the dog. Hiero of Syracuse was fed sweet foods by apes; Semiramus was fostered by birds; Midas was nourished by ants that put morsels of food into his mouth. Habia, king of the Tartessians, and Telephus, son of Hercules and Pelias in the Greek myth, were both suckled by deer; Paris and Orion, by bears; Aegisthus, by a goat; Rursus Sandrocotto of India, by a lion; Gordius of Lydia, by birds. Recently delivered mares refreshed the infants Croesus, Xerxes, and Lysimachus. These extraordinary foster parents were portentous omens of future greatness.[9] The city of Damascus is said to derive its name from Ascus, who was nourished by Dama, a doe, but this story likewise may be symbolic, since Ascus was a giant and the giants were nourished by Dame Mother Earth. In the Bible the deer represents maternal affection as well as timidity. In America in 1521 an Indian slave told his Spanish masters that the natives of Carolina had domesticated deer which furnished them with milk and cheese, but his story is questionable.

The goat, one of the earliest domesticated animals, served frequently as wet nurse to gods and heroes. Zeus and his offspring Dionysus, Asklepios, the god of medicine, and Aegisthus, slayer of Agamemnon, are only a few of these. The goat symbolized copious endowment with the good things of life, and Zeus rewarded the nymphs who took care of him with one of the horns of Amalthea, the goat that nourished him. This is the *cornu copeia*, "horn of plenty." The Bedouins of Israel still resort to the use of goat or sheep when a human wet nurse is needed but not available, and the goat tribe Anazeh derives its name from the fact that its progenitor was reared on goat's milk.[10] The Hebrew Talmud ascribes strength, endurance, and pluck to the goat and believes milk fresh from the goat's udder relieves heart pains and milk from a white goat posseses special curative properties.[11] Goats as wet nurses have been observed worldwide. One observer saw how devoted such a goat became to a Basuto child; another described how Hottentots tied their nurslings under the goats' bellies so that they could feed there.[12]

Because milk does not keep well once it is separated from the animal and because the act of suckling was believed to aid digestion in infancy, medical writers beginning in the eighteenth century began to advocate nursing children directly at the udders of goats. Goats were easier to obtain and cheaper than human wet nurses; they were safer from disease and were better in many other respects. Although cows' milk was almost exclusively used in early American infant feeding, William Potts Dewees, who wrote the first American pediatric treatise in 1825,[13] called attention to animal milks and pointed out that the English praised asses' milk; nevertheless, he preferred milk of goats. He then compared the chemical constituents of milk from cows, women, goats, asses, sheep, and mares. In 1816 Conrad A. Zwierlein, after listening to women at a fashionable European resort deploring their difficulties with wet nurses, wrote a book called *The Goat as the Best and Most Agreeable Wet Nurse*, which he dedicated to vain and coquettish women, as well as to sick, tender, and weak ones. Goat feeding then became very popular for a while until it was attacked on various grounds and fell into disfavor. In 1879 it was revived in the children's hospitals of Paris, especially for syphilitic infants.

Asses were also favored as animal wet nurses. These reduced infant mortality in the Parisian hospitals even better than goats.[14] Besides, since they had a better moral reputation than goats, the children were less apt to acquire a libidinous character. Nothing was more picturesque than the spectacle of babies, held under the bellies of the asses in the stable adjoining the infants' ward, sucking contentedly the teats of the docile donkeys.[15] Asses' milk, strenuously recommended by the ancient physicians, was esteemed as of sovereign benefit in rooting out most grievous distempers. It was recommended not only in the diet, but as a component of many remedies as well. A sacred anchor with divine qualities, it was considered the best antidote against poisons. Hippocrates, Galen, Aretaeus, Alexander of Tralles all praised it, especially for consumption. Galen believed that milk should be consumed instantly and so ordered the animals brought to patients' bedsides. He taught that its nature, like that of semen, is altered at once by open air. Friedrich Hoffman, whose opinion was highly regarded in scientific circles of the eighteenth century, explained that milk, like other liquids, possesses a subtle spirit with a strengthening or invigorating quality which should not be allowed to fly off with its warmth.[16] These ideas, once scientific, are still carried over into folklore. It was always a mystery how the body heat was maintained; so vital qualities were accorded to animal heat. Not long ago a patient of mine told me that when she was a baby, she used to drink milk right from the cow "with the animal heat still in it." Once cold, the milk was not wholesome.

Pigs, too, were domesticated at an early stage of civilization. They also served frequently as wet nurses, but the pig was socially persona non grata. A Breton peasant woman discovered about the year 1900 that babies thrived when fed directly from sows and tried to induce the medical profession to use them, but without success.[17] In 1748 William Cadogan derided as an insult to the honor of womankind the prevalent custom of giving a little piece of roast pig to the newborn to suck in order to cure it of its mother's erratic longings. Emblems of filthiness, swine and even swinebreeders were always social outcasts. The pig, being sacred to Osiris and the moon, was taboo to the ancient Egyptians; leprosy was the lot of humans who sinned against this dietary restriction.[18]

In Arequipa, Peru, children are fed, in addition to mother's milk, milk from goats, mares, and other animals. The milk from a black burro is a good tonic, and dog's milk gives a good stomach. Twin myths reminiscent of Romulus and Remus are widespread throughout South America. The Campa of ancient Peru had such a legend in which the twins, the sons of the creator, were brought up by jaguars. One of these twins, Chaingavane, became a great culture hero.[19] Tiri, a similar divine hero of the Yuracares of Bolivia, likewise suckled a jaguar.[20]

Occasionally, a North American Indian father had to bring up an unweaned infant. In 1830 such a Cheyenne father killed buffalo cows that were nursing calves and, cutting off the udders, gave them to his child to suck as if they were nursing bottles. Female deer and antelopes served the same purposes. A similar incident was related about an Arapaho chief.[21]

In art an ancient painting at Herculaneum depicts Telephus sucking a hind, and there are many representations from different periods of Zeus nursed by Amalthea. There is a beautiful French painting entitled *The Soldier as Nurse*, which shows a sheep acting as

wet nurse with a tenderhearted soldier holding the animal so that a
small child can suck greedily at the udder. Authors also used the
theme effectively: Vergil in his description of Romulus and Remus
in the *Aeneid*; Longus in the fifth century *Daphnis and Chloe*; Ibn
Tophail in a twelfth-century Arabic tale called *Hai Ibn Yokdhan*; and
many others before and since. Fairy tales also introduce the
theme—for instance, the suckling of Genovesa by a deer. The story
so often retold about the wolf child is best exemplified by Mowgli in
Kipling's *Jungle Book*. Only one example of a dog as wet nurse has
been found in the literature.[22]

Not only were children nursed by animals, but animals were
nursed by women. This was done for many different reasons: to
feed young animals; to relieve the women's engorged breasts; to
prevent conception; to promote lactation; to develop good nipples;
and for other health reasons. The custom occurred among the
ancient Romans and Persians, as it still occurs among Neapolitans
and roving Gypsies of Transylvania and in Germany, the Society
Islands, New Zealand, Australia, Sumatra, Thailand, Japan, and
South America. Travelers observed women in British Guiana nursing not only their own children of different ages, but also their
four-footed brethren just as obligingly and with equal tenderness.
So, too, among the Macusis and Arecunas; the latter brought up
children and monkeys together. The monkeys were like members
of the family. Other four-footed animals that were nursed were
opossums, pacas, agoutis, peccaries, and deer. Sometimes when
there were too many children born in rapid succession, grandmothers were impressed into nursing duty, and the older women
suckled young mammals of various sorts as well as children.
According to report, the Kamchadales of Kamchatka brought
young bears into their homes in order to have the women nurse
them. The purpose was twofold: to profit from the bear meat when
the bear was grown and to profit from the sale of the bear's gall,
which was highly prized as a medicine.[23] Dr. Richard Beaudry, who
lived among the Ainu for a time, relates that the Ainu have an
annual bear festival at which a bear is sacrificed. They capture a
bear cub that is then suckled by the Ainu women, for the animal
must be raised thus to be suitable for sacrifice.[24] About thirty or
forty years ago a book entitled *Ursula* appeared. It is a true story of
a family living in a Canadian lumber camp where a she-bear was
killed and her cub found. Since there was no milk available, the
foreman's wife nursed the bear cub with her own little daughter,
and the latter was named Ursula.[25]

Among numerous tribes the dog was the preferred adoptee, and even in Canada Indian squaws often suckled young dogs. As a matter of fact, although the dog did not serve as wet nurse as often as other animals, it seems to have been the favorite animal used to suck the breasts of women. One observer remarked that the Pima Indians withdrew their breasts sooner from their own infants than from young dogs.[26] In Siberia in 1821 a pestilence wiped out all the animals except for two tiny puppies so young they had not yet opened their eyes. A woman nursed them at her own breasts along with her children and had the happiness to see the dogs become the progenitors of a new canine race.[27] In the South Sea islands puppies and piglets seemed to predominate as milk siblings. In Persia and in Turkey young dogs were put to the breasts to toughen the nipples to make them better for the infant to suck on, and nurses in Turkey used suckling puppies to maintain their milk supply when they had to travel by sea from distant villages to the capital. In Dauphiné, France, where children were nursed two and a half to three years to prevent another pregnancy, if the child died too soon, the mother suckled either another child or a puppy for the same purpose. A doctor there discovered that the puppies developed rickets, which was cured when they received canine milk again, and he consequently recommended dog's milk as a cure for rickets in children.[28] I have known midwives who advocated the use of puppies to suck the breasts of mothers for one reason or another in my own practice in Philadelphia. Popular home medical books such as Aristotle's famous *Experienced Midwife* and the *Women's Secrets* of Albertus Magnus, reaching back in origin as far as the sixteenth century and reprinted in America from 1753 to the present day in many English and German versions,[29] recommended a woman or a puppy to "draw" the mother's breasts, especially when a golden necklace or small steel ingot worn between the breasts during pregnancy had failed to prevent "curdling" of the milk from too much blood accumulating in the breasts. In 1799 Friedrich Osiander reported that young dogs were suckled by women in Göttingen to disperse obstinate breasts nodules,[30] and Dewees, the first American pediatric author, in 1825 advised regular application to the breasts of a young but sufficiently strong puppy immediately after the seventh month of pregnancy to harden and confirm the nipples, improve breast secretion, and prevent inflammation of the breasts. The puppy's sucking efforts, if started early enough, prepared the nipples for the future assaults of the child. For women too modest to make use of a puppy and so unfortunately organized as to lack nipples altogether or have them very short or sunken in, he recommended drawing them out daily with a large tobacco pipe. By 1847 general aversion to the use of sucking animals must have been manifest to him because that year, in the ninth edition of his treatise, he conceded that the mouth of a puppy to draw the breasts was no better than that of a nurse or other person skilled in this operation. A skilled woman could regulate the force necessary in sucking the breast, but a pup was more easily procured. He then reported a case in which bleeding, purging, fasting, and hot vinegar fomentations had been needed to prevent breast abscess in a newly delivered woman, while the child itself had been wet-nursed; however, the next time the same woman became pregnant, a pup drew her breasts several times a day until after she was delivered, so that by the time the child needed her breast, there were good nipples for it to take hold of.[31]

Piglets and little lambs were also used in this country. There was an old Negro granny in Tennessee who had a reputation for drawing breasts at a nominal fee, but when such a skilled professional was not at hand in that area, mothers suffering with "caked breasts" whose infants were unable to empty the engorged organs employed a small baby pig or a puppy for this purpose. In one case, the piglet, squealing for its milk, followed the woman in and out of the house.[32]

The dog served womankind in many other ways. The living dog just laid upon the painful breasts could do good service. Cut up and bound to the head of a melancholy woman, it could cure her depression; and a suckling dog cooked with wine and myrrh was a help against epilepsy. Cooked dog meat could also make sterile women become fertile.

There is a Rowlandson political cartoon showing the celebrated statesman Fox, candidate for office in the Westminster election of 1784, as a fox fostered at the breast of his sponsor, the Duchess of Devonshire.[33] It is called *Political Affection*. This striking caricature played upon what must have been a familiar image to the voting public by showing that crafty animal nursed by a woman. Even more curious is the story told by Lucian of Samosata in Syria in the second century A.D. about a breed of serpents at Pella in Macedonia so tame and gentle that children took them to bed, women made pets of them, and they would draw milk from women's breasts like infants.[34]

There is also an Italian fable that attributes wasting in nurslings to a snake's sucking the mother's breasts dry at night while putting its tail in the infant's mouth to keep it from crying. The Slovakians believed that if no milk formed in the mother's breast, she was hexed, a word derived, perhaps, from Hecate, Greek goddess of witchcraft. In such a case the child, along with its mother, was placed under a cow which had just recently borne a calf, a few drops of milk were squirted on the child's face, and then the child, its face still wet, was put to the mother's breast, which had first been smoked and washed with brandy and milk.[35] Hecate, as Artemis or Diana, the wild huntress, was worshiped by the Laconians on Taygetus, where she milked lionesses for the gods.[36] The nymphs on Cretan Mount Ida, a mountain associated with the great mother goddess Rhea, fed Zeus on honey and goat's milk. Honey and milk then became symbolic of immortality.

This study of the folklore of animals in infant feeding may help to unravel the mystery in some of the traditional beliefs and behavior often met in modern medical practice. To take an example from my own practice, a mother was plagued recently by an infant with digestive problems and constant fretting. An allergist might have placed the child on a modern hypoallergenic formula, very likely without any relief. When the grandmother recommended goat's milk, I immediately acquiesced, with the happiest result. The child is now content, and the parents sleep well at night. Although the child obviously is not allergic to the goat's milk, I am convinced that the element of family faith in the traditional curative value of goat's milk was a determining factor in bringing about the child's contentment and a happier family.

NOTES

1. Hermann Bruning, *Geschichte der Methodik der Künstlichen Säuglingsernährung* (Stuttgart: Enke, 1908), p. 7.

2. E. Schlieben, *Mutterschaft und Gesellschaft* (Staude: Osterwieck A. Harz, 1927), p. 25.

3. James G. Frazer, *The Golden Bough*, 3d ed., 12 vols. (London: MacMillan and Co., 1936), Part V:2, 138.

4. Benjamin Lee Gordon, *Medieval and Renaissance Medicine* (New York: Philosophical Library, 1959), p. 93.

5. Deut. 32:14; Prov. 27:27.

6. Isidore Singer, ed., *Jewish Encyclopedia*, 12 vols. (New York and London: Funk and Wagnalls, 1901-1906), III, 520.

7. Samuel X. Radbill, "Child Hygiene among the American Indians," *Texas Reports on Biology and Medicine*, 3 (1945), 428.

8. W. M. Feldman, *The Jewish Child* (London: Bailliere, Tindall & Cox, 1917), p. 191.

9. Alexandri ab Alexandro, *Genialium Dierum*, 2 vols. (Leyden: Hackiana, 1673), I, cap. 21, 536.

10. Touvia Ashkenazi, "Hygiene and Sanitation among the Bedouins of Palestine," *Harofe Haivri*, 1 (1946), 149.

11. *Jewish Encyclopedia*, V (1903), 686.

12. Heinrich Ploss, *Das Kind in Brauch und Sitte der Völker* 3d ed., 2 vols. (Leipzig: Th. Grieben's Verlag [L. Fernau], 1911), I, 506.

13. William Potts Dewees, *Treatise on the Physical and Medical Treatment of Children* (Philadelphia: Carey and Lea, 1825), p. 47.

14. *Medical Record*, 24 (1883), 176.

15. *Sanitarian*, 20 (1889), 323.

16. Frederich Hoffman, *Treatise of the Extraordinary Virtues and Effects of Asses' Milk* (London, 1754).

17. *Philadelphia Medical Journal*, 5 (1900), 236.

18. Frazer, *op. cit.*, p. 25.

19. *Journal of American Folklore*, 59 (1946), 550.

20. Rushton M. Dorman, *Primitive Superstitions* (n.p., 1881), p. 93.

21. Radbill, *op. cit.*, p. 428.

22. Bruning, *op. cit.*

23. H. Ploss, *Das Weib in der Natur- und Völkerkunde*, ed. Max Bartels, 3d ed., 2 vols. (Leipzig, 1891), II, 411.

24. Byrd H. Granger (University of Arizona), personal communication.

25. Robert Rosenthal (St. Paul, Minn.), personal communication.

26. Ploss, *op. cit.*

27. Dr. O. v. Hovorka and Dr. A. Kronfeld, *Vergleichende Volksmedizin: Eine Darstellung volksmedizinischer Sitten und Gebräuche, Anschauungen und Heilfaktoren, des Aberglaubens und der Zaubermedizin*, 2 vols. (Stuttgart: Strecker & Schroeder, 1908-1909), I, 101.

28. *Medical Times*, October 28, 1876, p. 48.

29. *The Works of Aristotle*, new ed. (New England, February, 1813); Jacob Sala, *Kurzgefastes Weiber-Buchlein: Enthält Aristoteli und A. Magni Hebammen-Kunst*, (Somerset, Pa, 1813); *Nutzliches und sehr Bewahrt Befundenes Weiber Büchlein, Enthält Aristotelis und Alberti Magni Hebammen-Kunst: Für Mutter und Kind*, (Ephrata, Pa., 1822).

30. Ploss, *op. cit.*, II, 411.

31. Dewees, *op. cit.*, p. 53.

32. E. G. Rogers, *Early Folk Medical Practices in Tennessee* (Carthage, Tenn., 1941), p. 37.

33. J. G. Witkowski, *Curiositées médicalles, Litteraire et Artistiques sur les Seins et L'Allaitment* (Paris: G. Steinheil, 1898), p. 164.

34. Walton Brooks McDaniel, *Conception, Birth, and Infancy in Ancient Rome and Modern Italy* ("Sunnyrest," Coconut Grove, Fl., 1948), p. 33.

35. Hovorka and Kronfeld, *op. cit.*, II, 602.

36. Karl Wyss, "Die Milch im Kultur der Griechen und Römer," *Religionsgeschichtliche Versuche und Vorarbeiten*, XV Band, 2 Heft (Giessen, 1914,) p. 44.

The Mole in Folk Medicine: A Survey From Indic Antiquity to Modern America

I

JAAN PUHVEL, *University of California, Los Angeles*

Folklore is by definition oral tradition, a transitory product with all the hazards to survival implicit in Horace's saying *semel emissum volat irrevocabile verbum,* "a word, once uttered, is lost without recall." Only modern collectioneering, from written page to recorded tape, has largely conferred instant and literal preservation on matter which in earlier days could hope to linger on only in terms of the vague persistence inherent in a self-contained oral transmission itself. The folklore of antiquity is thus an elusive subject for recovery, dependent for immediate preservation on the occasional learned encyclopedist of curiosa. Unfortunately that kind of writer emerged only rather late and in Rome rather than Greece, Pliny the Elder being a suitable epitome. In early Greece historical lore (for example, Herodotus) was not alien to what might be called folktale tradition, but the genre developed fairly soon into the more hardheaded Thucydidean variety, and it never had much use for the more superstitious varieties of folk tradition to begin with.

Folk medicine being a part of folklore, the same strictures apply. Yet folk medicine has a further dimension in that it impinges also on folk religion, and the latter is an area worthy of separate appraisal. For folk medicine proper, Greek literary sources are once again wanting, because Hippocratean iatrics outstripped the strictly popular kind almost as fast as Thucydidean historiography left Herodotean legendry behind. But for folk medicine as a religious phenomenon we are not without means of interpretation in the more general terms of Greek religion.

We have now reduced our dichotomies to the opposition between folk religion and "official" religion in ancient Greece. Those tags are interchangeable with the more technical ones, *chthonian* versus *olympian*. Olympian religion is the canonic, codified variety of the well-known Greek deities after whom nowadays American rockets and warheads are named, very much a matter of atmosphere and space. Chthonian is the soil-oriented cult of fertility and subterranean powers, with black victims sacrificed in a pit, rather than white ones hoisted on altars. The chthonian element is a continuous religious underground which now and then wells up in the so-called mystery religions and pieces of which are sometimes habilitated and grafted onto the formalized olympian cults. Folk medicine should be preeminently a local chthonian matter; yet the Greek medical tradition is well formalized in official terms from the beginning: in the Catalogue of Ships in the *Iliad*, the Greek physicians Makhaon and Podaleirios are sons of Asklepios and hail from Trikka in Thessaly in the north of Greece. In general, Apollo, that multifunctional Greek god who is the plague-shooting archer of the *Iliad*, functions also as the patron of healing under the well-known principle ὁ τρώσας ἰάσεται, "he that wounds shall make whole." But the medicinal aspect is mainly invested and specialized in Apollo's son Asklepios (later latinized as Aesculapius), who is the lord of the great healing centers of classical Greece, Epidauros on the eastern Peloponnesus and Hippocrates' native island of Kos off the west coast of Asia Minor. Coupled with such a pan-Hellenic setting is the myth, the life story of Asklepios as son of Apollo and the mortal maid Koronis, a daughter of the Lapith Phlegyas from Thessaly. After conceiving Asklepios, Koronis betrayed Apollo's divine favors by consorting with a mortal man. Apollo shot her dead, extracted the fetus of his son from the mother's corpse, and assigned him to the wise centaur Kheiron to be educated. Asklepios became a famed healer, equally adept at spells, potions, herbs, and surgical incisions. Yet hubris got the better of him, and when he set about reviving the dead, Zeus cut him down with his thunderbolt. Thus Pindar tells the tale in his Third Pythian Ode, adding the exhortation μή, φίλα ψυχά, βίον ἀθάνατον σπεῦδε, τὰν δ' ἔμπρακτον ἄντλει μαχανάν, "dear soul, do not strive for immortal life, but exhaust the resources of the feasible."

This myth is replete with significance. Asklepios is the divine patron of healing, the lord of the curative sanctuaries, and yet he is no olympian god but a semidivine Thessalian whose life can be recounted from beginning to end. What this means is that he is a cyclical chthonian dying god embodying birth and rebirth, a subterranean kind of Thessalian daimon, a local bush leaguer from the north who happened to make good in the chthonian fringes of the olympian establishment and had the good fortune to be canonized by the mythographers and sung by the likes of Homer and Pindar.

But we can define this subterranean daimon from Trikka even more closely. The name *Asklepios* is derived from the ancient Greek word for the rodent mole, σκάλοψ or ἀσπάλαξ (the latter with metathesis), and modern Greek dialects of the islands of Imbros and Samothrace in the northern Aegean Sea still name the mole ἀσκάλπας. This explanation, first advanced by the Belgian scholar Henri Grégoire in the late 1940s,[1] is bolstered by the equally impressive archaeological discovery that the circular *tholos*, or underground incubation structure of the sanctuary at Epidauros, had the interior layout of a molehill. Thus, despite the later religious propagandists of Epidauros such as Isyllos, the builders of the *tholos* must have been conscious votaries of a chthonian healing cult featuring a deity who was theriomorphically a mole and whose origins were in the northern soil of Thessaly. Thessaly was, incidentally, still notorious for its moles in later antiquity, when the Romans took a rather more sinister view of the animal as being noxious rather than beneficent; thus, Pliny (*Natural History*, Book VIII, 104) quotes Varro to the effect that a whole town in Thessaly had been undermined by the subterranean burrowings of moles.

In Greek folk religion, however, as discernible in its formalized survivals, the mole-god Asklepios was not only totally beneficent; he was explicitly the healer in polar opposition to the plague shooting Apollo Smintheus. Σμίνθος was a Greek term for a rather ratty variety of mouse, and the association of rats with plague is well known. By contrast, then, the mole appeared as the "blind rat," the denoxified, chthonian permutation of the Apollonian plague animal. Archaeological evidence for this relationship has been found in excavations on Larissa, the acropolis of Argos in the eastern Peloponnesus, where terra-cotta figurines of mice or rats from about 700 B.C. appear with blindfolds or lying on their backs with bellies slit open and eyes bandaged. These objects point to some kind of sacrificial ritual involving rats and their sightless permutations.

In a synchronically sideways look from ancient Greece west to Italy and east across the Indo-European continuum of Anatolia, Iran, and India, there is little that engages one's attention in ancient Rome. There may have been a divinatory role for the rat, which would have tied in with another of the traits associated with the imported Apollo, and even the name *sminthe* is common in Etruscan onomastics. Possibly the Roman consul in 340 B.C., Publius Decius Mus, was in reality a Campanian named *Dekis Smintiis or the like who had translated his name into Latin.² The mole (*talpa*) gets medical attention only beginning with Pliny, and even then largely in connection with his discussion of the *magicae vanitates*, the superstitions of the Persian Magi, to whom the mole allegedly was *animal religionum capacissimum*, the beast most loaded with supernatural properties (*N.H.*, XXX, 19-20).

In view of Pliny's information it is curious that no significant mole cult is attested for ancient Iran. In ancient India, on the other hand, there is a set of data which are compellingly analogous to the Asklepios traditions of Greece. In view of the gap that exists in Anatolia and Iran, it is difficult to credit diffusionary influences, and polygenesis is ruled out by the peculiar complexity of the data. Thus we are probably in the presence of nothing less than an ancient Indo-European genetically reconstructible mythologem involving the theriomorphic divine manifestations of the rat and the mole.³ Thus, to juxtapose: Apollo the Rat (Smintheus) is the plague-bringing archer (Loimios) who shoots beasts and men (*Iliad* 1.50), but he is also a healer (Paieon) of men and cattle. His son Asklepios the Mole is purely a healer. Apollo is also known as Loxias (compare λοξός, "slanting, oblique") and is the god of incantations and poetry. The Vedic Indic god Rudra (the later Śiva) is an archer who kills cattle and men (*Rig-Veda* 1.114.10), but he also heals them (*RV* 1.43.6, 1.114.1). His animal is the mole (*ākhú-*), plentifully attested in the Vedas. Rudra is also known as Vaṅku (*RV* 1.114.4), which means "totterer," the one with the slanting gait, like the Greek Loxias. Rudra's son Gaṇeśa, who is his hypostasis with an epithetal name ("Lord of the Troop"), is the patron of poetry and also has the *ākhú* association. It thus appears that we are dealing basically with an Indo-European ambivalent archer-god who could either hurt or heal and whose animal manifestation was accordingly either rat or mole. The same god was characterized as having a slanting gait, apparently a theriomorphic trait relating to the movement of rodents. One function of the same deity was the patronage of incantations and by extension poetry, and this aspect was hypostasized in India as the son Gaṇeśa of the god proper. In Greece a hypostatic offshoot was specialized, at least in Thessaly, as healer alone and hence appropriated the mole exclusively. It is typical of Greece that Indo-European mythical survivals are to be found in the largely chthonian folk religion of the provinces rather than in the full glare of the olympian superstructure and are only secondarily integrated with the new synthesis.

The mole as the animal incarnation of the divine healer thus has remote roots in Indo-European antiquity. In Greece it made a great, though only recently fully credited, career as the chief patron of healing, and in the Western world Asklepios-Aesculapius has become, to use Karl Kerényi's expression, the "archetypal image of the physician's existence." Thus we can now tell our own M.D.'s that they are not historically leeches; they are rather all moles.

NOTES

1. H. Grégoire, R. Goossens, M. Mathieu, *Asklèpios, Apollon Smintheus et Rudra: Études sur le dieu à la taupe et le dieu au rat dans la Grèce et dans l'Inde*, Académie Royale de Belgique, Classe des Lettres, Mémoires, Tome XLV, fascicule 1 (1949); cf. H. Grégoire, *Le Flambeau*, 32 (1949), 22-54; *La Nouvelle Clio*, 3 (1951), 397; *ibid.*, 10-12 (1958-1962), 219-221.

2. Cf. J. Heurgon, *La Nouvelle Clio*, 3 (1951), 105-109.

3. Cf. R. Goossens, *La Nouvelle Clio*, 1 (1949), 4-22; *op. cit.* in n. 1 above, pp. 127-173.

The Mole in Folk Medicine:
A Survey From Indic Antiquity
to Modern America

II

WAYLAND D. HAND, *University of California, Los Angeles*

As anyone who has worked in the field of modern folklore knows, it is difficult to trace ongoing traditions back more than two or three hundred years and almost impossible to pursue leads all the way back to classical and Indic antiquity. In this folk medical study encompassing this tremendous time span, the two collaborators have been struck mainly by the general similarities in the way the mole has been associated with healing in the Indo-European continuum, seemingly from time immemorial. Details of the creature's healing office vary at different times in history and in different parts of the Western world, but the evidence, wherever encountered, points to the almost universal favor in which the mole was held as an agent of healing. With the skill of a classicist, and as a scholar trained in comparative Indo-European linguistics and mythology, Professor Puhvel has traced out the reverence shown the lowly rodent in earliest recorded history. In this portrayal the mole emerges almost as a divine being.

This vision of the mole has continued to modern times, though with a somewhat different emphasis. The divine attributes have been almost completely lost, but there has emerged from the time of Pliny the figure of a mysterious subterranean creature, almost a chthonic seer and divinity.[1] Because of its existence in the earth itself, the animal is connected in the folk mind with death and the realm of the dead[2] and likewise with the devil, witches, and magical powers.[3] In France the mole is thought to embody the powers of

both good and evil.[4] The supposed blindness of the creature, a view
established in classical times[5] and persisting to the present,[6] its
sheltered and solitary life, and its acute sense of hearing[7] have
invested the mole, in popular fancy at least, with divinatory
powers,[8] but particularly with the power to predict death.[9]

The most striking attribute of the mole in modern as well as in
classical times, however, is its supposed healing virtue. The blood,
flesh, viscera, skin, teeth, feet, and claws are used for a whole range
of diseases and ailments, as we shall see later. This is not unusual,
of course, because many other creatures—animals, birds, reptiles,
and even fish—figure in organotherapy, as Höfler and others have
shown.[10] Yet over and above any other animal, the mole is so highly
prized as a healer that people coveting the healer's art have seized
upon the creature as a sacrificial animal.[11] The vital healing essence
of the mole is secured either by suffocating or strangling the
animal in one's hands, plunging one's finger into the live animal's
body, biting off its head or its paw, or tearing the creature apart for
the healing applications of its warm and quivering flesh.

Before we proceed further with an exploration of these matters,
it is essential that we have before us the full text of what Pliny says
about the mole in doctrines and false faiths spread westward from
Persia into Greece and Rome by the magi. Pliny writes in his
Natural History, Book XXX, chapter vii, sections 19 and 20, as
follows:

> It should be unique evidence of fraud that they (the Magi) look upon
> the mole of all living creatures with the greatest awe, although it is
> cursed by Nature with so many defects, being permanently blind, sunk
> in other darkness also, and resembling the buried dead. In no entrails
> is placed such faith; to no creature do they attribute more supernatural
> properties; so that if anyone eats its heart, fresh and still beating, they
> promise powers of divination and of foretelling the issue of matters in
> hand. They declare that a tooth, extracted from a living mole and
> attached as an amulet, cures toothache. The rest of their beliefs about
> this animal I will relate in the appropriate places. But of all they say
> nothing will be found more likely than that the mole is an antidote for
> the bite of the shrewmouse, seeing that an antidote for it, as I have said,
> is even earth that has been depressed by cart wheels.

The strongest European attestations of the throttling of moles to
gain their healing virtue are to be found in the folklore of France,
Germany, Czechoslovakia, and Lithuania, but this sacrificial act is
also encountered in Transylvania, Austria, Switzerland, Spain,
England, Scotland, Holland, Belgium, Sweden, and elsewhere[12]—
that is to say, in countries that most immediately came under the

sway of medical knowledge and lore that moved northward into
Europe from the classical and Mediterranean lands in the early
Christian centuries. The folklore of Czechoslovakia, France, Germany, and other European countries contains details on how the
creature is killed, whether in both hands;[13] between one's fingers;[14]
in the left hand;[15] with the left thumb, as in Czechoslovakia;[16] and
the like. Often the process of smothering is very gentle, and it is
prescribed that the creature simply be held until it dies, as in Scotland.[17] In French and German traditions where the healing hand is
acquired in infancy, the creature is placed in the child's hand and
gently done in, or it is left to smother in the infant's swaddling
clothes.[18] In parts of Czechoslovakia the deed had to be performed
by a posthumous child.[19] In the central part of France it was
believed in the first decade of the present century that to acquire
the healing gift, a youngster must have killed seven moles in his
hand before being able to eat a rich soup,[20] and in other places the
gift was acquired by a child under seven or an otherwise virtuous
person.[21]

A bloody ritual act is often involved, particularly when the
animal is strangled and crushed or impaled on the healer's finger;
when it is cut open, torn apart for warm visceral applications to
swellings, excrescences and the like; or when a paw is bitten off for
medical or talismanic purposes while the creature is still alive.[22]
The ritualistic transfer of power is clearest, of course, in cases
where the healer's finger, the "murderous digit" (le doigt meurtrier)
is left in the animal's body overnight.[23] Other ritualistic aspects
involve carrying out the transfer of power at special phases of the
moon, on various church holidays,[24] or at other times of the year.[25]
A wide range of ailments is supposedly cured by what the French
call la main taupée, "the mole-hand."[26] Included are sores, wounds,
swellings, boils, abscesses, cancer, skin diseases, scrofulous conditions, and the like;[27] sore throat, fever, ague, colic in man and
beast;[28] fits and convulsions;[29] felons, bone growths, goiter, toothache;[30] and even perspiring hands.[31] The use of the mole in curing
scrofula in various parts of Slovakia, Moravia, and Bohemia
amounted to a ritual. For example, the animal had to be taken
before Saint George's Day, in some places after sunset,[32] and
disposed of by strangulation or tearing off the right front leg;[33]
sometimes the animal was even set free after its healing offices had
been secured by a godfather.[34] As cures for this dread disease,
baking the creature's heart and feeding it to the sufferer[35] and
having the patient bathe in water in which a mole had been bathed
were unusual in Czechoslovakia and not encountered elsewhere.[36]

Another more or less ritualistic act involving the mole as an agent
of healing is the drinking of the creature's blood, a treatment
reported from Lithuania for the cure of epilepsy, itself a magically
induced ailment,[37] and from France, where the blood was imbibed
only three-quarters of a century ago to cure drunkenness.[38] Mole's
blood, however, is applied for various maladies[39] and has been
since the time of Pliny, apparently, when it was sprinkled on the
delirious to restore them to their senses.[40] In France and England
within the present century, the blood of a mole was applied to
warts, wens, corns, and other excrescences.[41] It was also used
against bed-wetting in France, where a thread soaked in the creature's blood was worn as a necklace.[42] In more recent times in
Czechoslovakia, mole's blood was smeared on a patient to cure
scrofula.[43] In the western part of France near Poitou, blood was
instilled in the ear to cure deafness,[44] and in Puy de Dôme it served
as a specific to restore lost virility in man.[45] The application of the
warm viscera of a mole to cure felons, wens, and other growths is
reported from Slovakia and England, where the animal was killed,
cut in half, and applied to the ailing part.[46] In Lithuania the
exposing of the viscera was accomplished in a more ritualistic and
brutal way, namely, by tearing the creature in half. The warm parts
were then applied to patients suffering from rheumatism.[47] The
crushing of a mole's liver between the hands and its utilization in an
ointment to cure scrofula, as reported in Pliny,[48] of course points to
later sacrificial uses of the animal's vital parts. It is interesting to
note that Höfler has devoted a whole section on the use of a mole's
liver in modern organotherapy.[49] In Swabia early in the century the
boiled flesh of a mole was rubbed on the scalp to cause hair to
grow.[50] Just as the viscera, vital parts, and flesh of the mole were
applied to the human body in various kinds of curative measures,
so was the creature's skin. In France the skin was made into a
skullcap or bonnet and worn against fits and convulsions, particularly those caused by dentition.[51] In England the skin was wrapped
around the limbs and other parts to prevent cramp.[52]

The amuletic uses of moles' paws, claws, and teeth to aid dentition
and cure toothache and other maladies is a subject so broad and
involved that it deserves special treatment. Lack of time forbids
more than a cursory treatment here. Once more, sacrificial elements are apparent in the way the feet and claws were gained. In
Germany the paws were bitten off the living creature in an almost
omophagous ritual;[53] in France, around Liège, they were torn
out[54] or cut from the living creature,[55] a practice also noted from
Moravia and England.[56] In most cases these appendages were sewn

into a little sack and worn about the neck, or they were carried exposed, as in parts of Germany and Austria.[57] In England, not only were bags of moles' feet carried to prevent rheumatism and to avert toothache, but as late as 1910 they were also hanging on the mantlepiece as a cure for toothache, especially in Herefordshire.[58] I am unable to find modern cases in Europe of the extracting of teeth from a living mole for the cure of toothache, as described by Pliny,[59] but this hazardous act is reported from Kentucky, as I shall show later. In Swabia at the end of the century a mole's tooth worn on the chest in a sack was supposed to cure the gout.[60]

The mole also figured in veterinary medicine and in animal husbandry, especially in Lithuania, where horses were stroked with a live mole to keep them healthy and fat.[61] Moles were also killed in one's hand for the same purpose and were choked to death with the right hand to make the horses breed well.[62] In Bohemia one went into the fields before daybreak, caught a mole, opened it up, and rubbed the viscera on the stomach of the horse and on the manger, too, to make the animal thrive.[63] In Normandy a white mole taken into one's hand conferred the power to cure the colic in horses simply by touch.[64]

With European folk medical lore concerning moles before us, we can now look at these same manifestations in American folk medicine. Even though the traditions have been nowhere nearly so well preserved here as in Europe, one can nevertheless discover a considerable amount of related material—enough, at least, to warrant the title of this joint paper.

The smothering to death of a mole in one's hands is encountered in the Pennsylvania German tradition, among the southern whites, and also, sporadically, to be sure, and derivatively, in the American Negro tradition. These beliefs have been recorded from the early 1890s and continue through the first half of the present century. Bone felons, for example, were treated by those who had squeezed a mole to death or, as this act is often phrased, by those who had "allowed a mole to die in their hands."[65] This cure was practiced in the Pennsylvania German tradition, in Maryland,[66] and in Kentucky.[67] Risings—that is to say, swellings of any kind—receive a simple treatment in the white tradition of North Carolina and in the tradition of the southern Negro they are rubbed by someone who has smothered a mole.[68] Warts are cured the same way in North Carolina,[69] but in Taney County, Missouri, the sufferer smothers the mole and holds it above his head for a moment.[70] This act of holding the mole over the head, reminiscent of an Anglo-Saxon custom of waving the animal, is found in a curious Alabama cure, encountered nowhere else in the literature, so far as I know, European or American: "Catch a live mole, hold it between your hands above your head for an hour and you will gain the healing powers that will allow you to cure milk leg."[71] In the Alleghenies in the early 1890s, sprains were cured with the interrupted pressure of a hand that had squeezed a mole to death.[72] Headache, not encountered elsewhere in cures of this kind, is also cured by a hand in which a mole has been left to die, but only in North Carolina, so far as I can discover.[73] In the Negro tradition of Baltimore in the early 1890s, one could cure any pain if a mole were caught and allowed to die in one's hand.[74] From Europe the requirement of innocence in the healer has made its way to America. In Maryland around the 1920s, for example, it was believed that the mole must be killed by the hand of a child under two years of age. Another informant says that three moles must be killed by a child under seven.[75]

The folk medical use of the mole's bodily parts in America is scant, except for the creature's paws. For epilepsy, a magical disease, it is recommended in the Pennsylvania German country that the heart of the living mole be given to the patient.[76] Mole's blood for the cure of baldness in the mountain white tradition of North Carolina is reminiscent of a similar practice noted from Swabia earlier in this paper.[77] A curious belief about mole's flesh, rare and in the learned tradition, is found in Illinois: "If you boil a mole in an earthen pot and use this liquid when washing your hair, your hair will turn white."[78] This notion appears to have been handed down in the *Egyptian Secrets*, a nineteenth-century publisher's forgery purporting to derive from the writings of Albertus Magnus. That this magical quality of the mole's flesh is perhaps old is documented by a prescription in a sixteenth-century English redaction of the work, which claims that rubbing a black horse with a mole will turn its coat white.[79] The skin of a mole was worn in Illinois as recently as 1965 by those wishing relief from rheumatism.[80]

About the only part of a mole that is widely used in American folk medicine is the creature's paw. First of all, in different parts of the country it is worn as an amulet to ward off disease and to secure health and longevity.[81] It is most widely used, however, in childhood diseases, from cholera infantum and croup[82] to colds and whooping cough[83] and to teething and the convulsions that often accompany it. In the southern states, where the custom of placing a mole's foot around a child's neck is most prevalent, and as far west as Indiana, the foot is most generally suspended on a string, but it may also be enclosed in a bag or sack.[84] A mole's right front foot is prescribed in the Blue Ridge Mountain country, but in the neighboring state of Maryland it is the left hind foot, and the entry suggests the use of the foot itself as a teething instrument.[85] In Kentucky the tooth of a live mole was actually rubbed over an aching tooth to cure the pain as late as the 1930s.[86] Earlier in this paper I noted the use of teeth from a living mole for this purpose, as reported from the time of Pliny.

The only connection between the mole and deaf-mutes and other kinds of speechless humans is a measure reported from Illinois in the 1960s, wherein it is advised that a tongue-tied child wear a mole foot in a bag around its neck as a cure for the impediment.[87] The mole as a cure for deafness and speech defects is known in Europe, particularly in France.[88]

The comparisons that have been made between European and American folk medicine in modern times with regard to traditions involving the mole in curative practice accord pretty well with the transmission of other kinds of folk medical lore to these shores. Indeed, what has happened in the case of this one item of folk medicine is rather typical of what happens in folk belief and custom in general in the process of transmission across the Atlantic. For that matter, it mirrors what happens in folklore generally when a considerable time span, as well as changing patterns of culture, is involved. However, this is not really the problem before us. The more difficult part of this venture in a historical and comparative study is to trace the continuity of the tradition from ancient to modern times and from the classical lands to northern Europe.

This problem is made doubly difficult by the fact that folklore as such and folk medicine were not collected much before the eighteenth century. The principal exertions in this field of study actually did not come into full flower until the nineteenth century, and scholars of our own day are still trying assiduously to redress this neglect with last-minute efforts, as it were, to see that representative categories of material, at least, are turned up.

Through the courtesy of Professor Charles H. Talbot, the eminent historian of medieval medicine, I have been able to trace a continuing tradition of the mole as healer from the time of Pliny the Elder forward for some centuries, but the tradition is far from robust. Pliny's nephew, known as Pliny the Younger, transmitted at least three prescriptions involving moles that in their fundamental aspects were to live on until the present time. We read, for example, of the ashes of a mole mixed with honey and applied for boils and abscesses.[89] In a second cure for eruptions of the skin, the liver of a mole was ground between the hands, smeared on the neck, and left for three days without washing.[90] Finally, the heads of moles were cut off and ground up with earth thrown from the molehill and then fashioned into lozenges and kept ready in a box for all kinds of apostematic ailments.[91] In the fifth century Sextus Platonicus recommended that the entire mole be used to rub the neck for glandular swellings.[92]

In the first half of the fifth century, Marcellus of Bordeaux, drawing on the two Plinys and other sources, including contemporary local practitioners, repeated the first two prescriptions from Pliny the Younger cited above[93] and counseled the roasting of a mole for a head cold or catarrh. The roasted mole was supposed to be reduced to a powder and mixed with pepper and basil. This was given in wine in a bath in which the patient had never bathed before nor would ever be likely to bathe in again.[94] For glandular swellings a mole's liver was squeezed in the hands and applied to the throat.[95] I have not made much of the use of earth from a molehill, which is fairly common in modern European folk medical practice, but Marcellus prescribes an unusual remedy for nervous pains in the ligaments. "From three heaps of earth which moles throw up in their molehills," he writes, "one takes as much as one can grasp with the left hand three times, that is, nine handfuls, mixes this with vinegar, and kneads it up, applying it, where necessary, with healing efficacy."[96]

In the *Leech Book* of Bald, compiled about the middle of the tenth century in England, there is a prescription for pain in the fatty part of the belly which directs the sufferer to catch a dung beetle seen throwing up earth, wave it strongly in the hands, and then throw it over the shoulder without looking back after having thrice uttered the incantation "Remedium facio ad ventris dolorem." In a learned note, Cockayne has conjectured that the Anglo-Saxon author actually was talking about a mole rather than a dung beetle.[97]

At the end of this development before the Middle Ages, in which moles were variously squeezed, waved in the air, and the like, comes a purported cure for cancer, ascribed to Paracelsus, who flourished in the early sixteenth century. It has come down in a nineteenth-century chapbook known as the *Egyptian Secrets,* ascribed to Albertus Magnus, who, of course, predates Paracelsus by three centuries:

Secret Remedy of the Great Theophrastus Paracelsus
for Healing the Cancer

This celebrated remedy is composed as follows: "When a human being takes hold with his right hand of a live mole, and keeps the mole so long with a tight grip until it dies, such a hand obtains by dint of this miraculous proceeding, such marvelous power that cancer boils, repeatedly rubbed, by moving up and down with this hand, will break open, cease to form again, and entirely vanish."[98]

It is difficult to say whether the above prescription is new in the long line of popular treatises connected with the famed Bishop of Ratisbon or whether it stems from some earlier folk or literary tradition. The fact that this specific cure is not found in the sixteenth-century *Boke of Secretes* published in London (1560)—that is to say, in Paracelsus's own time—makes one wonder about this nineteenth-century recipe. Since I do not have access to the long line of *grimoires* connected with Le Grand Albert nor to the prolific German treatises in this tradition, I am in no position to say whether this derelict nineteenth-century item was the sole influence on modern medical traditions concerning the mole as an agent of healing. At any event, in the give-and-take between folklore itself and folk literature, one must not foreclose the possibility that the throttling of the mole fed into the chapbook tradition from earlier oral sources. The general sacrificial and sacral use of the creature—evisceration, biting off of the appendages, and amuletic uses—all these things speak for an ongoing tradition of reverence for the creature as a healer.

As a working hypothesis, pending a closer look at old and obscure literary sources, one must look at the rich corpus of folk medical items recovered in modern oral tradition, particularly in Europe. Folk medicine, I believe, constitutes a prime source of information for historical reconstructions such as the one we have undertaken today. That the published folklore record is rarely complete and never continuous need not deter us, really. This very lack of a precise line of descent of the various things we study should, on the contrary, only win us over with renewed dedication to the necessity of historical and comparative scholarship. Folklore, along with mythology, I need not remind you, has always stood in the forefront of disciplines committed to the study of cultural history—history in its broadest and most mysterious sweeps.

NOTES

1. Pliny, *Natural History*, ed. T. E. Page, E. Capps, W. H. D. Rouse, L. A. Post, E. H. Warmington, et al., 10 vols., Loeb Classical Library (Cambridge, Mass. and London, 1938-1962), XXX, vii, 19-20. (Hereafter *NH*; cited throughout by book, section, and lines.)

2. Max Höfler, *Die medizinische Organotherapie und ihr Verhältnis zum Kultopfer* (Stuttgart, Berlin, Leipzig, n.d.), p. 113. Cf. Pliny, *NH*, XXX, vii, 19. In France the

expression *être taupé* means "dead and buried." See Eugène Rolland, *Faune populaire de la France*, 13 vols. (Paris, 1877-1911), VII, 25, no. 14.

3. Hanns Bächtold- Stäubli and Eduard von Hoffmann-Krayer, *Handwörterbuch des deutschen Aberglaubens*, 10 vols. (Berlin and Leipzig, 1927-1942), VI, 11-12. This is hereafter cited: *HDA*. See also H. F. Feilberg, *Bidrag til en Ordbog over Jyske Almuesmål*, 4 vols. (Copenhagen, 1886-1914), II, 620, s.v. *muldvarp*.

4. Robert Morel and Suzanne Walter, *Dictionnaire des superstitions* (Bibliothèque Marabout, n.d.), p. 225.

5. Pliny, *NH*, XI, ii, 139; XXX, vii, 19.

6. Rolland, VII, 28, no. 20; 29, no. 22; Paul Sébillot. *Le Folk-Lore de France*, 4 vols. (Paris, 1904-1907), III, 11; *HDA*, VI, 8-9.

7. Pliny, *NH*, X, lxxxviii, 191; Rolland, VI, 28, no. 21; *HDA*, VI, 9.

8. Pliny, *NH*, XXX, vii, 19.

9. Rolland, I, 14, no. 5; *HDA*, VI, 15-16; E. and M. A. Radford, *Encyclopaedia of Superstitions*, 2d rev. ed, Christina Hole, ed. (London, 1961), p. 235.

10. Höfler, *op. cit.* Höfler's work is organized according to the medical use of various animal parts, but there is an orderly survey of the different animals involved and an excellent index.

11. I have devoted considerable space to the mole as a sacrificial animal in my forthcoming article on "Animal Sacrifice in American Folk Curative Practice" in the *Bulletin of the History of Medicine*.

12. The true geographical spread of this phenomenon would no doubt show a much wider diffusion of this folk medical belief and custom than I have been able to trace out in this paper. That it is also known outside of Europe in modern times would accord with the general presuppositions of the present study, particularly the broader Indo-European configurations charted by Professor Puhvel. I note, for example, that the strangling of a mole to cure swollen tonsils is reported from Syria; see Dr. O. v. Hovorka and Dr. A. Kronfeld, *Vergleichende Volksmedizin: Eine Darstellung volksmedizinischer Sitten und Gebräuche, Anschauungen und Heilfaktoren, des Aberglaubens und der Zaubermedizin*, 2 vols. (Stuttgart, 1908-1909), II, 13.

13. Rolland, I, 13-14, no. 3; William George Black, *Folk-Medicine: A Chapter in the History of Culture*, Publications of the Folk-Lore Society, XII (London, 1883), p. 16; *HDA*, VI, 20.

14. Sébillot, III, 49.

15. *Ibid.*, pp. 48-49.

16. Josef Čižmař, *Lidové lékařství v Československu* [Folk medicine in Czechoslovakia] 2 vols. (Brno, 1946), I, 165, 219.

17. Black, p. 161.

18. Sébillot, III, 49.

19. Čižmař, I, 219.

20. Sébillot, III, 48-49.

21. Sébillot, III, 48.

22. J. Elisonas, "Mūsu krašto fauna lietuviu tautosakoje" [Our land's fauna in Lithuanian folklore], in *Musu Tatosaka* [Our folklore], V (Kaunas: Lithuanian Folklore Commission, 1932) p. 198; Sébillot, III, 48; Rolland, VII, 29, no. 23; Höfler, p. 113; Adolf Wuttke, *Der deutsche Volksaberglaube der Gegenwart* 3d ed., Elard Hugo Meyer, ed. (Berlin, 1900), p. 307, par. 451.

23. Sébillot, III, 48; Rolland, VII, 30, no. 23.

24. Sébillot, III, 48.

25. *Ibid.*

26. *HDA*, VI, 20.

27. Wuttke, p. 315, par. 466; Elisonas, p. 198; *HDA*, VI, 20; Hovorka and Kronfeld, II, 401; Sébillot, III, 49; Elisonas, p. 198; Čižmař, I, 165.

28. *HDA*, VI, 20; Roland, VII, 29-30, no. 23; Hovorka and Kronfeld, II, 13; Sébillot, III, 49; Čižmař, I, 219.

29. Rolland, I, 13-14, no. 3; VII, 31, no. 23; Čižmař, I, 219.

30. Wuttke, p. 315, par. 466; *HDA*, VI, 20; Sébillot, III, 48; Rolland, VII, 29, no. 23; Čižmař, I, 219.

31. Sébillot, III, 49; Rolland VII, 34, no. 25; *HDA*, VI, 20.

32. Čižmař, II, 133.

33. *Ibid.*, 134.

34. *Ibid.*

35. *Ibid.*, II, 133.

36. *Ibid.*, II, 132.

37. Elisonas, p. 198.

38. Rolland, VII, 34, no. 25.

39. *HDA*, VI, 19; Sébillot, III, 49.

40. Pliny, *NH*, XXX, xxiv, 84.

41. Sébillot, III, 49; Rolland, VII, 34, no. 25; Ella Mary Leather, *The Folk-Lore of Herefordshire* (Hereford and London, 1912), p. 84; Radford and Hole, p. 235.

42. Rolland, VII, 34, no. 25.

43. Čižmař, II, 133-134.

44. Rolland, VII, 34, no. 25; Sébillot, III, 49.

45. Rolland, VII, 35, no. 25.

46. Hovorka and Kronfeld, II, 501; Leather, p. 84; Radford and Hole, p. 235.

47. Elisonas, p. 198.

48. *NH*, XXX, xii, 38.

49. *Organotherapie*, pp. 180-181, no. 25.

50. Hovorka and Kronfeld, II, 762.

51. Rolland, VII, 31-32, no. 24.

52. Radford and Hole, p. 235.

53. Wuttke, pp. 124, par. 167; 393, par. 601; Höfler, p. 113. Höfler says that this is done against the elfin demons of disease.

54. Sébillot, III, 49; Rolland, VII, 29, no. 23.

55. Rolland, VII, 32-33, no. 24. In the Ardennes the claws were clipped and carried in a sack around the neck to aid in teething.

56. Hovorka and Kronfeld, II, 334; Čižmař, II, 134; Black, p. 161.

57. Hovorka and Kronfeld, I, 292-293, who reproduce a life-size likeness of the amulet. Paws in metal jewelry clasps are pictured in Liselotte Hansmann and Lenz Kriss-Rettenbeck, *Amulett und Talisman; Erscheinungsform und Geschichte* (München, 1966), pp. 87, figs. 187-188; p. 226, fig. 750.

58. Radford and Hole, p. 235; Leather, 82. In Denmark the teeth of a mole were placed in the child's drink to promote teething. Cf. Feilberg, I, 620.

59. *NH*, XXX, vii, 20.

60. Wuttke, p. 356, par. 534.

61. Elisonas, pp. 198-199.

62. *Ibid.*, p. 196.

63. Wuttke, p. 451, par. 711.

64. Rolland, VII, 30, no. 23.

65. Edwin Miller Fogel, *Beliefs and Superstitions of the Pennsylvania Germans,* Americana Germanica, no. 18 (Philadelphia, 1915), p. 293, no. 1551; E. Grumbine, *Folk-Lore and Superstitious Beliefs of Lebanon County* (Papers and Addresses of the Lebanon County Historical Society, III, 1905-1906), p. 280.

66. Annie Weston Whitney and Caroline Canfield Bullock, *Folk-Lore from Maryland,* Memoirs of the American Folklore Society, Vol. 18 (New York, 1925), p. 83, no. 1707.

67. Daniel Lindsey Thomas and Lucy Blaney Thomas, *Kentucky Superstitions* (Princeton, N.J., 1920), p. 97, no. 1105.

68. Wayland D. Hand, ed., *The Frank C. Brown Collection of North Carolina Folklore,* 7 vols. (Durham, N.C., 1952-1964), Vol. 6, *Popular Beliefs and Superstitions from North Carolina,* 299, no. 2314; Newbell Niles Puckett, *Folk Beliefs of the Southern Negro* (Chapel Hill, N.C., 1926), pp. 378-379.

48 WAYLAND D. HAND

69. Hand, VI, 320, no. 2479.
70. Vance Randolph, *Ozark Superstitions* (New York, 1946), p. 130.
71. Ray B. Browne, *Popular Beliefs and Practices from Alabama*, Folklore Studies, IX (Berkeley and Los Angeles, 1958), p. 80, no. 1351. Healing power gained in the same way is also applied for the healing of sore breasts. *Ibid.*, p. 42, no. 630. Cf. Walter Gregor, *Notes on the Folk-Lore of the North-East of Scotland*, Publications of the Folk-Lore Society, VII (London, 1881), p. 123.
72. *Journal of American Folklore*, 7 (1894), 111.
73. Hand, VI, 207, no. 1587.
74. *Journal of American Folklore*, 5 (1892), 111.
75. Whitney and Bullock, p. 83, no. 1708.
76. Thomas R. Brendle and Claude W. Unger, *Folk Medicine of the Pennsylvania Germans*, Proceedings of the Pennsylvania German Society, vol. 45 (Norristown, Pa., 1935), p. 106.
77. Hand, VI, 122, no. 849; *North Carolina Folklore*, 18 (1970), 12, no. 184.
78. Harry Middleton Hyatt, *Folk-Lore from Adams County, Illinois* (Memoirs of the Alma Egan Hyatt Foundation, New York, 1935), p. 143, no. 295a.
79. *The boke / of secretes of Albartus Mag / nus, of the vertues of / Herbes, stones and / certaine beastes* (London, 1560), n.p. [78].
80. Harry Middleton Hyatt, *Folk-Lore from Adams County, Illinois*, 2d ed. (New York, 1965), p. 259, no. 5747.
81. Thomas and Thomas, p. 107, no. 1252; Hyatt, 2d ed., p. 195, no. 4551; Puckett, p. 316.
82. Hyatt, 1st ed., p. 208, no. 4338; Madge E. Pickard and R. Carlyle Buley, *The Midwest Pioneer: His Ills, Cures, and Doctors* (Crawfordsville, Ind., 1945), p. 77; John W. Allen, *Legends and Lore of Southern Illinois* (Carbondale, Ill., 1963), p. 83.
83. Hyatt, 2d ed., p. 277, no. 6087; "Oklahoma Writers' Project" (MS of the Oklahoma Historical Society, n.d.), pp. 44-45.
84. *West Virginia Folklore*, 12 (1962), 31; *Journal of American Folklore*, 12 (1899), 273 (Maryland); *North Carolina Folklore*, 18 (1970), 8, no. 58; Browne, p. 24, no. 327 (Alabama).
85. *Kentucky Folklore Record*, 9 (1964), 130 (Virginia); *Journal of American Folklore*, 12 (1899), 273 (Maryland).
86. Elza E. Fentress, *Superstition of Grayson County* (Kentucky) (M.A. thesis, Western State Teachers College, Bowling Green, Ky., 1934), p. 89, no. 151.
87. Hyatt, 2d ed., p. 334, no. 7194.
88. Rolland, VII, 30, no. 23.
89. *Plinii secundi iunioris*, edidit Alf Önnerfors (Berlin: Corpus Medicorum Latinorum, III, 1964), p. 71, lines 8-9.
90. *Ibid.*, lines 9-10.
91. *Ibid.*, lines 10-12.
92. Höfler, p. 181.
93. Marcellus, *Über Heilmittel*, hrsg. Max Niedermann, 2d ed. Eduard Liechtenhan, trans. Jutta Kollesch und Diethard Nickel, 2 vols. (Berlin: Akademia-Verlag, 1968), I, Chap XV, no. 81 [p. 260].
94. *Ibid.*, pp. 91-92, sec. 2, lines 29-[35].
95. *Ibid.*, Chap. XV, no. 81 [p. 260].
96. *Ibid.*, Vol. II, Ch. XXXV, no. 18 [p. 595].
97. The Rev. Oswald Cockayne, ed., *Leechdoms, Wortcunning and Starcraft of Early England*, 3 vols. (London, 1864-1866), II, 319, n. 2: "Our Saxon must have had Talpam or 'Ασπάλακα before him in this sentence; but he names the *Scarabaeus stercorarius*."
98. Albertus Magnus, *Egyptian Secrets* (n.p., n.d.) p. 15.

Miraculous Restoration of Lost Body Parts: Relationship to the Phantom Limb Phenomenon and to Limb-Burial Superstitions and Practices

DOUGLAS B. PRICE, M.D., *Georgetown University School of Medicine*

In this paper[1] we will attempt to show that the folklore theme of loss and restoration of body parts, especially the limb, constitutes a metaphorical or symbolic presentation of the phantom limb phenomenon. We will also demonstrate that stories with the motif of loss and restitution contain information about superstitious beliefs and practices regarding the burial of amputated parts.

We will give first a rather complete description of the phantom limb along with certain related clinical data. We will then present several miracles concerning the restoration of lost body parts and discuss the relationship of these miracles to the phantom limb phenomenon and to limb-burial superstitions and practices. This will be followed by a brief general discussion that includes some historical implications of the miracles.

CHARACTERISTICS OF THE PHANTOM LIMB

Almost every individual who has lost a limb or a part of one feels at one time or another that some portions of the missing part are still present. This subjective sensory and psychological experience is generically referred to as the phantom limb phenomenon (PLP) or simply as the phantom limb (PL). Most commonly associated with and found in cases of removed limbs, phantoms occur also in cases of loss of the eye, ear, nose, facial tissue, tooth, larynx, breast, penis, testicle, and possibly anus and rectum. The topics treated in this paper, however, are related primarily to the loss of extremities or their parts.

Since 1871, when S. Weir Mitchell, the American neurologist and novelist, created the term *phantom limb* to designate the phenomenon,[2] there have been about four hundred reports on the subject. Although there are considerable variations in the findings from these studies, certain descriptive aspects of PLs have been reported often enough to be considered characteristic. It is mainly from these frequently noted aspects that the following description of the PLP has been derived;[3] occasional references to more unusual data are also included.

PL sensations usually are not felt immediately after the individual awakes from the anesthesia or after the limb has been severed, although the person may be quite unaware of the loss. PL sensations as such usually begin within a matter of a few days after removal of a limb. Some investigators, however, have noted a considerable interval—up to many years—between the loss and the commencement of painful PL sensations.[4]

PL sensations are abnormal in character. Amputees describe these paresthesias in various ways: itching, tingling, numbness, pricking, formicating, pins-and-needles, electric shock, shooting, pulsating, cramping, biting, stinging, burning, stabbing, or crushing. The paresthesias are not present constantly or continuously. They vary in intensity from the mildly annoying to the very painful; most investigators report a preponderance of the mildly irritating variety and a small percentage (1 to 10 percent) of the severely painful type. It is often reported that in an occasional case the PL pain is identical with that experienced before amputation.

Usually only the more distal and prominent aspects of a removed limb are felt; for example, most individuals with an amputation of a leg at mid-thigh level are aware only of the toes (especially the big toe), the sole, the heel, or the dorsum of the foot; a smaller percentage of thigh amputees feel also the two malleoli or the whole foot and the knee; and only a very few report feeling the missing leg in its entirety. A similar pattern is found in arm amputees, although a phantom of an entire missing hand is more common than one of an entire foot. Thus, the typical PL consists of the perception of certain anatomically prominent aspects of a missing limb with gaps or holes between them and the stump. (See figure 1.)

The size of the PL is frequently the same as that of the real limb; rarely is it larger.[5] *Telescoping*, a phenomenon that consists in the gradual shrinking in size of the PL and its withdrawal and location

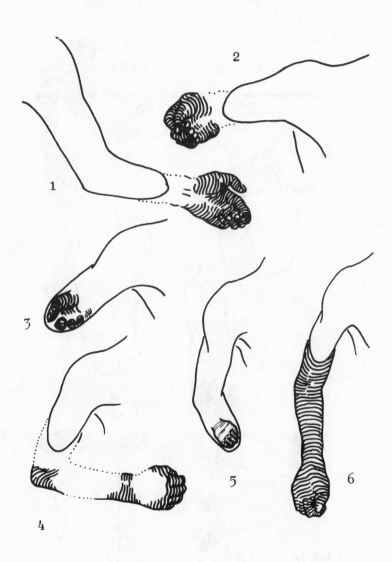

Figure 1.
(Continued on next page.)
(Legend on page 53.)

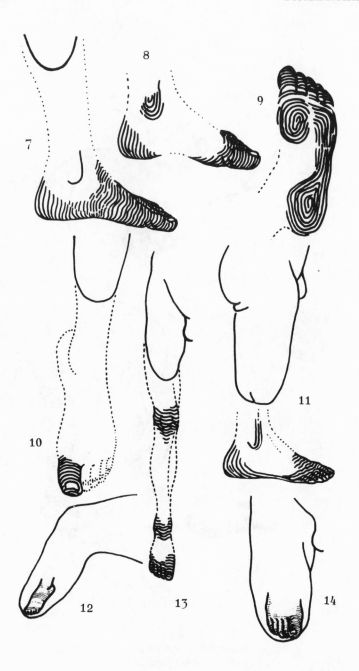

Figure 1 (pp. 51 and 52).

Some of the commonest phantom types.*
1-6, arm amputations; 7-14, leg amputations. Perceived missing parts indicated by hatching.

1. Mid-lower. Hand normal distance from stump. Most of hand and outline of wrist (styloid processes) perceived. Fingers slightly flexed; thumb sl. adducted.
2. Mid-upper. Normal-sized hand telescoped close to stump. Fingers clenched, digging into palm; thumb adducted.
3. Mid-upper. Normal-sized hand telescoped and completely withdrawn into stump. Fingers, thumb, and thenar eminence perceived. Fingers and thumb sl. flexed.
4. Mid-upper. Part of hand and elbow, most of wrist perceived. Normal distances from stump. Fingers and thumb sl. flexed. Arm in mid-flexed position.
5. Mid-lower. Smaller than normal hand telescoped into stump. Most of hand perceived. Fingers and thumb sl. flexed.
6. Mid-upper. All of missing parts perceived. Normal distances from stump. Fingers and thumb sl. flexed; arm in sl. flexed position.
7. Above-ankle. Toes, sole, instep, heel, dorsum of foot, and outline of medial malleolus perceived. Normal distance from stump.
8 & 9. Above-ankle. Toes, ball of foot, lateral sole, heel, and medial malleolus perceived. Normal distance from stump. Foot in sl. adducted position.
10. Above-ankle. Normal-sized big toe perceived. Farther than normal distance from stump because foot in equinus position, i.e. hyper-flexed.
11. Mid-thigh. Parts perceived as in 8 & 9, and lateral malleolus in addition. Foot telescoped near stump.
12. Above-ankle. Smaller than normal foot telescoped within stump. All of foot and ankle perceived.
13. Mid-thigh. Toes, ball of foot, ankle, and knee perceived. Normal distances from stump. Normal or laterally twisted position.
14. Mid-thigh. Smaller than normal distal portion of foot telescoped within stump.

*From Kauko Solonen, "The Phantom Phenomenon in Amputated Finnish War Veterans," *Acta orthpaed. scand.*, suppl. 54, 1962. Used with the kind permission of the author and Munksgaard International Publishers Ltd.

within the stump, is well known, though not reported by all investigators (See figure 1, nos. 2, 3, 5, 11, 12 and 14).

Voluntary movements of the PL are experienced by about 50 percent of amputees; some individuals, however, do not attempt to move the PL for fear of producing pain. Voluntary movements are most frequent in the beginning, but often their execution becomes difficult and their range of motion limited with the passage of time. Occasionally, voluntary movement may involve an amplitude of excursion greater than is possible for a normal limb; the imaginative amputee may accomplish even greater feats, such as placing his phantom hand in front of his body, then passing it through the thickness of his body to his back.[6]

Involuntary PL movements occur less frequently than those of volition. But in many cases the PL is in a fixed position, as in the case of a phantom hand in which the fingers are clenched and dig into the palm.

Although amputees frequently rely, especially at the beginning, on their visual and tactile senses to correct the perceptually based conviction of the presence of an absent limb, the PL may possess visual and tactile qualities; for example, some individuals who have lost a limb from gunshot wounds report that the PL seems to be full of holes, just as the limb actually was after the injury—"the last moment of corporeality," as some authors call it. This perception may not be tactile or visual in nature, but rather the individual's way of interpreting or reporting the gaps in his PL.

Definite instances of PLs which involve tactile sensations are, however, known: in one case, the phantom hand felt smooth on the volar surface, rough on the palmar;[7] in another case, a man felt in a phantom finger the former constriction of a wedding ring that had become so tight that it had had to be removed some time before the amputation of his hand;[8] and in a third case, a man felt a corn on his phantom little toe, where there actually had been a corn.[9]

The PL may rarely incorporate visual sensations: in one man's case, the PL was "yellowish—like the hand of a dead person"; in that of another, the PL was pale blue, "as if gangrenous."[10] Occasionally, an amputee feels that there is a clear line of demarcation between perceived and unperceived parts of the missing extremity. Sensations of temperature of the PL seem to be distributed equally among the ranges of cool (or cold), warm (or hot), and normal.

There is some evidence that the PL may continue or reappear throughout the life of an amputee. Some amputees have experienced definite PL sensations for as long as fifty years; still, durations are quite variable, with the PL paresthesias usually fading away gradually from awareness.

Especially at the beginning, amputees frequently "forget" that they are missing a limb. For example, a leg amputee may get out of bed and start to stand up after placing his "feet" on the floor. As he begins to fall, he realizes he has forgotten the loss of his leg. There is some question whether automatic acts of this kind depend on the presence of PL sensations at the time of the event or are manifestations of the perduring nature of the individual's body image.[11]

In a typical amputee, the PL manifests a wide variety of changes: the paresthesias may change in type, intensity, or frequency; a given part may be perceived as more prominent at one time than at another; the range and ease of movement of the PL may change; and in telescoping, the distance of the PL from the stump is variable. These and other alterations occur under many different conditions, such as emotional stress, involvement with psychologically significant persons, strenuous physical activity, wearing of a prosthesis, micturition, defecation, orgasm, or change in weather conditions.

What has been described so far may fairly be called the typical PL of the amputee. There is, however, another aspect of the PLP that has been delineated and described in some recent reports. This aspect is seen more obviously in several conditions other than amputation, such as in aplasia and other congenital limb abnormalities,[12] in paralysis of the limbs during spinal anesthesia[13] and from spinal cord injury,[14] and in limb loss and deformity resulting from leprosy.[15]

We have called this aspect of the PLP the "natural" PL because it corresponds, generally speaking, to a normal limb—that is, it replicates the integrity, size and shape, sensations, and functional capacities of a normal limb.[16] The natural PL seems to be a mental impression rather than a sensory experience. In cases of leprosy and congenital limb abnormalities especially, a patient's impression of having normal extremities, despite actual severe mutilations or deformities or absence of the limb, occurred most often when the individual was engaged in activities that involved the use of the extremities, for example, wood carving, crocheting, plowing or digging, or throwing a ball.

There are few systematic studies of the dreams of amputees. The reports we have read and our studies indicate that most amputees at the beginning dream of themselves as having complete, intact bodies; about a year or two after the loss they first begin to dream of themselves as lacking the limb. There are, however, references to amputees who have continued to dream of themselves with complete bodies for as long as thirty-two years. The complete-body dream of the amputee may be due to the persistence of a normal body ego or body image, but this dream-content may result from the simple but significant wish to be physically complete and whole.

Although there is still disagreement about the etiology of the PLP, a majority of investigators believes that the phenomenon is the result of two main factors: (1) abnormal impulses originating in the severed nerve ends, resulting in an imbalance in the activity of certain neural fibers;[17] (2) the persistence of the body image, a factor which incorporates psychological, emotional, and social elements.[18] Suddenness of loss was until recently thought generally to be a necessary factor in the production of PL sensations; but the PLP has been found to be associated with cases of slowly occurring loss, such as frostbite,[19] gangrenous sloughing of major parts of limbs,[20] and digital shortening (that is, loss not associated with surgical amputation) in leprosy.

THE FOLKLORE MOTIF OF THE RESTORATION OF LOST BODY PARTS

Relationship to the PLP

There are a number of myths, legends, miracles, and märchen which contain as a principal or incidental event the magical or miraculous restoration of a missing body part. This motif includes the loss and restoration of limbs, head, lips, tongue, nose, eye, penis, and visceral organs. The theme is found in folklore and mythology the world over, from ancient to modern times. Except for the head and visceral organs, the body parts considered in these stories correspond to those with which the PLP is associated.

When we first examined some of these stories (in English or in summary form), we noted that in many cases the restoration was described in a straightforward manner. But in a few cases there were present some elements that seemed to be either quite incidental, selective, and facultative or vaguely reminiscent of the PLP.

Since a large number of legends of this motif occur in the medieval Marian collections and in the lives of the saints, we decided to examine examples from this genre to determine whether they contained any allusion, direct or indirect, to the PLP.[21] For this analysis, we collected versions of five main stories primarily from these collections; two involved the leg (or foot), two the hand, and one the face.[22] Of the total of forty-eight legends analyzed, twenty-six were in Latin; nine in French (various dialects); five in English (Middle and Early Modern); and two each in Greek, Italian, Spanish (Castellano), and Portuguese (Gallego).[23] All of the stories concerned an event which occurred in the period from the seventh to the fifteenth centuries; almost all the accounts were written before the sixteenth century. There was one additional miracle which took place in the modern period, namely, about 1640.

Some of these miracles, though basically the same because of a common source, contained elements which involved the appearance, functions, or other attributes and aspects of the restored part; these elements varied from story to story and often from version to version. Analysis of these attributes and aspects showed them to correspond frequently to known characteristics of the PLP.

To demonstrate this finding, we will present two miracles that show a high degree of correspondence. The story will be summarized, but the passages which concern the restoration will be given in full (in quotation marks).

The first miracle was written about 1110 by Guibert de Nogent (1053-1124).[24] We have examined eighteen versions, seven of which definitely derive from Guibert's original account.

Near Grenoble, an oxherd named Peter lost the flesh and bones of one of his lower legs and the flesh of the thigh from the sacred fire, that is, ergotism. Later, the thigh bone was accidentally knocked from the hip joint; Peter hid this bone in a wall of a church in Viviers which was dedicated to the Virgin Mary and renowned everywhere for its miracles. One night, the Virgin and Saint Hippolytus appeared to Peter in a dream. At the command of the Virgin, the Saint, picking up the once scattered, now divinely consolidated, parts of the leg, began to join them to Peter's body. During this engraftment, Peter was tortured by severe pains. When he awoke, he told the household about his dream. It was found that Peter's new leg was "entirely insufficient in strength because of infantile softness and was not suitable in size. The man's leg differed from the old in that there seemed to be present a composition very different from the roughness and coarseness of the other leg; nor in any way could it match the old leg for supporting the body. The miracle remained incomplete (limped) for an entire year." At the end of the year, the Virgin and Hippolytus appeared again to Peter in a dream. "The Saint touched the newly molded limb and supplied all that was lacking in last year's creation, except the softness of the skin and the appearance of newness; the leg was shaped to resemble very closely the old." Peter was asked if he could tell whether his old limb or another one had been grafted on him. "He answered that he did not know. 'I cannot twist myself this way and that to look around because of the newness of the leg itself.'" But he told the people that if they found a scar on it, then they would know that it was the leg he once had. They looked closely and soon saw the signs of the wound.

The outstanding element mentioned in connection with the first restoration of the limb is the pain Peter experienced during the engraftment. On the basis of our analyses of the forty-eight miracles, we have concluded that the element of sensation or pain in the restored part either during or after the restoration corresponds basically to the typical aspect of the PL, namely, (painful) paresthesias. This conclusion is based on the following reasoning. The PL is basically a sensory phenomenon. A reference in a story to sensation or pain in a limb during or after its restoration more clearly implies the existence of a PL than does the more primitive and concrete symbolism involved either in the mere witnessing of the restoration by the amputee in a dream or vision or in the inspection of the restored limb by bystanders in reality. The definite presence of the element of sensation in the restored part in twelve of the miracles (representing three of the five main stories) permits the consideration that those versions embody a case history of a PL.

The qualities and aspects of Peter's initially restored limb also suggest strongly that Guibert was describing, not a newly created leg, but an instance of a PL, as is shown by the following matching of the elements with aspects of the PLP outlined in the first section:

1. Insufficient strength = fear of moving PL, or absence of voluntary movement of PL, or incomplete PL, i.e., "gaps and holes";
2. Softness = yielding sensation, i.e., involuntary PL movements;
3. Unsuitable size (which in context implies small size) = telescoped PL;
4. Different texture = tactile or visual PL sensation;
5. Inability to support the body = same as 1 or 2.

Although some of the elements are matched with less well-known aspects of the PLP, for example 4, the correspondence of other elements, particularly 3, is to frequently described aspects. Elements 1, 2, and 5 may, of course, refer metaphorically to the real insubstantiality of a PL, that is, to the actual inability of a PL to support the body.

The second restoration resulted in a leg that very closely resembled the old—it had the identifying mark of an old scar—but the leg had several qualities related to newness: the softness of the skin, the appearance of the leg, and the inability of Peter to twist his body. These elements may be equated with aspects of the PLP; for instance, the scar corresponds to the "last moment of corporeality" or to a visual aspect of a PL, and Peter's inability to twist himself corresponds to a fear of moving a PL or an absence of voluntary movement.

Overriding these individual correspondences, moreover, is the common quality of newness, which represents the newness of change. In the second restoration, the change would be from a tele-scoped PL to one of normal size and shape, a natural PL. The quality of newness suggested by the deficiencies of the first restora-tion, taken as a group, may similarly represent the change from a painful PL (in the dream as well as, probably, in consciousness) to a painless, telescoped PL.

The next story concerns a miraculous leg restoration which occurred in Spain around 1640; it is the most recently dated restoration miracle we have come across. The following summary and extracts are from an account of it written by Christopher Davenport, better known as Father Franciscus a Sancta Clara (1598-1680).[25]

Because of an infirmity of his right leg, Miguel Juan Pellicero had an amputation of his leg at the General Hospital in Zaragoza in January, 1638. The amputated leg was buried in the hospital cemetery. Because of the pain in the remaining part of his amputated leg, Miguel fre-quently anointed the scar with oil from a lamp in the Chapel of the Virgen del Pilar. One evening, he went to bed early and immediately fell asleep. A little while later, his parents went into his room and found him asleep—but he had two legs. They awakened him and asked him how that happened. He did not know but said that he had a dream: he was in the Chapel of the Virgen del Pilar and was annointing the scar; he therefore believed that it had been done by the Virgin. (. . . there was a marvelous apparition of the Blessed Virgin that he had in his sleep and the truth of the promised event makes indubitable the truth of this vision. [P. 70]) After finding the identifying mark that Miguel said should be there, all identified the leg as the same one which had been amputated. "After the restoration, Miguel was not able immediately to put his foot down firmly, for the sinews and toes of his foot were drawn together and held fast. (The restored toes were not yet mobile nor extended but were grown together [as if] into a fist and could not be used. [P. 72]) He did not feel the natural heat in his leg, and the color was that of death; nor did it match the other leg in length and thickness. The leg was weak and deformed. Miguel still had some pain. Three days after the restoration, by another miracle the natural heat was com-municated to the restored leg, the sinews and the toes were extended; finally, the leg came to match the other, and its forces and firmness were recovered."

The phrase "the pain in the remaining part of his amputated leg [*dolor in residuo cruris amputati*]" closely parallels the designation of PL pain then in use by medical writers: "the remaining pain of an amputated limb (leg) [*dolor residuus membri (cruris) amputati*]."[26] Although the distinction is clear both in the original and in the translation, the parallelism of the phrases raises the question whether Franciscus (or the author of the *Epitome*) was acquainted with the PLP; that Franciscus was is suggested but not established.[27]

Each of the defects of Miguel's initially restored leg may be matched with an aspect of the PL as follows:

1. Inability to put foot down firmly = fear of moving PL or absence of voluntary movement of PL;
2. Sinews and toes drawn together and held fast (like a fist) = PL toes hyperflexed and laterally cramped together, i.e., PL in cramped or vicelike position;
3. Immobility of toes and inability to use toes = PL in fixed position; absence of both voluntary and involuntary movement of PL;
4. Absence of natural heat = cool or cold PL;
5. Color of death = visual aspect of PL;
6. Lack of match in length and thickness, i.e., from the context, shortness and thinness = telescoped PL;
7. Leg weak = PL sensation of numbness or same as 1;
8. Leg deformed = PL in abnormal position or "gaps and holes";
9. That Miguel still had pain = continuation of PL pain or decrease in severity of PL pain;
10. Scar = "last moment of corporeality" or visual aspect of PL.

The changes in the leg after three days may also be equated with aspects of the PLP:

1. Warmth = warm PL;
2. Extension of sinews and toes = voluntary or involuntary PL movement;
3. Matching of new leg with old = change from telescoped PL to natural PL;
4. Recovery of strength and firmness = absence of fear of moving PL; ability to make voluntary PL movements;
5. All the changes taken as a whole = same as 3.

It is unusual to find in the miracles a restoration performed in two stages; in fact, in many of the versions based on Guibert's story, the restoration is presented as a single act, even though various elements that pertained to the restored part were retained or new ones included. Nevertheless, these two stories present in highlight the varying degrees of correspondence to the PLP that we have found in twenty-one of the stories;[28] each of the five main legends was represented in this finding. If this were the only positive finding, it alone would provide, we believe, a clear and firm case for the metaphorical representation of the PLP in the restoration-of-body-part motif; but there is further evidence that supports this hypothesis.

Relationship to Limb-Burial Superstitions

In addition to the stories which present the PLP in metaphorical terms, there are others which contain a different kind of data which we also believe relates to the PLP. An example is a legend included in the life of Saint John of Damascus (ca. 645-ca. 750) written by John, Patriarch of Jerusalem (d. 966).[29] The following summary and extracts are from a version that had been drawn from fragments of Arabic manuscripts and subsequently embellished.

> John of Damascus was falsely accused by Leo, Emperor of Constantinople, of writing a letter of treason. The Caliph of Damascus ordered John's right hand amputated. This was done, and the cut-off hand was placed high up in the forum. "When evening came, John suppliantly sent a request to the Caliph to this effect: 'My pains are becoming intense and they have become unbearable for me. And the sharpness of my pain [the shooting pain, ἡ τῆς ἀλγηδόνος ἀκίς] will not let up as long as my cut-off hand hangs in the air. Give orders, therefore, that as a favor it be given me so that I may bury it beneath the earth and the great pain will abate.' The tyrant yielded immediately to his request and the hand was given to the just man. John carried his hand to his oratory, where he prostrated himself flat before a holy image . . . of the Mother of God. He placed his cut-off hand against its previous juncture and began to pray to her, shouting with groans and tears, 'Come, then, as quickly as possible, and cure my hand. . . . may the right hand of the Most High heal my right hand.' While tearfully saying this, he fell asleep. [In his sleep], he saw the holy image of the Mother of God gazing at him with merciful and cheerful eyes and saying, 'Lo, your hand has been healed [has become healthy]. . . .' Awakening and being healed, he then examined, more carefully than was needed, his cut-off hand and, seeing it healed, he rejoiced. When the neighbors heard his joyful singing, some Saracens immediately accused him of fraud and asserted that his right hand had not been cut off at all but someone else's, say a slave's hand or a servant's, and that they who had been ordered to cut it off had exchanged the punishment for money. John was summoned and ordered to show the cut-off right hand. When he had shown it, God's Mother had also seen to it that there barely appeared [v.l. there appeared on the surface] a line marking the cut, which showed a genuine amputation."

There are several elements unrelated to the restoration that suggest strongly the PLP; these elements are connected with John's request that his amputated hand be returned to him. The basic meaning of the request is unambiguous: John believed not only that the unbearable and increasingly intense (shooting) pain was due to the fact that his severed hand was hanging in the air in the forum, but also that the pain would be relieved by burial of the hand.

These sentiments of John's will sound familiar to those acquainted with American superstitions about amputation, for the belief underlying the sentiments is identical to those now currently and popularly held beliefs that concern the origin of the PLP, namely, superstitions which attribute phantom pain or paresthesias to faulty, careless, or improper disposal of amputated parts.[30] To be specific, John's statement parallels closely those superstitions in which the pain or paresthesia that follows amputation is not stated but implied to be phantom in type, as in the following example from Kentucky:

> When a finger, a toe, or an arm is amputated, it should be buried in a straight position; otherwise the patient will suffer pains from cramp. Secrecy should be observed in the burial of the amputated member.[31]

Although the pain in this example is not explicitly stated to be phantom in type, there can be no doubt that the phrase "pains from cramp" refers to the frequently described sensations of a PL, just as our alternative translation of the phrase "shooting pain" in John's request describes a typical PL paresthesia. The example and other variants like it have the same basic reference to the PLP as have the superstitions in which the reference is explicit, as it is in the following example:

> If a member of the body has been amputated and the owner suffers in that member, it is because the amputated part has not been properly buried. To cure the pain, the member must be dug up and properly buried. Sometimes it is twisted, or a finger or toe is doubled up, and if this is straightened out, the pain ceases.[32]

On the basis of the close similarity of John's sentiments and presently held superstitious beliefs, we infer that John's pain was of the phantom type. This inference is supported by certain aspects of the story.

When John received his hand, he took it into his chapel; while he was beseeching the Mother of God to cure his hand, he placed the severed hand against his wrist-stump. These actions and the content of his prayers may be interpreted as representing John's wish for the restoration of his hand. This would not be an unusual desire, since restoration of the lost part is consciously wished for by the amputee in some of the miracles. In John's case, however, the interpretation overlooks the fact that John did not ask directly that his hand be restored, nor—what would seem to be the most appropriate or natural request—did he ask that the amputation wound or the stump be healed; he asked only that his hand be healed. Reference to healing of his hand occurs three times in the story before the restoration occurred. These facts argue that no confusion between hand, wound, and stump existed in the mind of the author. The hand, then, that John wished healed was a phantom hand, and the pain described in his request to the caliph, therefore, logically referred to pain in a phantom hand.

John's gesture of placing his amputated hand against the stump may also be symbolic of the PLP if we take the gesture to represent, in terms of the visual, John's impression that his hand was still in the place where it always had been, that his hand was still part of his body. The fact that there is no mention in the story that his hand was ever buried may be slight confirmation of this interpretation.

Thus, although there is no explicit statement that John continued to feel the presence of his hand after it had been severed and despite the fact that the site of his pain is not given, it is a reasonable deduction, based on current clinical and folklore data, that John was suffering from a painful phantom of his hand. This deduction is substantiated by an element in the story irrelevant to the restoration but relevant to the PLP, namely, the postrestoration scar; this element corresponds to those aspects of the PLP which were related to the scars in Peter's and Miguel's cases. In John's case, the scar may also constitute a symbolic reference to the division between perception of a part by abnormal sensation and perception of a contiguous part by normal sensation.

We see, therefore, in John's case the occurrence of a painful phantom of the hand soon after amputation; through the intervention of a therapeutic dream, this painful PL was converted into a natural phantom of an entire missing hand.

In addition to the importance of this legend as it relates to the PLP, there are probable historical implications in the connections between early medieval beliefs about physiological effects of burial of amputated parts and twentieth-century American superstitions which link the PLP to "proper" disposal of removed parts. Further study of the miracle and other folklore genres is necessary before the implications and their significance can be elucidated in a more complete way than we have been able to do.

Relationship to Limb-Burial Practices

While analyzing these miracles for metaphors and symbols of the PLP, we noted that information about burial of amputated limbs was given directly in many of them. The three miracles given here may serve as examples.

In two of the legends, burial of the amputated part is mentioned: in Miguel's case, which occurred in 1638, his leg was buried in the hospital cemetery; in John's case, which occurred in the seventh or eighth century but was recorded in the tenth century or later, burial of his severed hand was intended. In the version of the legend about John given here and in the other versions as well, the presentation of the intention to bury the hand is straightforward and unembellished; this manner of presentation implies that burial of a separated body part was practiced from at least the eleventh century on.

The frequent and rather casual references to burial of amputated limbs in Franciscus's text suggest further that burial of limbs was not uncommon by the early seventeenth century.[33] That burial of Miguel's limb was in a hospital cemetery is of some additional interest.[34]

In Peter's case, which occurred in the early part of the twelfth century, the separated femur was hidden by Peter in a hole in a wall of the church. This detail was retained in four of the seven versions that were definitely based on the original account, although in several cases, it was a tibia that separated and was hidden, and in one version the alteration included actual burial.[35] We interpret the hiding of a bone in a church wall as a metaphorical equivalent of a "proper" burial of an amputated limb. Thus, in addition to the symbolism of burial inherent in the act of hiding a bone in a church, these references to disposal of separated bones or flesh may constitute implicit allusions to a superstitious belief similar to the one presented directly in the legend about John; these allusions may have been readily understood by the medieval reader or hearer of the stories.

In versions of two of the remaining three main miracles, there also are references to burial of limbs. Thus, there is contained in the restoration stories considerable information about limb-burial practices. This contrasts distinctly with the paucity of data on the subject in several other literary genres we have examined, including the medical and surgical literature of the corresponding and later periods. From our work on the history of the PLP, we know of only three works in which burial of an amputated limb is mentioned, each instance being given as a passing remark in connection with a case of the PLP.[36] Also, in a philosophy dissertation written in 1693 there is a comment on the frequent practice by surgeons of preserving amputated limbs.[37] We assume that the preservation was done so that the limb could be kept for burial with the individual when he died.

In closing this section, we can only note here that the medieval restoration stories appear to be one of the few sources of historical information about a social custom which has many implications, especially in regard to early body-image phenomena.

DISCUSSION

In this study we found what we believe to be metaphorical, symbolic, or implied allusions to the PLP in forty-one (that is, about 85 percent) of the forty-eight miracles analyzed. In some of the stories, such as the ones presented here, the allusions seem related clearly and definitely to the PLP; in others, the references are obscure, indirect, or minimal. Cursory analysis of restoration stories from other folklore genres shows similar findings, although allusions to the PLP seem to be more frequent in miracle stories than in other types.

While these findings are not suitable for statistical evaluation, they are, we believe, in quantity sufficient and in meaning clear enough to permit the conclusion that the folklore motif of loss and restoration of body parts represents a common mythologem that often embodies the PLP.

The PLP was not described as a clinical entity until late in the Renaissance,[38] although the survival of amputees is attested centuries earlier.[39] On the basis of the nearly universal occurrence of the PLP as reported in modern studies, it may be reasonable to assume that some of these earlier surviving amputees did experience PL sensations, possibly in the clinical configuration known today.[40] That they did is strongly suggested by the results of our analyses of the medieval and other restoration stories. On the basis of those positive findings, we believe that the PLP was presented metaphorically and symbolically in folklore long before the first scientific report and description of it appeared in print.

In this communication, we are not able to present fully the circumstances, probably best seen in the medieval miracles, under which folklore transformed an amputee's PL from a natural occurrence into a magical or miraculous limb-restoration.

In regard to the motif of loss and restoration, it seems clear that to the medieval amputee and his reporter (who may also have been his confidant), the reality of the PL sensations and the reality of the dream of a complete body were so phenomenologically close and in principle so alike as to make the restoration of a lost body part also a reality. The central importance of the dream (or vision) in the miracles is related primarily to the medieval author's attempt to explain the PLP; for this reason, we do not believe that the frequent inclusion of the dream in these miracles was simply a literary or folklore device, nor that the dream was clearly a derivative of Aesculapian incubation rites.

Because of lack of space, we also can only refer—without documentation—to what we see as an historically extended interplay of scientific thinking and folk belief regarding the general topic of loss and restitution of external body parts. Before the sixteenth century, there was a long period, ending at about the close of the fifteenth century, of scientific opinion that the reunion of body parts was impossible; this period overlaps another, from the twelfth through the fifteenth centuries, of greatest interest in their miraculous restoration. After the sixteenth century, there is an overlapping of three periods: a period of scientific demonstration of successfully reuniting minor body parts (nose, finger) and transplanting parts (cock's spur to the comb) and of studying regeneration of limbs and other body parts in species of *Amphibia* and *Mollusca*; a period of scientific and scholarly interest in restoration miracles; and a period when no new limb-restoration miracles appear in the Marian and hagiographic literature.

Coming midway between these coinciding and overlapping periods, in the middle of the sixteenth century, are the first reports of the PLP in scientific literature. The dividing lines between the scientific and folklore trends are not clear-cut, but the interplay between the two trends seems evident and supports the primary hypothesis presented in this paper.

CONCLUSIONS

From this correlative study of folklore and clinical data, we draw four main conclusions:

1. Stories of the restoration of lost limbs and other external body parts (with the probable exception of the head) are to be considered as a common mythologem that frequently represents or embodies the phantom limb phenomenon.
2. The history of the phantom limb phenomenon begins with the earliest restoration stories.
3. Burial of severed body parts was practiced early in the Christian era.
4. Superstitious beliefs that assign the cause of phantom limb

pain or paresthesias to improper disposal of the amputated limb extend back at least to the tenth or eleventh century.

This study demonstrates, we believe, the validity of the following remarks of George Santayana:

> We sometimes speak as if superstition or belief in the miraculous was disbelief in law and was inspired by a desire to disorganize experience and defeat intelligence. No supposition could be more erroneous. Every superstition is a little science, inspired by the desire to understand, to foresee, or to control the real world. . . . A miracle is so far from being a contradiction to the causal principle that it is primarily a better illustration of that principle than an event happening in the ordinary course of nature. . . . A developed mythology shows that man has taken a deep and active interest both in the world and in himself, and has tried to link the two, and interpret the one by the other. Myth is therefore a natural prologue to philosophy, since the love of ideas is the root of both. Both are made up of things admirable to consider.[41]

NOTES

1. The contents and therefore the title of this paper vary somewhat from the paper prepared for presentation at the conference. Lack of time there did not permit our giving the section on limb-burial superstitions, their relationship to the PLP, and their clinical implications and applications. These subjects will be considered in another article.

2. S. Weir Mitchell, "Phantom Limbs," *Lippincott's Mag. Pop. Lit. and Sci.*, 8 (1871), 563-569.

3. Specific references to frequently reported aspects of the PLP will not be cited; at least one of the following references applies to these aspects: Macdonald Critchley, "The Body-Image in Neurology," *Lancet*, 1 (1950), 335-341; Jack R. Ewalt, Guy C. Randall, and Harry Morris, "The Phantom Limb," *Psychosom. Med.*, 9 (1947), 118-123; J[oseph] A. M. Frederiks, "Occurrence and Nature of Phantom Limb Phenomenon Following Amputation of Body Parts and Following Lesions of the Central and Peripheral Nervous System," *Psychiat. Neurol. Neurochir.*, 66 (1963), 73-97; W. R. Henderson and G. E. Smyth, "Phantom Limbs," *J. Neurol., Neurosurg. and Psychiat.*, 11 (1948), 88-112; Lawrence C. Kolb, *The Painful Phantom: Psychology, Physiology and Treatment* (Springfield, Ill.: Charles C. Thomas, [1954]); S. Weir Mitchell, *Injuries of Nerves and Their Consequences* (Philadelphia: J. B. Lippincott & Co., 1872), chap. 14, pp. 342-368; Paul Schilder, *The Image and Appearance of the Human Body* . . . (New York: International Universities Press, Inc., 1950), pp. 63-70; Kauko A. Solonen, "The Phantom Phenomenon in Amputated Finnish War Veterans," *Acta orthopaed. scand.*, suppl., 54, 1962; Erwin Steter, "Zur Phaenomenologie des Phantomgliedes," *Deutsche Zeitsch. f. Nervenheilk.*, 163 (1950), 141-171.

4. O[tfrid] Foerster, "Über das Phantomglied," *Med. Kl.*, 27 (1931), 497-500.

5. Stetter, *op. cit.*

6. F. Lobligeois, "Auto-Observation d'Illusion des Amputés," *Monde Méd.*, 37 (1927), 873-878.

7. Water Riese, "Über die sog. Phantomhand der Amputierten," *Deutsche Zeitsch. f. Nervenheilk.*, 23 (1928), 270-281.

8. Jean-Martin Charcot, *Leçons du Mardi à la Salpêtrière. Policliniques. 1888-1889.* (Paris: Bureaux du Progrès Médical, 1889), pp. 447-460, (lesson 1, June 18, 1888).

9. A[rthur] M. Blood, "Psychotherapy of Phantom Limb Pain in Two Patients," *Psychiat. Quart.*, 30 (1956), 114-122. (Blood presents some interesting variants and clinical aspects of superstitions about disposal of amputated limbs.)

10. Riese, *op. cit.*

11. William B. Haber, "Observations on Phantom-Limb Phenomena," *Arch. N. and P.*, 75 (1956), 624-636.

12. Sidney Weinstein and Eugene A. Sersen, "Phantoms in Cases of Congenital Absence of Limbs," *Neurol.*, 11 (1961), 905-911.

13. James E. Miles, "The Phantom Limb Syndrome Occurring during Spinal Anesthesia: Relationship to Etiology," *J. nerv. ment. Dis.*, 123 (1956), 365-368; Stephen J. Prevoznik and James E. Eckenhoff, "Phantom Sensations during Spinal Anesthesia," *Anesthes.*, 25 (1964), 767-770.

14. Ernest Bors, "Phantom Limbs of Patients with Spinal Cord Injury," *Arch. N. and P.*, 66 (1951), 610-631.

15. Douglas B. Price, "The Phantom Limb in Patients with Leprosy" (in preparation).

16. Stetter, an amputee himself, in his excellent paper, *op. cit.*, has subsumed the characteristics of the natural PL under the term *das Phantomgliederlebniss*, "the phantom limb experience." Weinstein and Sersen, *op. cit.*, refer in passing to a "natural" phantom in one individual with aplasia of an upper limb.

17. W. Noordenbos, *Pain: Problems Pertaining to the Transmission of Nerve Impulses Which Give Rise to Pain* (Amsterdam: Elsevier Publ. Co., 1959), chap. 19, pp. 150-164.

18. Schilder, *op. cit.*

19. Marianne L. Simmel, "Phantoms in Patients with Leprosy and in Elderly Digital Amputees," *Am. J. Psychol.*, 69 (1956), 529-545. (One case of frostbite is mentioned. In this study—the only other investigation of the PLP in leprosy patients besides ours—Simmel did not find any PLs associated with digital shortening in thirteen patients. This contrasts with our study, in which twenty-three out of thirty-five patients with shortened digits had PLs; nineteen were natural and four were typical. Out of a total of forty-two patients, four patients (three with digital shortening and one with an amputation) did not have any PLs.)

20. François Nicolas Marquet, *Observations sur la Guérison de Plusieurs Maladies Notables Aigues, et Chroniques;* . . . (Paris: Chez Briasson, 1750), pp. 141-145.

21. Stith Thompson, *Motif-Index of Folk-Literature;* . . ., rev. and enl. ed., 6 vols. (Copenhagen: Rosenkilde and Bagger, 1953-1958). In this work, especially vol. 2 under "Magic Powers and Manifestations," a number of references to stories concerning the restoration of lost body parts are given. As far as general examples of the motif are concerned, this index is invaluable; yet it is insufficient as a source of references to medieval stories, especially in Latin but also in the vernacular other than English. For the present study we used the following works: Albert Poncelet, "Miraculorum B. V. Mariae quae Saec. VI-XV Latine Conscripta Sunt Index Postea Perficiendus," *Analecta Bollandiana*, 21 (1902), 241-360 (sometimes available separately); Alfred Mussafia, "Studien zu den mittelalterlichen Marienlegenden," *Sitzungsberichte d. phil.-hist. Classe d. Kaiser. Akad. d. Wissensch. (Wien)* [five articles], (I) 113 (1886), 917-994; (II) 115 (1888), 5-92; (III) 119 (Abh. IX) (1889), 1-66; (IV) 123 (Abh. VIII) (1891), 1-85; and (V) 139 (Abh. VIII) (1898), 1-74; H[arry] L. D. Ward (Vol. II) and J[ohn] A. Herbert (Vol. III), *Catalogue of Romances in the Department of Manuscripts in the British Museum*, Vols. II and III (London: Printed by order of the Trustees, 1893 and 1910); John Esten Keller, *Motif-Index of Mediaeval Spanish Exempla* (Knoxville, Tenn.: University of Tennessee Press, [1949]). (Material from this index was incorporated in the revised edition of Thompson's *Motif-Index*. Keller has misread some of the exempla concerning amputation, e.g., V411.3 (Enx. 295), p. 63, and thus some are incorrectly categorized.)

22. Stories of the loss and restoration of the eye and the tongue were not included in this survey because there is insufficient clinical information about phantom eyes and tongues on which to base an analysis of correspondence between

elements in the stories and PL aspects. The lack of clinical information on phantom eyes is regrettable because stories of the loss and restoration of eyes are the most common and perhaps the only representatives of the motif (other than tales about replacement of the head) in American Indian folklore.

23. We are presently finishing a monograph-length treatment of this study, which has been going on for several years in collaboration especially with Neil J. Twombly, S. J., professor emeritus of Latin, Georgetown University, Washington, D.C.; Mary R. Price, my wife; and Mary Chamberlain, Ph.D. I am deeply grateful to these individuals, for the testing of my hypothesis was possible only through their interest and efforts in translating, respectively, the miracles from the Latin, Greek, and Italian; the French; and the Spanish and Portuguese. I am also very grateful to Father Twombly for his knowledgeable scrutiny of all the translations, for his careful reading of this paper and his numerous suggestions that improved it, and for the example of his scholarship and keen logic. Thus, the editorial "we" in this section reflects the collaborative nature of the work.

24. Guibert de Nogent, *Liber de Laude Sanctae Mariae*, in his . . . *Opera Omnia* . . ., ed. Luc d'Achéry (Lutetiae Parisiorum: Sumptibus Ioannis Billaine, 1651), pp. 304D-306E (Caput XI). Reprinted in *Patrologiae Cursus Completus* . . . *Series Latina* . . ., ed. J[acques]-P[aul] Migne, 221 vols. (Parisiis: Apud Garnier Fratres, 1879-1890), 156, cols. 568-572.

25. Franciscus a Sancta Clara, *Religio Philosophi Peripati Discutienda; in qua offertur Epitome Processus Historiae Celeberrimi Miraculi, a Christo Nuperrime Patrati, in Restitutione Tibiae Abscissae & Sepultae, ab Aristotele in suis Principiis Examinati* (Duaci: Typis Baltasaris Belleri, 1662), pp. 150-162 (*Epitome*). Except where noted in the text, we have taken the story from the *Epitome* which closes the work. Daniel Turner, *The Art of Surgery:* . . ., 4th ed., 2 vols. (London: Printed for C. Rivington, J. Lacy, and J. Clarke, 1732), II, 504-509. Turner adds to the end of this edition of his surgical treatise an abstract of Franciscus's *Religio*. We are grateful to Richard J. Durling, Ph.D., of the Institut für Geschichte der Medizin und Pharmazie, Christian-Albrechts-Universität, Kiel, for bringing the Turner reference to our attention. It was from this work that we learned of Franciscus's *Religio*. After we had presented the version of this paper at the conference, we had the opportunity to read the earlier and briefer comments on the miracle which Franciscus first published in 1652 in a work under the name of Francis Coventry (Franciscus Coventriensis), one of his several pseudonyms: Franciscus a Sancta Clara, *Paralipomena Philosophica de Mundo Peripatetico* in his *Operum Omnium Scholasticorum et Historicorum* . . ., 2 vols. (Duaci: Ex Typographia Baltazaris Belleri, 1665-1667), II, 36, cols. 1 and 2, and 70, col. 2. This account confirmed several conjectures we made while analyzing the account in the *Religio*. There are also important differences in the two accounts; we note here only one: in the *Paralipomena*, there is no indication that the restoration was imperfect for three days. Franciscus first heard of the miracle probably in 1649, perhaps 1650, in Paris from several individuals who had been in Spain at the time of its happening. Since over a decade had passed since the miracle, it is unlikely that imperfections would have been included in an oral account of the event. Moreover, at the time of writing the *Paralipomena*, Franciscus had not yet seen the *Epitome*, which was an official resume of the judicial proceeding, called *Processus*, held to investigate the event and conducted by the Spanish Inquisition in 1641. It was this body that declared the event a miracle.

26. Douglas B. Price and Neil J. Twombly, *The Phantom Limb: An Eighteenth Century Latin Dissertation: Text and Translation, with a Medical-Historical and Linguistic Commentary*, Languages and Linguistics Working Papers no. 3 (Washington, D. C.: Georgetown University Press, 1972), pp. 39-40.

27. After completing his education in France, Franciscus returned to England, where he soon became "remarkable for his learning." (*Dictionary of National Biography*, s.v. "Christopher Davenport"; John Berchmans Dockery, *Christopher Davenport, Friar and Diplomat* (London: Burns & Oates, 1960), p. 25. To judge from some of his writings, he was especially well read in philosophy but also in scientific

and occult fields. With this background and these interests, it would not be unreasonable to expect that he had come across one of the twenty or so published reports on the PLP, five of which were in works by philosophers and one in Martin Schoock's tract on ecstasy, a subject which Franciscus treats in his *Paralipomena* (pp. 72ff). Internal and circumstantial evidence—too lengthy to document here— indicates he could have read two of these reports.

28. None of the versions of any of the five main stories was exactly the same as any other. Since there were also variations in the elements concerning the restored parts, the finding in twenty-one stories of elements that can be equated with the PLP cannot have been the result of simple copying from earlier versions, although this is the case in some of the stories. There is evidence in some of the accounts that the author was familiar with the psychology of the amputee. On that basis, we conjectured that these authors were personally acquainted with the PLP.

29. John [VI], Patriarch of Jerusalem, βίος τοῦ Ὁσίον Πατρός Ἡμῶν Ἰωάννου τοῦ Δαμασκήνου ..., in *Patrologiae Cursus Completus ... Series Graeca ...*, ed. J[acques]-P[aul] Migne, 166 vols. (Parisiis: Apud Garnier Fratres, 1857-1866), 94, cols. 439D-460C (VII-XX).

30. From folklore and clinical sources, published and unpublished, we have collected some thirty-nine American variants of this superstition; in eleven, PL type of pain or paresthesia is implied or understood, and in twenty-eight, the phantom nature of the sensations is stated or indicated in explicit terms. We are greatly indebted to Wayland D. Hand for his supplying over the years many of the references to these superstitions from the materials he has been collecting for his Dictionary of American Popular Beliefs and Superstitions.

31. Daniel L. Thomas and Lucy B. Thomas, *Kentucky Superstitions* (Princeton, N.J.: Princeton University Press, 1920), p. 93, no. 1059.

32. Annie W. Whitney and Caroline C. Bullock, comp., *Folk-Lore from Maryland*, Memoirs of the American Folklore Society, vol. 18 (New York: American Folklore Society, 1925), p. 93, no. 1875.

33. Franciscus a S. C., *Religio*, pp. 1, 10, 16, 46-47, 74, and title page.

34. From our visits to five leprosy centers (two each in the Pacific and South America and one in the Caribbean), we learned that burial of amputated major limbs in the hospital cemetery was usual. One patient who had amputated his own great toe in the hope of stopping the spread of his case of lepromatous leprosy buried the toe at the edge of the cemetery. The practice in these leprosariums contrasts with the usual disposal by incineration in modern general hospitals. That there is some current general interest in hospital practices regarding disposal of dismembered body parts is attested by a question on the subject sent recently to Ann Lander's *Advice* column (*Washington Post*, Aug. 2, 1973).

35. In this version, written in the early fifteenth century, the component was altered in an unusual way: "... all the bad flesh and all the rotted flesh ... fell off him and he had them buried" (Jean Mielot, *Miracles de Nostre Dame*, ed. George F. Warner [Westminster: Nichols & Sons, 1885], pp. 38-40 [XLI]).

36. Joh. Nicolas (i.e., Johann Nikolaus) Binninger, ... *Observationum et Curationum Medicinalium, Centuriae Quinque* (Montbelgardi: Typis Hyppianis, 1673), p. 142; Johann Bohn, ... *De Officio Medici Duplici, Clinici Nimirum ac Forensis*, ... (Lipsiae: Apud J. Friedericum Gleditsch, 1704), p. 233; Joannes Scultetus (i.e., Johann Schultes), Χειροπλοθήκη *seu ... Armamentarium Chirurgicum XLIII. Tabulis ...* (Ulmae Suevorum: Typis & impensis Balthasari Kühnen, 1655), p. 18. (First published 1653.)

37. Johann Jacob Wunderlich, *Paradoxa Sensatio, sive Dolor Membri Amputati* (Master's diss., Tubingae: Typis Georg-Henrici ReisI, 1693), pp. 12-13. In interposing the concept of sympathy as a possible explanation of paradoxical sensations, i.e., the PLP, Wunderlich stated: "Certainly surgeons, to whatever school of thought they belong, religiously preserve such [amputated] members from decay, suspending them in smoke and making them quite dry." Despite a long and still continuing search, neither corroboration nor elucidation of this remark of Wunderlich's has

been possible. Examination of many works on surgery, medicine, embalming, burial and social customs, and general and specific histories has failed to turn up any reference to a custom of preserving limbs around the seventeenth century. (We appreciate the many hours Ms. Hanna S. Fields has spent examining nonmedical sources). The negative finding of this search agrees with the opinions of the following historians of medicine (surgery) or science as expressed in personal communication in 1972 or 1973: Allen G. Debus, Ph.D., Richard J. Durling, Ph.D., Professor Mirko Drazen Grmek, Professor Pierre Huard, Jerry Stannard, Ph.D., Owen H. Wangensteen, M.D., and Leo M. Zimmerman, M.D.

Still, the practice described by Wunderlich is very similar to an event which took place in Adoua, Abyssinia, in 1839 and which was recorded by one Doctor Antoine Petit: three prisoners of war were each punished by the amputation of a hand and a foot. The amputated parts were placed on an iron plate, similar to that used for making bread, and cooked over a fire. After the flesh was dried, the parts were to have been kept in butter until the individual died, when they would be buried with him. This practice was done so that the individual could rise again whole on the universal day of judgment (Antoine Petit, "Note A" in [Charlemagne]-Théophile Lefebvre, *Voyage en Abyssinie Exécuté Pendant les Années 1839 [à] 1843* . . ., 6 vols. in 8 [Paris: Arthus Bertrand (Preface: 1845-)1851], I, 2d pt., pp. 369-379).

38. Paré has universally been acknowledged to be the first to describe the PLP (Ambroise Paré, *La Maniere de Traicter les Playes Faictes tât par Hacquebutes, que par Fleches:* . . . [A Paris: Par la vefue Iean de Brie, 1551], fol. 59 recto). During our work on the history of the PLP, however, we discovered what may be an earlier reference by Girolamo Fracastoro (Hieronymus Fracastorius, *De Sympathia et Antipathia Rerum Liber Unus* . . . [Venetiis (Colophon: apud heredes Lucaeantonij Iuntae) 1546], fol. 17 recto).

39. Bernard J. Ficarra, "Amputations and Prostheses through the Centuries," *Med. Rec.*, 156 (1943), 94-97; 154-156; and 239-240. Norman T. Kirk, "The Development of Amputation," *Bull. Med. Libr. Assoc.*, 32 (1944), 131-163.

40. The fact that visual elements are often included in the descriptions of the restored limbs in the miracles may indicate a greater optical component in PLs of medieval amputees than is the case today.

41. George Santayana, *The Life of Reason or the Phases of Human Progress. Reason in Religion* (New York: Charles Scribner's Sons, 1945), pp. 22 and 51. By kind permission of the publisher.

A New Approach to the "Old Hag":
The Nightmare Tradition Reexamined

DAVID J. HUFFORD, *Memorial University of Newfoundland*

It is my intention that this paper should make two major points beyond its immediate subject matter. The first is that folklore research can make direct contributions to the solution of specific medical problems. In other words, there is an important place for medical "applied folklore" work.

The second point is that research into folk belief, including folk medicine, often misses information of great importance as a result of an overly deductive approach. Practically all studies of belief begin with quite a heavy burden of assumptions, often implicit, which act to filter out certain kinds of data. Three such assumptions are especially distorting: (1) that statements which do not appear to allow for materialistic interpretation may be rejected out of hand; (2) that "the folk" are always poor observers and consistently confuse subjective with objective reality—a confusion which the scholar can unravel rather easily at second hand; and (3) that informants therefore cannot maintain memorates separate from legends (this leads to an underemphasis on von Sydow's important distinction between memorate and legend).[1] All of these positions have something to recommend them for use at some point in research, but when used *in the field*, they completely spoil objectivity. It is such assumptions that have often prevented field-workers from gathering such essential information as the actual success and failure rates of folk healers, since it has generally been thought that this data can be extrapolated from the extent to which their methods resemble orthodox therapy. What is needed is a more rigorously empirical approach to the collection of data. We should suspend our disbelief and not start wondering immediately what *really* happened—that is, what would be an explanation we would accept. When an informant relates a bizarre but believed experience, we should try to ask some of the questions that his friends and neighbors might, as well as those that occur to a university professor.

Now to the main subject of this paper. In Newfoundland there is a group of traditions centering on what is locally called "the Old Hag." Like most terms that exist largely in oral tradition, *Old Hag* refers to more than a single thing, but it does have a well-defined core of meaning. It primarily refers to certain kinds of dreams and dreamlike experiences, all of them unpleasant, which are sometimes seen as pathological. However, most bad dreams are not included under this heading. Those that are, usually exhibit some of the following characteristics: being chased by an evil creature; being crushed; falling; and "being unable to wake yourself up." This last point is often mentioned and seems to indicate that these are lucid dreams[2]—that is, that the sleeper is aware that he is sleeping. A belief that one can *really* be killed in these dreams is often stated. People generally report that when awakened from such a dream, they are exhausted and drenched with sweat.

More often Old Hag refers to the following experience: (1) waking up during the night (or occasionally the experience occurs before sleep); (2) hearing and/or seeing something come into the room and approach the bed; (3) being pressed on the chest or strangled and therefore feeling suffocation; (4) being unable to move or cry out until either being awakened by someone or finally breaking through the feeling of paralysis, at which point all of the sensations usually cease. As with the dream, there is often cold sweat, palpitations, and exhaustion. The victim is almost invariably lying on his back during the experience and is convinced that he has been awake throughout. These are the same basic features described in Tillhagen's essay "The Conception of the Nightmare in Sweden"[3] and Ernest Jones's *On the Nightmare*,[4] two of the best-known works on the subject, and it is obvious that the Old Hag is part of the Nightmare tradition. The one point that neither Tillhagen nor Jones stresses is the insistence that this is a waking experience rather than a genuine dream.

In Newfoundland there are also many statements about who is most likely to have the Old Hag, or to be "hag-ridden" or "ag-rog,"[5] and when. But there is no general agreement on this except for the omnipresent condition of lying on one's back, and the reports do not come heavily from one sex or age group. There is more consistency about causation: the most common naturalistic explanation is poor circulation. Jones provides a very useful recapitulation of eighteenth- and nineteenth-century medical opinion on the Nightmare,[6] and the local naturalistic explanations correspond closely to this outdated material.

Newfoundland tradition also supplies some supernatural explanations of the Old Hag. Most common is the idea that an ordinary person can hag another for spite. A malicious person can accomplish hagging by performing certain ritual acts, such as saying the Lord's Prayer backward before going to bed. Occasionally it is said that the one likely to do the hagging is actually a witch. Least common is the belief that the Old Hag may be a ghost.

Naturally, tradition supplies a number of ways of preventing the Old Hag. These are very similar to the common protections against witches: sleeping with a Bible or knife under the pillow or turning one's shoes out from the bed at night. But by far the most common preventative is simply to avoid sleeping on one's back.

The Old Hag tradition is widely distributed in Newfoundland and is known to many younger people as well as their elders, but not all in either age group know and understand it. Nonetheless, the knowledge of the tradition has been general enough that a ballad composed in the 1920s by Johnny Burke, a local broadside man, could contain the following lines:

> For her skirts are so tight around the hips, Jennie,
> It's no wonder she got the old hag.[7]

After I had obtained this general picture of the Old Hag, I decided to employ the approach that I suggested at the beginning of this paper: to suspend my tendency to disbelief and attempt to seek out the experience itself, rather than the tradition only. In this way I was trying the most parsimonious hypothesis: that the statements by informants refer with fair accuracy to an actual phenomenon which has been experienced by a number of people, rather than to traditional elaborations on mundane dreams. The fact that the great majority of the narratives containing clear descriptions of the event are memorates rather than other kinds of legend suggested that this approach would be useful. The accounts is Jones's book, *On the Nightmare*[8] and Heinrich Roscher's essay "Ephialtes,"[9] also supported my hypothesis, although their interpretations did not fit my observations.

In order to test the hypothesis, I composed a questionnaire on the Old Hag that ran in an order roughly opposite to the one previously circulated by the Memorial University of Newfoundland

Folklore and Language Archive.[10] The first three questions were "Have you ever awakened during the night to find yourself paralyzed, that is, unable to move or cry out?"; "Are you aware of anyone else having had such an experience?"; and "Describe as many of the features of this experience as you can." I then asked for general information, such as the length of time involved, frequency, manner of termination, and so forth. This ambiguous portion of the questionnaire contained twelve questions. Then the final questions were "Define the Old Hag"; and "Have you ever known anyone who had the Old Hag?" These were the only references to the term *Old Hag* in the questionnaire. I administered the questionnaire to university classes in the following way: having obtained the instructor's permission, I arrived unannounced and simply stated that I wished to administer a questionnaire; I then presented the questions orally, waiting until everyone had finished answering before proceeding to the next one. In this way I intended not only to avoid suggesting answers, but also to separate information concerning the occurrence of the event from the knowledge of the tradition.

Although I do not yet have an adequate sample to justify any strong statistical statements, my preliminary results may be summarized as follows: of those questioned about one-sixth have had the experience themselves; about one-fourth have either had it or heard of someone else who has; about one-half know something about the Old Hag tradition; of those who have had the experience themselves, about one-half do not know the Old Hag tradition (that is, they were unfamiliar with the term *Old Hag* and were not aware of others having had the experience). Of these latter individuals a number reported complete Old Hag experiences, with the ugly creature, suffocation, and so forth. Other interesting information came to light through the questionnaire, but this disclosure was the most dramatic.

To me these results are quite astonishing. Based on the questionnaire findings, subsequent interviews, and research in both folklore and psychiatric literature, the following picture emerges: (1) accounts of the Old Hag or Nightmare center on an actual experience which is adequately described, generally without elaboration, by the informants themselves; (2) this is a far more common experience than the literature suggests; (3) the obvious explanation that tradition has shaped or even created this experience is not correct, and the opposite seems to be true—a recurring human experience has given rise to and shaped the tradition.

At this point the next logical step was an effort to find out how local or widespread this peculiar situation might be. As mentioned above, both Jones and Roscher provide a number of reports. Most of these are quite old, reaching back to classical antiquity, and they are mostly of a very sophisticated or even literary nature. In order to extend the picture beyond this material, I looked for connections between the Old Hag and other folk traditions which might refer to the same experience. Some were obvious.

A few reports from the field in Newfoundland together with a considerable mass of etymological data[11] make it clear that there is a genetic relationship between the Old Hag in Newfoundland and traditions of witches riding on people. Although I have not seen this connection discussed by folklorists, it is difficult to imagine that it has not been noticed before. Thompson seems to have missed it in the *Motif-Index*,[12] for there are no cross-references between his "Nightmare" numbers (F471.1.ff) and his "Witch rides on person . . ." number (G241.2.). Nonetheless, the existence of the connection is undeniable when enough of these witch accounts are read. The more elaborate accounts involving magical bridles and the transformation of the victim into a horse[13] do not provide much help, but a good many witch-riding memorates have no such fantastic details and consist of the same sort of material given by Newfoundlanders when they speak of being hagged. Two excellent examples of this kind of narrative are found in Dorson's *American Negro Folktales*,[14] where they are indexed under the witch-riding motif number.

The connection of the Old Hag experience with some ghost tales is now also clear. In Hand's Volume VII of the *Brown Collection*,[15] for example, there are several notes that refer to ghost stories that do not contain the word *nightmare* but describe the experience. Especially useful instances are Hand's references to the "Lineback Ghost" in the "Tales and Legends" portion of Volume I of the *Brown Collection* and to Hudson's 1934 article on the "Bell Witch" in the *Journal of American Folklore*.

Outside of folk tradition, interestingly, the same experience has turned up regularly in the popular literature on flying saucers and other weird phenomena. For example, John Keel comments at considerable length on such reports in his book *Strange Creatures Out of Space and Time*,[16] in which he uses the term "Bedroom Invaders" without showing any awareness of the older traditions. Besides providing some very intriguing material for analysis in connection with the Old Hag, these examples illustrate some of the important questions about the relationship of popular printed materials to folk belief.

It should be noted that the search for these accounts is not an easy one. In addition to the absence of cross-references between Nightmare and witch-riding stories, there is a frustrating lack of description of informants' subjective experiences of both hauntings and witch riding. Such a major work as Kittredge's *Witchcraft in Old and New England*[17] does not have a single description of witch riding or Nightmare, although it makes numerous references to both. Many collections which might have been expected to contain texts of Nightmare or witch-riding—for example, Hyatt's *Folk-Lore from Adams County, Illinois*[18]—instead occupy themselves solely with cures and preventives. Most of these difficulties appear to result from the collector's assumption that he was dealing with fiction. They are further aggravated by the constant failure of many authors of all kinds to distinguish clearly between the word *nightmare* as it is often used today to cover all bad dreams and the "classical" sense in which Jones and others use it.

Despite these difficulties, I have managed to bring together enough memorates of the Nightmare experience (using *Nightmare* as the most general term) to feel safe in making the following statements about the distribution of the phenomenon: (1) the experience is widespread, at least throughout Western culture; (2) it has been regularly reported for more than two thousand years;[19] (3) it has been attached to a variety of narrative frameworks too numerous to give here, but regardless of the framework, the experiential features have remained basically the same; (4) this consistency of detail, apparently rather independent of tradition, is the most surprising and difficult feature to account for.

As far as I am aware, there are just two fairly accessible explanations of the Nightmare and, therefore, of the related traditions given above; and one or the other of these two is generally offered even today. The first is the outdated medical opinion already mentioned. This ranges from indigestion, as in Scrooge's explanation in *A Christmas Carol*,[20] to various kinds of neurological and circulatory "stagnation." Jones does a good job of dispatching this school of thought by pointing out that the factors usually brought forward for these ideas, such as going to bed with a full stomach, are often present without Nightmare, and just as frequently Nightmare can be shown to occur when they are absent.[21] Although such explanations are therefore inadequate, they still appear in serious works— for example, Nathaniel Kleitman's important *Sleep and Wakefulness.*[22]

Jones's explanation is far more ingenious and has gained fairly wide circulation.[23] Although my understanding of Nightmare coincides with Jones's on the crucial point that we are dealing with a real experience, there are several other points in his interpretation with which I must take issue. Put very briefly, these points are the following: (1) the Nightmare is a class of genuine dream experiences; and (2) it can always be interpreted in sexual—specifically feminine, masochistic, genital, and repressed—terms. Such an interpretation is hardly a surprise coming from a classical psychoanalytic writer like Jones. However, my research provides counterevidence on both points. First, (and compressed as much as possible) the evidence that this is not a dream rests on these factors: (1) the victims state that they were not dreaming; (2) the event always takes place in a setting identical to the victim's real situation, usually his bedroom; (3) perceptions are clear, and there is none of the ineffable, evanescent quality usually associated with dreams; (4) some reports include corroboration of the victim's visual perceptions while in this state; and (5) those who discover individuals being hagged and awaken them sometimes report seeing that their eyes are open during the event.

Stating that the Nightmare is some altered state of consciousness other than a sleep dream is, I realize, not immediately very informative.[24] But ruling out ordinary dreams as the source does at least redirect our attention. There are several features in the Nightmare experience which suggest that an altered state of consciousness might have been spontaneously produced. In order to see these features, we must first take a brief look at just what conditions have been found to lead to such states. Very useful for this investigation is Arnold Ludwig's article "Altered States of Consciousness,"[25] which provides a concise list of these conditions. Ludwig prefaces the list with the observation that "there seems to be an optimal range of exteroceptive stimulation necessary for the maintenance of normal, waking consciousness, and levels of stimulation either above or below this range appear conducive to the production of ASC's . . ." (as altered states are often called).[26] It is reduced levels which occur in the situations reported to produce Nightmare. Ludwig's first specific condition is "*Reduction of exteroceptive stimulation and/or motor activity.*"[27] Here he notes such things as highway hypnosis, experimental deprivation states, and hypnagogic and hypnopompic states. The fact that Nightmare almost always occurs when the victim is lying on his back either preparing for sleep or, occasionally, reading[28] indicates that this sort of reduction is practically always present. Voluntary motor activity stops; visual stimulation ceases when the eyes close; auditory stimulation is usually at a very low level; tactile stimulation quickly becomes redundant and is lost; internal sensations of strain are less likely because of the more general and even support of the supine position. If a person stays this way for very long without passing into normal sleep, he will soon approximate quite closely the conditions of experimental sensory deprivation.

Another pertinent condition given by Ludwig is *"Decreased alertness or relaxation of critical faculties."*[29] This is, of course, generally the case when one is preparing for sleep and is not uncommon while reading, as shown by the phenomenon of "reading trance."

Finally, Ludwig mentions *"Presence of somatopsychological factors,"*[30] among which he lists hyperventilation. I have inferred that hyperventilation is often present in Nightmare from the fact that those who have the experience often report a feeling of suffocation and great difficulty in breathing, but those who have observed others having Nightmare often report that the victim was breathing very heavily. Hyperventilation is characterized by "overbreathing" together with a sense of suffocation caused by the resulting chemical imbalances. It does not appear that hyperventilation is always present, but when it is, we might expect it further to alter consciousness and intensify the experience.

Many of the reports I have collected from Nightmare victims include statements that strongly suggest ASCs. These include disturbances of time sense; anomalous emotions; changes in body image, including out-of-the-body feelings; some perceptual changes, usually observed as an increase in clarity; and the hallucination. It is also significant that whenever a victim offers an analogy to explain his sensations better, he chooses clearly altered states other than dreams. I have, for example, received comparisons to hallucinogenic drug experiences, gasoline sniffing experiences, and the experience of being unable to come out from under anesthetic after surgery.

So much for my reasons for doubting Jones's position that Nightmare is a class of genuine dreams. Concerning his sexual interpretation I would simply note that many of the reports do not contain anything that appears to be sexual content, either repressed or overt, nor does the assumption of its existence appear to make the experience more understandable. Therefore, Jones's interpretation does not seem sound on grounds of parsimony when one looks at the general run of the material. Additional arguments against this aspect of Jones's interpretation, from a different quarter, may be found in J. A. Hadfield's *Dreams and Nightmares.*[31]

If one accepts, then, that Nightmare is an ASC other than ordinary dreaming, the first logical place to look for related

phenomena is the hypnagogic state, the period between wakefulness and sleep, which is just starting to be seriously researched.
Vogel, Fuolkes, and Trosman's article "Ego Functions and Dreaming During Sleep Onset"[32] provides a good introduction to this
state as studied in the laboratory and gives much data relevant to
the question, Is Nightmare a special class of ordinary hypnagogic
phenomena? Defining the hypnagogic state in terms of brain wave
activity and eye movement proceeding in four stages from waking
alpha wave activity through descending stage 2, these authors
report finding substantial dream ("defined as hallucinated dramatic episodes"[33]) in all four stages, contradicting claims that
dreams occur only during emergent stage 1 rapid eye movement
(REM) periods. This discovery appears promising, but they further
state that compared with REM dreams hypnagogic dreams "were
usually shorter, had less effect and were more discontinuous; that
is, more like a succession of slides than like a movie...."[34] This
would suggest that hypnagogic phenomena are, at least typically,
even less like Nightmare than are ordinary REM sleeping dreams.
Nonetheless, some of the material presented in their study does
suggest directions for further investigation relevant to Nightmare.

The direction which has so far proved most fruitful for my
attempts to pin down the Nightmare ASC has been the medical
literature on narcolepsy.[35] This is an illness of which the definitive
characteristic is a very strong and abnormally frequent drowsiness
and urge to sleep. This unavoidable sleep is sometimes frequent
enough to disrupt the sufferer's life thoroughly. Its auxiliary
symptoms are very interesting for our present purpose. These are
clearly described by Robert Yoss and David Daly in their paper
"Criteria for the Diagnosis of the Narcoleptic Syndrome."[36] From
their extensive study they present the following picture:

> Narcolepsy, cataplexy, sleep paralysis, and hypnagogic hallucinations
> make up the narcoleptic tetrad, but only 11 per cent of patients
> presented this complete picture. All patients had narcolepsy; 68 per
> cent had cataplexy; 24 per cent had sleep paralysis; 30 per cent had
> hypnagogic hallucinations.[37]

Cataplexy, briefly, is a "sudden decrease or loss of muscle tone,
which may be generalized or limited to certain muscles."[38] The
cataplectic attack is precipitated by strong emotion, such as laughing at a joke, and the victim apparently remains conscious through
the generally very brief attack. Some writers have suggested a
connection between cataplexy and sleep paralysis,[39] and they do
have some obvious similarities.

About sleep paralysis Yoss and Daly say:

> The incidence of sleep paralysis is low, and usually the episodes occur
> infrequently. The typical attack seizes the patient as he falls asleep at
> night or awakens in the morning. Suddenly he is aware that he cannot
> move or cry out; yet he feels awake. This may last only a few seconds
> or as long as a minute or two. The attack either terminates spon-
> taneously or will end if someone touches or talks to the patient.[40]

This is clearly a reasonable description of some of the most
important features of Nightmare.

The matter becomes even more startling in the authors' discussion of hypnagogic hallucinations:

> Some patients report visual or auditory hallucinations. . . . In many
> instances there may be concommitant sleep paralysis. Some authors
> describe the content of the hallucinations as unpleasant or even
> terrifying; this has not been our impression.[41]

Sleep paralysis with unpleasant hypnagogic hallucinations, then,
would seem to be practically identical to Nightmare. The statement
that the hallucinations are not always unpleasant is also consistent
with my findings. I have had many reports, perhaps one-half the
total, in which the element of the frightening hallucination was
absent. Those with the frightful attacker simply stand out because
they constitute the only single picture encountered repeatedly.

It is difficult to know just what to make of this unexpected
surfacing of the Nightmare, especially because the connection is
never made in the literature so far as I have been able to discover.
However, Yoss and Daly's statistics, taken with my preliminary
results, indicate that sleep paralysis (frequently with "hypnagogic
hallucination"), which was the definitive characteristic in my
questionnaire, occurred only slightly more often among their
sample of narcoleptics than it appears among Newfoundland
university students.[42] Yet the incidence of narcolepsy is less than
one-half of 1 percent in the total population.[43] This must at least
raise a serious question about the value of sleep paralysis and
hypnagogic hallucination as diagnostic indicators of narcolepsy,
though it can by no means rule out the possibility of some sort of
connection. This caution must be stressed because of some recent
work which suggests that there are differences between narcoleptics who show auxiliary symptoms and those who do not.[44] Allan
Resctschaffen and William Dement have offered an interesting
theory about the nature of the narcoleptic states. Very briefly, it is
that they are some sort of accidental triggering of the REM sleep
phenomenon.[45] One reason for this theory is the fact that there is

characteristically a loss of muscle tone during REM periods, and this loss could serve to explain the paralysis. Also, since it is known that dreams are very frequent during REM sleep, the theory could also provide a convenient explanation of the hallucinations. The primary objection to it is that which I raised earlier in arguing against Jones's treatment of Nightmare as a genuine dream phenomenon. Reschtschaffen and Dement make the following comment on this difficulty:

> The relation between narcoleptic symptoms and REM periods still leaves open the question of why the attacks of cataplexy should be experienced mostly during wakefulness and why sleep paralysis and hypnagogic hallucinations should be subjectively experienced as waking phenomena rather than aspects of ordinary dreams. This question is not yet answered. One hypothesis has proposed that in narcolepsy there is a failure of the mechanisms of wakefulness to inhibit REM sleep. Thus phenomena of REM sleep and wakefulness could occur simultaneously in narcoleptics.[46]

If this were true, the same would presumably have to be said about those otherwise normal people who experience Nightmare. Perhaps such an unusual event could be a result of the ASC to which I have ascribed Nightmare; or perhaps further research into this altered state will make the REM hypothesis seem less necessary for the understanding of Nightmare.[47] In any event, these facts from the narcoleptic literature strongly urge further inquiry into the apparent connections between the narcoleptic tetrad and the Nightmare and related traditions, from both the medical and the folkloristic points of view.

SUMMARY

The Old Hag, Nightmare, witch riding, and some other traditions are based on a recurring and real human experience which is widespread and frequent. Some of the features of this experience may be seen as logically arising from an altered state(s) of consciousness not yet fully described. Other features, especially certain details which show surprising consistency over space and time, are much more difficult to understand and still lack even a hypothetical explanation. An improved knowledge of the traditions, their distributions, and their exact relationship to the experience would be very valuable in connection with a number of medical matters. This value can now be demonstrated for narcolepsy and appears to have interesting potential for other kinds of sleep disturbances, such as *pavor nocturnis*.

NOTES

1. Carl. W. Von Sydow. "Popular Prose Traditions and Their Classification," in *Selected Papers on Folklore*, ed. Laurits Bǿdker (Copenhagen: Rosenkilde and Bagger, 1948), pp. 60-88. For a good recent discussion of the term *memorate*, see "Memorate," *International Dictionary of Regional European Ethnology and Folklore*, Vol. II, *Folk Literature (Germanic)*, ed. Laurits Bǿdker (Copenhagen: Rosenkilde and Bagger, 1965), pp. 195-196.

2. C. E. Green, *Lucid Dreams* (London: Hamish Hamilton, 1968), see especially pp. 45-50, 117-124.

3. Carl-Herman Tillhagen, "The Conception of the Nightmare in Sweden," in *Humaniora: Essays in Literature, Folklore, and Bibliography Honoring Archer Taylor . . .* , ed. Wayland D. Hand and Gustave O. Arlt (Locust Valley, N.Y.: J. J. Augustin, 1969), pp. 317-329.

4. Ernest M. Jones, *On the Nightmare*, The International Psycho-Analytical Library no. 20 (London: The Hogarth Press; Toronto: Clark, Irwin & Co., 1931, 1949).

5. The initial *h* sound is frequently dropped, producing "aig" or "ag," so that the connection with the word *hag* is not always recognized.

6. Jones, *op. cit.*, pp. 31-37.

7. John White, comp., *Burke's Ballads* (St. John's, Newfoundland: n.p. [1960]?), p. 24.

8. Jones, *op. cit.*, pp. 16-27.

9. Wilhelm H. Roscher, "Ephialtes: A Pathological-Mythological Treatise on the Nightmare in Classical Antiquity," in *Pan and the Nightmare*, Dunquin Series 4, ed. The Analytical Psychology Club of New York, Inc. (New York: Spring Publications, 1972), pp. 1-88. (Originally published in Leipzig in 1900.)

10. Memorial University of Newfoundland Folklore and Language Archive questionnaire Q70B, "Nightmare/Hag/Old Hag," the source of much of my initial information.

11. A great deal of local material came from the files of the "Dictionary of Newfoundland English" at Memorial University of Newfoundland. See also The Philological Society, *The Oxford English Dictionary*, 12 vols. (London: Oxford University Press, 1961), VII, 146-147.

12. Stith Thompson, *Motif-Index of Folk-Literature*, 6 vols. (Bloomington & London: Indiana University Press, 1955).

13. For example, see Emelyn E. Gardner, *Folklore from the Schoharie Hills, New York* (Ann Arbor: University of Michigan Press, 1937), p. 65.

14. Richard M. Dorson, *American Negro Folktales*, (Greenwich, Conn.: Fawcett Publications, Inc., 1967), pp. 238-245.

15. Wayland D. Hand, ed., *The Frank C. Brown Collection of North Carolina Folklore*, vol. 7, *Popular Beliefs and Superstitions from North Carolina* (4874-8569) (Durham, N.C.: Duke University Press, 1964), pp. 136-137.

16. John A. Keel, *Strange Creatures from Time and Space*, (Greenwich, Conn.: Fawcett Publications, Inc., 1970), pp. 188-194.

17. George L. Kittredge, *Witchcraft in Old and New England*, (New York: Atheneum, 1972), *passim*.

18. Harry M. Hyatt, *Folklore from Adams County, Illinois*, (New York: Alma Egan Hyatt Foundation, 1935). However, Hyatt does give some very interesting material on the experience in his book *Hoodoo—Conjuration—Witchcraft—Rootwork*, 2 vols., Memoirs of the Alma Egan Hyatt Foundation (Hannibal, Mo.: Western Publ. Inc., 1970), pp. 135 ff.

19. See especially Roscher, *op. cit.*, pp. 3-44, and Ludwig Laistner, *Das Rätsel der Sphinx*, (1897).

20. Charles Dickens, *A Christmas Carol and The Chimes*, (London: Oxford University Press, 1923), p. 28. ("You may be an undigested bit of beef, a blot of mustard, a crumb of cheese, a fragment of an underdone potato. There's more of gravy than of the grave about you. . . .")

21. Jones, *op. cit.*, pp. 37-39.

22. Nathaniel Kleitman, *Sleep and Wakefulness*, (Chicago and London: University of Chicago Press, 1963), p. 280.

23. For example, see Rossell [*sic*] Robbins, *The Encyclopedia of Witchcraft and Demonology*, (London: Bookplan for Paul Hamlyn Ltd., and New York: Crown Publ., 1959), pp. 355-358.

24. For discussion of the problems of defining and using the concept of altered states of consciousness see Charles Tart, ed., *Altered States of Consciousness*, (New York: John Wiley & Sons, 1969), *passim*. See especially Tart's "Introduction", pp. 1-6.

25. Arnold M. Ludwig, "*Altered States of Consciousness*," in Tart, *op. cit.*, pp. 9-22.

26. *Ibid.*, p. 10.

27. *Ibid.*, pp. 10-11.

28. Dorson, *op. cit.*, p. 239.

29. Ludwig, *op. cit.*, p. 12.

30. *Ibid.*, pp. 12-13.

31. J. A. Hadfield, *Dreams and Nightmares*, (Baltimore: Penguin Books, Inc. 1971), 177 ff.

32. Gerald Vogel, David Foulkes, and Harry Trosman, "Ego Functions and Dreaming During Sleep Onset," in Tart, ed., *op. cit.*, pp. 75-91.

33. *Ibid.*, p. 77.

34. *Ibid.*

35. I am indebted to Carl Thompson, a psychologist in the Department of Behavioral Science of the Pennsylvania State University College of Medicine at The Hershey Medical Center, for the suggestion that I look into the literature on narcolepsy for leads relating to Nightmare.

36. Robert E. Yoss and David D. Daly, "Criteria for the Diagnosis of the Narcoleptic Syndrome," *Proceedings of the Staff Meetings of the Mayo Clinic*, 32, no. 2 (June 12, 1957), 320-328.

37. *Ibid.*, p. 320.

38. *Ibid.*, p. 325.

39. For example, see Allan Rechtschaffen and William C. Dement, "Narcolepsy and Hypersomnia," in *Sleep: Physiology and Pathology*, ed. Anthony Kales (Philadelphia and Toronto: J. B. Lippincott Co., 1969), pp. 119-130.

40. Yoss and Daly, *op. cit.*, pp. 325-326.

41. *Ibid.*, p. 326.

42. The existence of sleep paralysis without narcolepsy has been mentioned before. For example, see Kleitman, *op. cit.*, pp. 236-237.

43. Robert E. Yoss and David D. Daly, "Narcolepsy," *Archives of Internal Medicine*, 106 (July-December, 1960), p. 169.

44. Rechtschaffen and Dement, *op. cit., passim*.

45. *Ibid.*, p. 122-126.

46. *Ibid.*, p. 123.

47. I have found some other statements concerning Nightmare in the psychology of sleep literature, but these have tended to be brief, and a number of them contradict one another or, in some cases, my observations. For example, compare the statements concerning Nightmare referred to under that term in the index of Kales, *op. cit.*

The Interrelationship of Scientific and Folk Medicine in the United States of America since 1850

BRUNO GEBHARD, M.D., *Cleveland Health Museum*

A personal note: I am not a professional folklorist. I am a physician, a diplomate of the American Board of Preventive Medicine and Public Health with a great interest in medical history and folklore. I believe that medical folklore is not just a "footnote" in the history of medicine, as Louis C. Jones has suggested,[1] but an essential part of it. In my medical-school days I read, besides the then standard work of Hovorka-Kronfeld, Volumes III and IV of Richard Wossidlo's *Mecklenburgische Volksüberlieferungen*, which dealt with child care and rhymes for children.[2] Wossidlo's work is the classic publication for the Low German- (Plattdeutsch-) speaking common people in Mecklenburg, my home state.

I was an eyewitness to the rise of *Volksmedizin* and *Naturheilkunde* in the days of the Weimar Republic and the early years of Nazi government. Being declared "politically unreliable" in 1936, I emigrated to the United States the following year.

Richard M. Dorson is right in stating that "the first national state to make capital of folklore studies was the National Socialist government of Hitler,"[3] but folklore publications in those days were not just those trying "to document the Nazi concept of a 'Herrenvolk.'" A case in point is the *Atlas der Deutschen Volkskunde* (1930 to 1937). Regarding our special subject, the publication of Paul Diepgen titled *Deutsche Volksmedizin*[4] and that under the same title by Gustav Jungbauer[5] have stood the test of time and are reprinted in part by Elfriede Grabner in *Volksmedizin*, published in 1967.[6] Many of the German folklorists of the 1930s were members of the German youth movement. One of them was a leading adult educator and folklorist, Adolf Reichwein (1898-1944). His office at the Volkskunde Museum in Berlin served as a meeting place for German resistance leaders in the summer of 1944. Unfortunately, an undercover agent of the Gestapo was also present. Adolf Reichwein and others were executed on October 20, 1944.[7] It took another generation and more than twenty years to get folklore studies in Germany on a respected basis.

Little did I dream that my first job in 1937 in the United States as technical consultant to the Hall of Medicine and Public Health at the New York World's Fair 1939-1940 would involve me with American folk medicine.

The Maze of Superstition, located in the Hall of Man, covered nearly one thousand square feet. It was sponsored by the Bayer Company. The material was collected by Science Service of Washington, D.C. We exhibited about one hundred items. By making a slight detour at the entrance, one could avoid a huge ladder which was placed across it. An electric eye clocked those who passed under the ladder. The exit of the exhibit was marked by a giant wishbone gate.[8] In selecting the items to be exhibited, we had given preference to those in which women were expected to be more interested than men, but it turned out that the ratio of male to female visitors was one to one. An advisory committee was chaired by Howard W. Haggard from Yale. Members were Otis Caldwell, then secretary of the Agricultural Adjustment Administration, Henry E. Sigerist from Johns Hopkins, and the psychiatrists Gregory Zilborg and James F. Walsh, both of New York.

More important from the viewpoint of medical folklore research was a visitor reaction study carried on both in New York and at the San Francisco Fair in 1939 and 1940.[9] The New York study, financed by the Carnegie Corporation, had forty thousand participants; the one in San Francisco was operated by the Pacific Coast head office of the Metropolitan Life Insurance Company. The studies administered seven forms of tests, consisting of 225 questions, 69 of which dealt with superstitions and misconceptions about health (nos. 129-180). Questions were either multiple choice or true-false. The subject matter included wart removal remedies, rheumatism, night blindness, burn treatment, birthmarks, brain foods, hiccups, "feeding a cold," baldness, keeping the body alkaline, and several on tuberculosis and venereal disease.

The study was conducted by the National Institute of Health of the United States Public Health Service. Mayhew Derryberry, Ph.D., was the director. A detailed report in mimeographed form was published under the title "What The Public Knows about Health."[10]

Voting machines and I.B.M. immediate scoring machines were used. In San Francisco more women participated than men. One-third of the participants in New York were in the 17-21 age group. The main data of the analysis were as follows: the general public was best informed about cancer, to an equal extent in New York and San Francisco (92 percent); the lowest gross percentage of correct responses fell to questions about tuberculosis and venereal disease (57.2); superstitions and misconceptions put New York in the 72.6 bracket and San Francisco somewhat lower at 69.4. In other words, one-third of the questions were wrongly answered. In San Francisco the response to the anatomy and physiology questions was the poorest of all subject matter groups, namely, 57.1 percent. Regional differentiations were most apparent in the superstitions. This comes as no surprise to folklorists. It poses the interesting question whether the migration from the South into California in the last thirty years might have wiped out this difference. To our surprise the sex difference regarding superstitions was quite pronounced. The ratio of correct to incorrect answers, which showed significant differences in favor of women, was 17:14 for New York and 26:16 for San Francisco, an even higher proportion. On the other hand, men were better informed than women about advertising claims. The most unexpected figures came from a breakdown according to occupation in seven groups, from laborers and domestics to professionals. The tests showed that there was no difference between the professional health worker and the nonprofessional worker and, what is worse, that both groups shared equally incorrect answers by 30 percent. This reminds me of a remark by H. L. Mencken: "I am an agnostic, therefore very superstitious."

Unfortunately, because of contingencies of World War II, this study never got printed. It might be worthwhile to have a comparative study more or less thirty-five years later at a large state fair or a national convention attended by a good cross section of the American populace.

In hindsight I am sorry that we did not differentiate superstition clearly from folk medicine. Just as in scientific medicine, today's truth might be tomorrow's error; so-called superstition has often turned into a piece of rational folk medicine. I absolved myself from this sin of omission by presenting to the annual meeting of American Public Health Association in 1940 a paper entitled "Grandma Is Not Always Wrong."[11] I identified her not as the

perpetrator of "old wives' tales" but as a symbol of three genera-
tions living side by side and of all that is good in folk medicine.
Twenty-five years later my good friend W. W. Bauer took up this
theme in "Potions, Remedies, Old Wives' Tales: Medical Folklore
That Proves Why Grandma's Prescriptions Were Often Right"
(New York, 1965).

LAY MEDICINE PREFERRED TO FOLK MEDICINE

Today's scientists can fight over definitions just as bitterly as the
theologians of the Middle Ages. It is no wonder that the question of
what folklore is still remains unsettled. The division of folk
medicine into a natural, rational science and a magico-religious
healing art is generally accepted, but I would not limit the first
aspect to herbal healing, as Don Yoder does.[12] There is more to it
than purging, bloodletting, fasting, sweating, and so on. I prefer to
speak of both parts together as *lay medicine*, identical to what in the
last century was called domestic medicine. I grant that the term *lay*,
defined as not belonging to the clerics' guild, smacks of professional unionism and the haughtiness so often displayed by the
members of organized medicine, but I do not know of a better one.
I like to define lay medicine as the patient's—not the doctor's—
concept of health and disease and the cures applied in case of
illness or accident.[13] A person becomes a patient when he or she is
physically or mentally not at ease, regardless of age, education, or
social status. My definition goes along the same direction as
Hermann Bausinger's: "to attempt to trace the modification and
mutations undergone by folk culture in the industrialized and
urbanized world."[14]

AMERICAN MEDICINE IN THE NINETEENTH CENTURY

All during the nineteenth century, American students and physicians went to Edinburgh, Dublin, or London, to Paris, Vienna, and
Berlin for a sound medical education. Benjamin Rush (1745-1813)
gave this bit of advice to his students: "When you go abroad always
take a memorandum book and whenever you hear an old woman
say such and such herbs are good, or such a compound makes a
good medicine or ointment, put it down, for, gentlemen, you may
need it."[15] Around 1850, when California became a state, there
were few medical schools and few hospitals in the United States.
Ohio built a state penitentiary in 1815, long before it built a state
asylum. Medically speaking, the Civil War was a great disaster:
more men died from disease than from battle wounds. The Union
army, for example, had only half a dozen clinical thermometers.

After the war medical education improved. Introduction of embalming made year-round teaching of anatomy possible and thus put an end to body snatching. The quality of medical students was not the best—even in Harvard Medical School, where the head of the school declared in 1870 that "written examinations could not be given because most of the students could not write well enough."[16] Public and private support was meager. In 1891 the endowment funds for all medical schools was only half a million dollars; that for schools of theology came up to eighteen million dollars.[17]

DOMESTIC MEDICINE IN THE NINETEENTH CENTURY

What about the rank and file of medical practitioners and the people? When people got sick in nineteenth-century America, they stayed home, where they lived, where they were born, and where they would die. It was a far cry from our present-day reliance on "hospital medicine" (to use E. Ackerknecht's term) from birth to death.

Madge E. Pickard and R. Carlyle Buley have given us a classic picture in "The Midwest Pioneer: His Illness, Cures, and Doctors" (1946). In Abraham Lincoln's time infants died "by the grace of God" at the rate of twenty per hundred. Malaria was endemic in the Mississippi Valley, and so were many fevers, from typhoid to rheumatic. Newcomers were warned:

> Don't go to Michigan, that land of ills;
> The word means ague, fever, chills.[18]

Infectious children's diseases were thought inevitable and unavoidable. The tidal waves of Asiatic cholera during 1846-1851 and later yellow fever epidemics took many lives. In Cincinnati, out of a population of fifty thousand, nearly seventy-five hundred died. In Sacramento, of those who had not fled in time, every fourth became a victim of cholera. Yellow fever killed twenty thousand in New Orleans in 1878.[19]

About the practice of medicine around 1840 James Marion Sims (1813-1883) had this to say: "It was heroic, it was murderous. I did not know anything about medicine, but I had enough common sense to see that physicians killed their patients, that medicine was no exact science, that it proceeded empirically and that it was preferable to put one's confidence in to nature and not in to the dangerous skill of physicians."[20] Sims's opinion might be biased, since he was a very successful surgeon, but his opinions were shared by many lay people. And what did the people do?

The people helped themselves as they had done for centuries before. Medicine is older than the medical profession. All through the Middle Ages folk medicine and professional medicine walked the same way; they separated only after the universities in Europe took on medical education. In the United States medicine acquired academic status about four hundred years later, around the turn of our century. As Glenn Sonnedecker put it: "At no time has man abandoned self-treatment altogether and to American settlers remote from regular medical care, it seemed essential for survival itself."[21] Remedies were routinely available from places like the Drug and Family Medicine Warehouse of T. W. Dyott in Philadelphia. In a kind of pharmaceutical "survival kit," Benjamin Vaughn (1751-1835) recommends two dozen items. Eight of these are botanicals, including Peruvian bark and foxglove; six are chemicals such as calomel and tartar; and half a dozen are compound preparations, including laudanum. All during the nineteenth century, everyone was practicing some kind of medicine. In the South especially the planter's wife or the overseer was a surrogate doctor. Everywhere the pharmacist substituted for the hard-to-get and sometimes expensive physician, and midwives, besides just "catching babies," gave free advice. Family medical manuals had their place next to the Bible. Dr. John C. Gunn's *Domestic Medicine: or, Poor Man's Friend, in the House of Affliction, Pain, and Sickness* (Knoxville, Tennessee) was first published in 1832, and by 1885 it had 213 printings.

The development of sectarian medicine in the nineteenth century was as turbulent as that of academic medicine was slow. The followers of the homeopath Christian Friedrich Samuel Hahnemann (1755-1843) grew so quickly and extensively that half of the population preferred treatment with drugs in small doses and without bloodletting. Around 1900 there were still twenty-two medical colleges and a dozen journals flourishing under Hahnemann's name. In the same year his followers unveiled a magnificent monument on Scott Circle in Washington, D.C. The immigrants from Germany in the 1930s brought a revival of this branch of medicine, with Marlene Dietrich as their glamor girl.

Botanic medicine, the brainchild of Samuel Thompson (1769-1818) was favored for nearly thirty years, since it was closely linked with the Indian herb practice. It is estimated that at least one-third of Ohio's people were treating themselves or were treated according to botanic medicine. It was easy. For twenty dollars, no small sum, one could get Thompson's book, *New Guide to Health: or, Botanic Family Physician*. With it came a certificate which looked like a diploma.

Sectarian medicine was promoted with much religious fortitude. The regular doctors were accused of atheism and immorality. An Ohio agent for botanical medicine who doubled as a radical Methodist preacher was quoted as saying that "the practice of employing physicians to officiate in midwifery was so demoralizing that he believed that any woman who would willingly submit to have a Doctor to deliver her child would let the same Doctor afterwards get her with child, if he chose to do so."[22]

The "eclectic" physician, wavering between the old and new, claimed to prove all things and hold fast to that which was good. Near the end of the century the number of practitioners allied with the various schools was estimated at the following: old school (classical training), 73,028; eclectic, 9,703; homeopathic, 8,640; physio-medical, 1,553.[23] The turn of the nineteenth century also saw osteopathy and Christian Science gain adherents.

The health of the people in larger cities had worsened because of overcrowding. Sanitary reforms led by lay people worked for better housing, clean water and milk, and efficient health administration. In the rural districts health had improved. More people took advantage of smallpox vaccination. Malaria decreased as quinine and metal screens on doors and windows came into general use. The new science of bacteriology gave hope that tuberculosis could be reduced, if not eradicated. There was hope now that infectious diseases could be checked by immunization. The discovery of Xrays gave surgery a greater margin of success in operations and widened the scope for better diagnosis in internal medicine. But at the opening of the Phipps Clinic of Johns Hopkins in April 1913, Sir William Osler made this statement: "Still in the thaumaturgic stage of mental development, ninety-nine percent of our fellow creatures, when in trouble, sorrow or sickness, trust to charms, incantations and to the saints. Many a shrine has more followers than Pasteur; many a saint more believers than Lister. Less than twenty years have passed since the last witch was tried in the British Isles!"[24]

THE PRESENT

How widely folk medicine is practiced today in this country is hard to say. Surely folk medicine is not dead, but just how lively and active is it in, let us say, the third generation of city-born people? During our century the pharmaceutical industry and patent medicines have more or less taken over, with the eighty-seven-year-old Lydia Pinkham still selling well. Aspirin and vitamin supplements, pep pills and tranquilizers are today's leaders in folk medicine, and of course there is The Pill. One British observer remarked that American urine must be the most expensive in the world.

Research in folk medicine is increasingly carried out by non-medical people. In some ways anthropologists, sociologists, and folklorists are better qualified. We would like to suggest more collaboration with physicians for field studies in hospitals and clinics, in outpatient departments and state institutions. This was done on a limited scale in a Jacksonville, Florida, hospital. A social worker at the University of Florida interviewed seventy families in Lafayette County. She obtained forty different herbs "sworn by" more than one person who had used them effectively in recent years. Twenty-two of the forty found their usefulness confirmed in scientific publications. Other material was acquired directly from ward patients in the hospital by supervisory nurses. These findings confirmed that nine rusty nails in a pint of whisky, possibly "shine," is still a widely used home remedy. So is clay eating for "treating the worms" and starch eating for an easier pregnancy. New to me was the drinking twice daily of a tea brewed from Spanish moss to supplement the insulin injection required by a twenty-five-year-old Negro—a true blending of scientific and folk medicine.[25]

THE LIFETIME OF SPECIFIC FOLK MEDICINE ITEMS

For many years I have tried to get a chronology of specific beliefs and the practice of certain aspects of folk medicine—when and how they originated, how they became modified over the century, and their possible ending or limited circulation. Here are a dozen of them:

Case I: Fish is a brain food. This notion originated with the German physiologist Jacob Moleschott (1822-1893) and the contemporary philosopher of materialism Ernst Buchner as the slogan "Without Phosphorus—No Thought." Since fish contains a relative high percentage of phosphorus, it was recommended to increase brain power. Louis Agassiz supported this theory. In the 1920s Cleveland high school students learned this ditty:

> Fish is a brain food that is never said to fail
> I therefore recommend that you should eat a whale.

The lines add another superstition, since whales are not fish.[26] On October 28, 1973, the widely read comic strip "Nancy" by Ernie Bushmiller had with its illustration this copy: Nancy: "I am worried about my exams this afternoon." Sluggo: "Make a fish sandwich for lunch—fish is good brainfood"; whereupon she puts on her sandwich three sardines: "One for arithmetic, one for history, one for geography." A good example of comics as conservators and perpetrators of folklore.

Case II: Cooking in aluminum causes cancer. This fear sprang up after World War I, when aluminum replaced iron, copper, and enamel as kitchenware. Led by the dentist Charles Bett (Toledo, Ohio), a vast propaganda against aluminum swept this country. The Mellon Institute Bulletin 3, 1932 (Pittsburgh) reported extensive experimental studies proving that there was no carcinogenic effect of aluminum in cooking utensils.[27] It should have put all fears to rest—but did it?

Case III: Feed a cold and starve a fever. This false statement is heard daily by millions of television viewers. It appeared first in the writings of Celsus (ca. A.D. 50), who was not a physician, and then it appeared in 1478 in his printed works, which were widely read. It was challenged by the Dublin physician Robert F. Graves (1796-1853), who requested that the phrase "He fed fevers" should be put on his gravestone. Final proof came during World War II. Doctor Joseph I. Goodman (Cleveland) and Robert Garvin found that "administration of food does not raise the temperature and that hourly feedings of up to 5000 calories a day saved the life of many a soldier by not letting them starve to death."[28] For thirty years we have known that "Feed a cold, starve a fever" is wrong. How long will it still be quoted, advertised, believed in, and practiced?

Case IV: Not carrots, but radar. Many a scientist believed British statements during World War II that eating carrots prevents night blindness. It does it only to a minimal extent. The truth is that shrewd advisers of the War Cabinet circulated the rumor "that the successes of the R.A.F. were due to carrots in order to conceal from the enemy the fact that radar was used for the first time."[29]

Case V: Spinach is good for you. Introduced from Persia in the fifteenth century, a favored dish on fast days in Europe, spinach has been pushed by advertisements since 1900 and since 1930 by the pipe-smoking, spinach-eating Popeye the Sailor, created by E. C. Segar. Crystal City, Texas, which claims to be the spinach capital of the United States, erected a statue to honor Popeye in its central square. Spinach has little iron and robs the body of calcium.[30]

Case VI: Goldenrod causes hay fever. Not true. The main cause is the pollen of the very inconspicuous ragweed, which blooms at the same time as the very showy goldenrod. The English physician John Bostock discovered in 1819 that ragweed is the main culprit, but goldenrod is still blamed.

Case VII: Fluor is poison. Our body and our food contain fluor. Water fluoridation, proven successful in mass prevention of cavities, started in the United States in 1944. Opponents use the "poison" argument now in the same way it was used forty years ago against the addition of iodine to table salt to prevent goiter. Some patriotic groups like the Daughters of the American Revolution see it as a communistic intrigue, but, ironically enough, large cities in Russia plan to use fluoridated water.

Case VIII: Electric Heels: Yes; Electricity: No! Many of the Amish in Ohio will not use electric power but will put inside the heel of one shoe a zinc disc and inside the other a copper one, the mutual proximity of which produces a slight galvanic current and thus supposedly gives relief from rheumatic pain. "General" Jacob S. Coxey (1855-1951), of Veterans' March to Washington fame, was bedded down with severe rheumatism when he read about Louis Galvani (1737-1798). Coxey, then ninety years old, made himself a pair of electric heels, found that they gave him relief, and added this item, named Cox-E-Lax, to his other popular patent medicines. Coxey's electric heels are still sold for a handling charge[31] of $1.50 with the admonition: "We promise nothing, we guarantee nothing." The borderline between folk medicine, magic, and plain hoax is very thin.

Case IX: "Blood is a very special kind of sap." Goethe puts these words into the mouth of Mephistopheles, who is urging Faust to sign his pact with him in blood. McKenzie speaks of "the sanctity and potency of blood." Beliefs and misbeliefs about blood are innumerable. Medical columns of newspapers often carry letters concerned with the possibility of getting cancer through blood transfusion. Jehovah's Witnesses refuse blood transfusions on Biblical grounds (Lev. 17:11), and where medicine competes with religion, it loses. Decisions regarding blood collecting made by the armed forces in the early 1940s were not always based on scientific data but more often followed public pressure. Nevertheless, by 1947 separation of blood by race was stopped. But the television show "M*A*S*H" made quite a play of a white soldier's concern during the Korean War about getting the "wrong color blood" (November 10, 1973). Dressed up as a humorous affair, an old superstition was very likely revived for many viewers.

Case X: Boy or girl? For many years the Cleveland Health Museum has had a push-button exhibit that tries to explain and to convince visitors that the father determines the sex of the expected child. We often have women questioning this fact. Thomas R. Forbes points out rightly that it was natural to assume that fetal sex was controlled by the mother. Science took nearly two hundred years to lead up to the final discovery around 1900 of the genetic regulation of sex. For centuries women were blamed and "put aside" because they failed to produce a male heir.

Case XI: Fertility pebbles. Allan Roy Dafoe, M.D., who delivered the Dionne quintuplets in 1934, says "that hundreds of sterile women visited the famous Canadian quintuplets and took home one of the "magic pebbles in the courtyard in the hope of bearing a child"; one of them had been childless for as long as fourteen years and became pregnant within a year.[32] Dr. Dafoe also relates that Mrs. Dionne was quite embarrassed by the multitude of babies, since people would assume that it takes intercourse five times to produce five babies (personal communication).

Case XIII: Acupuncture. Used in China since 2800 B.C., acupuncture came to Europe through Jesuit missionaries. It was fashionable in France during the nineteenth century and again in the 1930s. It will be interesting to see how long the present enthusiasm in the United States will continue.

Folk medicine is surely not dead. It has been more and more replaced by aspirin, vitamin supplements, tranquilizers, pep pills, and The Pill. How effective is folk medicine? E. H. Ackerknecht estimates primitive medicine to be 25 percent objectively helpful; for folk medicine in the nineteenth century the figure might be 50 percent. Lauri Honko claims that the primitive medicine man was equally well qualified to act as a psychotherapeutic agent as the modern psychiatrist—that is, if not better qualified.[33]

Today too many people live in the gray zone of quackery, plain hoax, and humbug. The relationship of folk medicine and scientific medicine is a truly two-way street. Folk medicine has one advantage: it has no doubt; it believes. Scientific medicine moves from truth to error to truth—it must search and re-search.

NOTES

1. Louis C. Jones, "Practitioners of Folk Medicine," *Bull. N.Y. Acad. Med.*, 23 (1949), 492.

2. Richard Wossidlo, *Mecklenburgische Volksüberlieferungen* (Wismar, Rostock: Carl Hinstorffs Vlg., 1906-1931).

3. Richard M. Dorson, *Folklore and Folklife* (Chicago: University of Chicago Press, 1972), p. 16.

4. Paul Diepgen, *Deutsche Volksmedizin* (Stuttgart: Ferdinand Enke, 1935), p. 136.

5. Gustav Jungbauer, *Deutsche Volksmedizin* (Berlin and Leipzig: Walter de Gruyter, 1934), p. 248.

6. Elfriede Grabner, *Volksmedizin: Probleme und Forschungsgeschichte* (Darmstadt: Wiss. Buchgesellschaft, 1967), pp. 89-92, 200-222.

7. Annedore Leber, *Das Gewissen steht auf* (Berlin: Mosaik Verlag, 1954), pp. 60-62.

8. *Man and His Health: A Guide to Medical and Public Health Exhibits* (New York: Expositions Publications, 1939), pp. 73-74.

9. *Your Health: A Guide to the Medicine and Public Health Building* (New York: American Museum of Health, 1940), pp. 92-93.

10. M. Derryberry, A. Weissman, and C. G. Caswell, "What the Public Knows About Health," mimeographed (New York: American Museum of Health, Inc., 1942), pp. 67-99.

11. Catherine Mackenzie, "Child and Parent," *The New York Times Magazine* (October 6, 1940), p. 16.

12. Dorson, *op. cit.*, p. 197.

13. Bruno Gebhard, "Historical Relationship between Scientific and Lay Medicine for Present-Day Patient Education," *Bull. History of Medicine*, 32, 1 (1957), 46-53.

14. Richard M. Dorson, *op. cit.*, p. 43.

15. Clarence Meyer, *American Folk Medicine* (New York, 1973), p. 15.

16. Louis Lasagna, *The Doctor's Dilemma* (New York, 1962), p. 104.

17. R. H. Shryock, *Medicine in America* (New York, 1966), p. 77.

18. Madge E. Pickard and R. C. Buley, *The Midwest Pioneer* (Crawfordsville, Ind., 1945), p. 13.

19. Geddes Smith, *Plague on Us* (The Commonwealth Fund, 1941) pp. 15-23.

20. Erwin H. Ackerknecht, *Therapeutics: From the Primitives to the Twentieth Century* (Stuttgart: Enke Vlg., 1973), p. 119.

21. Glenn Sonnedecker, "Home Medication on the American Frontier," *Veroeffentlichungen d. Int. Gesellschaft f. Geschichte d. Pharmazie*, n.s. 38 (1972), 253-270.

22. James H. Young, *The Toadstool Millionaire*, quoted from *Belmont Med. Soc. Trans.* (1850), pp. 57-58 (New York, 1961), p. 52.

23. Ronald L. Numbers, "The Making of an Eclectic Physician," *Bull. History of Medicine*, 47, 2 (1973), 155.

24. Harvey Cushing, *The Life of William Osler* (Oxford: The Clarendon Press, 1925), II, 351.

25. Max Michael, Jr., and Mark V. Barrow, "Old Timey Remedies of Yesterday and Today," *T. Florida M. A.*, 54, 8 (1967), 779-784.

26. Gebhard, *op. cit.*, p. 49.

27. Magnus Pike, *Food and Society* (London: John Murray, 1969), p. 95.

28. Joseph I. Goodman and Robert O. Garvin, "Results of High Caloric Feeding," *J. Gastroenterology*, 6 (1946), 537-562.

29. Pike, *op. cit.*, p. 93.

30. Claudia de Lys, *A Treasury of American Superstitions* (New York: Philosophical Library 1949), p. 240.

31. *The Plain Dealer Magazine* (October 7, 1973).

32. De Lys, *op. cit.*, p. 216.

33. Lauri Honko, "Über die tatsächliche Wirkung der Volksmedizin," in E. Graebner, *op. cit.*, p. 497-508.

Shamanic Equilibrium: Balance and Mediation in Known and Unknown Worlds

BARBARA G. MYERHOFF, *University of Southern California*

The shaman is a paradoxical figure. His problem—and his profession—is one of equilibrium and mediation, and this balancing occurs simultaneously on several levels. Let us speak first about psychological equilibrium. The shaman must be a master of psychological control, for his profession requires continual and intense attainment of abnormal psychological states—magical activities, trances, and visions. Eliade (1960) is convincing in arguing against the view that shamans are often neurotic, unstable, or epileptic, for in the course of rigorous training and dedication, the individual who is perhaps initially neurotic learns to control his frenzy, to manipulate his proclivity to visions, fits, and trances, to use them in the service of his group. Thus, he can no longer be regarded as sick, and his profession constitutes his cure.

The shaman is above all a connecting figure, bridging several worlds for his people, traveling between this world, the underworld, and the heavens. He transforms himself into an animal and talks with ghosts, the dead, the deities, the ancestors. He dies and revives. He brings back knowledge from the shadow realm, thus linking his people to the spirits and places which were once mythically accessible to all. It is the special responsibility of the shaman to return to *illud tempus* on behalf of his people, to make his ecstatic journey through the assistance of animal tutelary spirits, to bring back information of the other realms to ordinary mortals. As mediator, the shaman travels back and forth and with exquisite balance, never becoming too closely tied to the mundane or to the supernatural. His soul leaves his body during trance states, and by means of a magical flight he rejoins that which was once a totality—man and the animals, the living and the dead, man and the gods. In this state of primordial oneness, all social, sexual, and age distinctions are set aside, and all is unity. It is a vision so ubiquitous that Eliade exclaims: "We have the right to assume that the mystical memory of a blessedness without history haunts man from the moment he becomes aware of his situation in the cosmos" (1960:73). And what is that situation? Above all it is the situation of barriers, separations, and loss of integration. In providing this integration, the shaman provides his magical cure. The shaman as a connector is bridging the primordial past and the mythical past with historical time. He is at the same time mastering psychological transitions, going from normality to states of possession and back. And in carrying out his cures, he accomplishes social equilibrium as well by establishing balance between the individual and his group, by reweaving the social texture that has been ruptured by illness and frequently by some violation of group norms that causes the sickened individual to be seen and treated as a deviant.

The shaman, then, is recovering and reestablishing equilibrium in many ways at the same time. As a connecting figure, he is at once the restorer of balance and the symbol of the possibility of balance. In his cosmic undertakings, his personal destiny mirrors his profession, and the microcosm and macrocosm are reunited by his activities.

I first became aware of the significance of the shaman's need for exquisite balance in my contact with the Huichol Indians of North Central Mexico several years ago. For some time I had been working with a Huichol *mara'akame*, or shaman priest, named Ramón Medina Silva. One afternoon, without explanation, he interrupted our sessions of taping mythology to take a party, Huichol friends and myself, to an area outside his home. It was a region of steep barrancas cut by a rapid waterfall cascading perhaps a thousand feet over jagged, slippery rocks. At the edge of the fall, Ramón removed his sandals and announced that this was a special place for shamans. He proceeded to leap across the waterfall, from rock to rock, frequently pausing, his body bent forward, his arms outspread, head thrown back, entirely birdlike, poised motionlessly on one foot. He disappeared, reemerged, leaped about, and finally achieved the other side. I was frightened and puzzled by the performance, but none of the Huichols there seemed at all worried. The wife of one of the older Huichol men told me that her husband had started to become a *mara'akame* but had failed because he lacked balance. I assumed that she referred to his social and personal unsteadiness, for he was alcoholic and something of a deviant. I knew I had witnessed a virtuoso display of balance, but it was not until the next day, when discussing this event with Ramón, that I began to understand more clearly what had occurred. "The *mara'akame* must have superb equilibrium," he said and demonstrated the point by using his fingers to march up his violin bow. "Otherwise, he will not reach his destination and will fall this way or that," and his fingers plunged into an imaginary abyss. "One crosses over; it is very narrow and, without balance, one is eaten by those animals waiting below."

I could not be sure whether Ramón was rehearsing his equilibrium or giving it public, ceremonial expression that day in the barrancas. In societies without writing, official statements about a person's status and skill are often made in dramatic, public, ceremonial form. Whether seen as a practice session or as a ritual, the events of the afternoon provided a demonstrative assertion that Ramón was a true *mara'akame* and, like all authentic shamans, a man of immense courage, poise, and balance. Those familiar with Castaneda's (1971) work will recall a strikingly similar display of virtuoso balance in one of his books. The description of Don Genaro leaping across rocks and cliffs suggests the same interpretation, a shaman's presentation of credentials as a mediator.

Many years before, I had witnessed a peculiar piece of behavior which I had not known how to account for but which suddenly fell into place as I contemplated shamans' public demonstrations of skill in balance. I had been working with a Luiseño Indian shaman named Domenico on a Southern California reservation.* He was an eccentric, and it was as usual difficult to distinguish the cultural from the psychological factors in his work. He was known far and wide for his curing skills. North Americans, Mexicans, Indians from other tribes, even Europeans came to him for an assortment of treatments and advice. Domenico was a consultant on weekends only. On Friday afternoons individuals would begin to gather, assembling in the dusty clearing before his little shack, bringing sleeping bags and pallets, wearing white to signal their faith in him. I was struck by the fact that early Friday afternoons, Domenico climbed to the roof of his shack and stood quietly without moving for long periods of time while he gazed toward the road with one leg pulled up and curled into the crook of the other. I assumed that he was looking for his clients, but even at the time it seemed odd

*For fuller description of this case see Myerhoff, 1966.

that he risked life and limb by standing on the fragile, tar paper-roofed little structure when he could have easily walked up a little hill behind his house for a better vantage point. Perhaps he thought it unseemly to appear overeager. I dismissed it. Later it occurred to me that he was balancing there. His culture and society were terribly disrupted at the time I met him. The people had been almost entirely dispersed or assimilated. Their beliefs were fragmented and vague. I believe now that there was no conscious intention in his action and that had I thought to ask, he would not have been able to explain what he was doing. In retrospect, it seems clear that he was demonstrating his mediating capacity by showing himself to be a specialist in balance.

Shamanic balance is a particular stance. It is not a balance achieved by synthesis; it is not a static condition achieved by resolving opposition. It is not a compromise. Rather it is a state of acute tension, the kind of tension which exists, as Gonzales put it, when two unqualified forces encounter each other, meeting headlong, and are not reconciled but held teetering on the verge of chaos, not in reason but in experience.* It is a position with which the westerner, schooled in the Aristotelian tradition, is extremely uncomfortable. Unlike the view of highest good as the golden mean, this view gives us few guidelines for action. Unfortunately, we westerners have come to feel that enduring this sort of tension is not really necessary, that somehow it is possible to allow one pole to exist and prevail without its opposite. We seek good without evil, pleasure without pain, God without the devil, and love without hate. But the shaman reminds us of the impossibility of such a condition, for he stands at the juncture of opposing forces, and his dialectical task is continually to move between these opposites.

The shamanic journey is in three phases. The shaman sets forth from the realm of the mundane; he then journeys to the supernatural and returns. Always the passage involves these three destinations or locations. His ultimate message is that there is yet the connection between the world as we know it now and the world which existed before Creation instituted the primordial divisions that destroyed the mythical paradisiacal past. Since that rupture, mortality—the human condition—is a state of division, separation, and loss that is symbolically mended by the shaman when he undertakes his magical flights. He himself creates unity and at the

*Rafael J. Gonzales, personal communication, Los Angeles, 1970.

same time stands for a continuing condition of unity between the known and the unknown world.

The shaman cannot fail to go nor fail to return and still be a shaman. He must venture out and come back, and the passage is a dangerous one fraught with peril. There is always the possibility of the loss of balance, either in not returning to this world or in being unable or unwilling to leave it. Entrances and exits are hedged with rituals and symbols, for these are points of potential disaster. The shaman travels to the edge of the social order each time he undertakes these journeys. He enters nonform, the underlying chaos of the unconceptualized domain which has not yet been made a part of cosmos by the cultural activity of naming and defining. With each crossing over he gains power, as do all persons who travel to the edges of order of the world, for as Douglas (1966) reminds us, such contacts with the boundaries of conceptualization are sources of power as well as danger. Shamans are liminal people, at the thresholds of form, forever betwixt and between.

It may be assumed that the shaman is continually tempted to remain in that other realm to which he alone has ready access, for a condition of prehuman bliss and unity is an essential ingredient of all paradises—Valhalla, Eden, Elysium—all names for the state which existed before the world began. There, there was no hunger, weariness, or appetite, and men knew no disharmony. They were innocent, sexless, without consciousness and undifferentiated. It was a condition which had to be left behind; and since then men have been mortal as we know them now, with all the burdens of being human—reproducing by copulation, eating, working, suffering, and dying—with the everlasting torment of the memory of what has been lost. It is the loss of bliss which occurs at the moment of primordial splitting, after which nothing can be the same.

Shamans must be dialecticians, agile and capable of maintaining exactly the right relations between the opposites they bridge. They may not value the rewards of one world over the other. The desire for wealth and position in the mundane realm and for perpetual ecstasy in the supernatural are threats to the shamanic enterprise. Imbalance is fatal, for it jeopardizes their precarious poise. This need for a sense of proportion and balance of values comes to us in many forms; it is variously inflected but constant in its meaning. Echoes of it can be found in folktales told, ironically, to children who understand them instinctively and thus need them less than we adults. This theme resonates throughout the fairy tale, "Jack and the Beanstalk." It can be read as a parable for the shamanic journey, a moral statement on the meaning of the shamanic passage in everyday life. Without conducting a formal analysis and without any intention of exhausting its riches, I shall interpret "Jack and the Beanstalk" as a moral tale which speaks to us of something we know and forget and relearn forever.

The story is redolent with shamanic symbolism. To begin, Jack is living outside of ordinary society, neither child nor man, fatherless, separated from his group socially and spatially, a young man not well connected in the world. Jack is foolish and spoiled. He is naive but recognizes the magic of the beans that are given to him in exchange for his family cow. Jack, a kind of *idiot savant*, intuitively realizes that the beans have mysterious powers incomparably more precious than the worldly worth of the cow. Jack has the power of the weak; he is wise and rich in spiritual terms while poor and ineffectual in the mundane realm. Like most liminal figures, his moral position is exalted and reverses his social position, which is lowly. The mother, with no understanding of this, is aghast at Jack's conduct. The beans are rejected as worthless, and Jack is punished by his mother. Subsequently he discovers the beanstalk grown from the discarded beans and responds to his irresistible call to climb it, though he is warned away from it. At the top, high amidst the leaves and clouds, Jack looks down toward the distant land. His house and mother are far below, tiny from this vantage point, and he is filled with wonder and delight at the perspective offered him at this great height. He has climbed the *axis mundi*, the world pole or tree of life, which penetrates the layers of the cosmos and connects the underworld and the heavens. He has accomplished the breakthrough in planes which is the goal of shamanic ascents. And he is rewarded by the view of the miniature world beneath. Such miniaturization allows one's eyes or mind to place vast spaces and objects in relation to one another. It is a vision only available to those somehow removed and elevated from the throbbing, absorbing details of everyday life. Jack at the top is in the supernatural realm, the abode of the Giant. The latter, in some versions, has become enormously wealthy by stealing property that once belonged to Jack's father. These are magical objects—a bag of gold that never empties, a goose that lays a golden egg, a lyre that sings. Such wondrous items are rightfully Jack's, and one at a time he steals them, or rather retrieves them, and brings them back to his mother. Jack and the mother are restored to a position of wealth and social importance, and Jack is recognized as a young man of intelligence and prospects, a respected figure. He is seen at the end of the tale, married, mature, completely settled. (In one version of the tale, Jack's entire family has achieved completeness, for the songs of the lyre have restored the father who was not dead but only ailing.)

And what has Jack brought back from the supernatural region of the Giant? The bag of coins is simple worldly wealth. The goose that lays the golden egg is a standard shamanic symbol of magical flight and rebirth. And the lyre is an orphic symbol, representing the shaman's ability to cure through song and myth, his voice raised in poetry and beauty.

What Jack has gained is very clear. He is grown and successful. He is a man and a man of the world, rooted and secure; but the beanstalk has been severed forever and with it, access to the supernatural world. To save himself, Jack had to cut it down; and now, at the end of the tale, he is a proper and ordinary citizen living out his life peacefully amidst his family and possessions. He retains mementos of his past gifts, visions, powers, and adventures. The goose is reminiscent of his capacity for flight and freedom, of rebirth and the immortality which was his when he made ecstatic flights to the world before Creation. And the lyre bespeaks his orphic gifts, his capacity for spontaneous song, his previous existence as an innocent and as a child. Jack, as shaman, has ceased to exist. He has lost his balance and become fixed in one of the worlds at the cost of the other. But this is not only the story of a shaman without equilibrium. It is a tale of every man. Different symbolic interpretations may emphasize different aspects of the adventure, but all have in common the telling of this sad triumph of the passage of youth into maturity and manhood.

A Jungian reading of the tale leads to an emphasis on Jack's going forth from his origins, leaving mother and home in an ascent which is separation, differentiation, and individuation. The bag of gold is Jack's worldly success, the bird stands for spiritual development, the lyre represents feeling—taken together they suggest a rounded, balanced human being. The Freudian reading stresses Jack's achievement of genital maturity, his vanquishing his fears of the overwhelming phallic power of the father figure, fantasized as a dangerous Giant. In resolving the Oedipus complex, Jack separates from his nurturant mother and is reconciled with his mortal father, properly reduced to human proportions. A Lévi-Straussian interpretation stresses the complex exchanges and meditations which occur between various oppositions—plant (beans) for animal (cow); culture (mundane realm) for supernatural (Giant's realm); male (father) for female (mother); mortality for eternity; worldly position for mystical vision; and so forth. Whatever emphasis one prefers, Jack is always bereft of his early gifts and no longer allowed to enter the timeless order. Domestic riches have been won at the cost of mystery and fantasy. Gaining maturity is often conceptualized as this exchange. The child, like the shaman, is an innocent who understands the language of the animals, a visionary and a poet who loses these gifts as he is socialized into the proper adult.

The conclusion of the story is foregone, for Jack has fulfilled his destiny. As a shaman he has failed, but as a boy he has become a man. Order is again prevalent; and fantasy, a vague recollection. The *axis mundi* has been felled and the worlds divided, to be retrieved henceforth through rare and precious glimpses afforded by other shamans.

The story is also about the relation of the individual to the social order, about a rite of passage wherein the microcosm and the macrocosm recapitulate each other, with the personal, subjective experience as another and parallel version of the supernatural event. "Paradise lost" is an eternally repeated event collectively and a unique event only in the experience of the individual. Loss of childhood and achievement of manhood is a restatement of the cosmic event in psychological terms.

Turner (1969) calls our attention to the aptness of the life cycle for remarking upon the replication of timeless, religious events as nonrepeating personal experiences. An adolescent's passage into adulthood allows us to make such statements about the inevitable nature of things, and the statements reconcile us to the inevitable outcome. The individual's destiny is enacted and presented in terms of eternal collective sequences, and the cosmic order is brought alive by being rendered in these individual, subjective terms.

Perhaps we are thus reconciled to our inevitable destiny—adulthood and the loss of fantasy and innocence. The story itself saves us from the total annihilation of childhood; the complete assault of the social order on our idiosyncratic and nonformed individuality is averted by the remembrance that at some point we saw things from a different perspective. Thus some part of ourselves remains alive with nostalgia, recognizing, perhaps even promoting, the former capacity for vision. We have with us still the lyre, the bird, the golden treasures which are magical mementos telling us that though we became what we were destined to be by biology and society, we are not utterly owned by that destiny; and so long as we have fairy tales and shamans, we need not be.

If Jack has lost his balance and all of us have made the transition from childhood to maturity, if our contemporary religions have only symbolic vestiges instead of practicing shamans, must we sadly admit that this was always our unfortunate but inevitable destiny? Perhaps not. Presently we find the various functions of shamans distributed among numerous specialists: priests, poets, artists, psychotherapists, teachers, and metaphysicians. Separated and fragmented in this way, the shamanic role loses its whole point, for the shaman's function is precisely that of integration. The retrieval of wholeness represented by the shaman's journey is impossible in these conditions, for no single specialist can attain the total vision of man as simultaneously part of the present world and the past, connected to his own childhood and to his social matrix, consisting of inseparable body and mind. That the retrieval of wholeness is itself curative is implied in the words *whole, Heil, heal, holy, healthy.* Restoration achieved through integration of individual and group, attitude and body, private and public belief is the foundation of all folk healing systems. Underlying them is the acknowledgment of a common causality for man and nature. The renewed interest in folk medicine is a practical matter, and at present we are facing the rediscoveries of the common basis of religion and medicine. The Western medical model is becoming more cognizant of this shared ground and increasingly looks to indigenous health practices as sources of information that may enlarge somewhat its view of health as merely the absence of illness. Modern medicine consisting of a system of meanings as well as a body of applied techniques may come to represent precisely that world view in which shamanism functioned originally, and human integration on all levels may yet reemerge as the goal and the ideal, with the result that shamans may be among us once more.

Grateful acknowledgment is hereby made to Deena Metzger, whose insights and interest were essential. The help of Pat Braun and Janet Dallet was also invaluable and most generous.

BIBLIOGRAPHY

Casteneda, Carlos. 1971 *A Separate Reality: Further Conversations with Don Juan.* New York: Simon & Schuster.

Douglas, Mary. 1966. *Purity and Danger: An Analysis of Concepts of Pollution and Taboo.* London: Penguin.

Eliade, Mircea. 1954. *The Myth of Eternal Return.* New York: Bollingen.

———. 1962. *The Two and the One.* New York: Harper Torchbooks.

———. 1964. *Shamanism: Archaic Techniques of Ecstasy.* Trans. W. R. Trask. Bollingen Series LXXVI. New York: Pantheon.

Lévi-Strauss, Claude. 1967. "The Story of Asdiwal." In *The Structural Study of Myth*. Ed. E. Leach; Trans. Nicolas Mann. London: Tavistock. Pp. 1-47.

Myerhoff, Barbara G. 1966. "The Doctor as Cultural Hero: The Shaman of Rincon." *Anthropological Quarterly*, 39, 2, 60-72.

———. 1974. *Peyote Hunt: The Sacred Journey of the Huichol Indians*. Ithaca and London: Cornell University Press.

Turner, Terence. 1969. *Oedipus: Time and Structure in Narrative Form*. In *Forms of Symbolic Action*. American Ethnological Society.

Wolfenstein, Martha. "Jack and the Beanstalk: An American Version." In *Childhood in Contemporary Cultures*. Ed. Margaret Mead and Martha Wolfenstein. Chicago: University of Chicago Press. Phoenix Books. Pp. 243-245.

California Indian Shamanism and Folk Curing

LOWELL JOHN BEAN, *California State University,*
Hayward

This paper describes the major sociological, and some of the philosophical, features of shamanism among Native Californians before European contact. Since I have elsewhere (Bean 1974) described the philosophical (existential and normative) postulates central to California shamanism and the place of shamans within the broader sociocultural contexts (Bean 1974b), in this essay I will concentrate on the following: (1) the place of the shaman in the cultures of Native California; (2) varying degrees of medical knowledge; (3) disease causation and sources of curative power-knowledge; (4) varieties of shamanic roles and malevolent uses of power; (5) the shaman as a professional and his acquisition of the status; (6) postcontact reactions to curing and shamanic roles; (7) conclusions.

THE PLACE OF THE SHAMAN

Shamans (better described for Native California as shaman-priests) were the principal religious functionaries among California groups, but they were often political administrators (chiefs) simultaneously. The position of shaman has not been fully appreciated in the ethnographic literature of California. It is necessary to see them as the principal philosophers, poets, artists, musicians, intellectuals, scientists, doctors, and psychotherapists because all of these roles were carried by them. They were invariably closely tied, as they still are on some reservations, to all the major sociocultural institutions. Gayton (1930) was the first to demonstrate just how shamans and chiefs worked closely together in political and economic affairs, and her observations among the Yokuts hold for most California groups. Shamans were integral to the political, economic, legal, moral, and religious institutions of their societies, as well as central to the aesthetic and healing arts.

Shamans served as mediators between the sacred and profane worlds; they defined the cosmology of the people and the nature of the afterworld. Characteristically, they went in "magical flight" to gain supernatural aid for their people, learned about the universe so they could aid the souls of the deceased in their journey to the land of the dead, and received instructions from the supernatural world on proper life-styles in the here and now, as well as diagnostic and curative techniques. Always they served as philosophers for their people, composing, interpreting, and performing in dramatic enactments many of the sacred happenings which served as cosmological guides for their people. The aesthetic development of poetic myth in southern California, the rich ritual paraphernalia of central California, and the expert use of native plants for medical cures found throughout California point to the crucial position of the shaman; they are also some of the contributions which served to provide people with avenues of power, enrichment, creative expression, and social service. In historic times they were the designers of new philosophical adjustments to the horrors of European contact (for example, the Bole Maru [Dreamer] Cult). Even now (1974) they are the focus of cultural identity for young and old alike, since they serve as culture heroes, culture brokers, and philosophers in context of rapid social change.

Where organized cults appeared in California, membership correlated with shamanic status, and women were generally excluded from access to the role (for example, in southern California) or reduced, at least formally, to curative and divinatory functions as men generally attempted to control and keep exclusive their access to the sacred. In historic times in certain groups this changed as people became disillusioned with traditional forms.

Since the shaman was seen as potentially dangerous and any misfortune might be attributed to his malevolency, this potential was used politically by chiefs and the power elite in almost all groups, either to tighten social control in their own societies or to protect people from the aggressiveness of other groups.

VARYING DEGREES OF MEDICAL KNOWLEDGE

Among all Native California groups there were clearly separate degrees of medical knowledge, practice, and roles available to individuals. There was a common folk medicine available to anyone—the treatment of usual maladies by simple techniques of therapy ranging from the use of herbs, sweating, massage, and bed rest to magical forms (for example, in songs and formulas) privately and/or commonly owned. More specialized forms existed, however; they increased in their degree of specialization as shamanic or doctoring roles were more associated with resources of supernatural power and formal education. Consequently, persons analogous to health aides, nurses, and diagnosticians were recognized, as were more advanced specialists whose occupational roles required years of specialized training, often in schools or through membership in secret societies.

These specializations were logically consistent with Native California concepts of how the universe was structured: power was arranged in various degrees. Hence, all social relationships and the acquisition and use of knowledge were similarly arranged hierarchically. All living things, for example, were organized from lower to higher life (and power) forms. Social classes contained elites, ordinary people, and poor people, and power resources were similarly organized. Consequently, differing degrees of power were available and/or explained by the connection an individual or group or species had with the various levels of the supernatural world (Bean 1974a).

Common people had residual power inherent to the species of man; thus they had knowledge of common uses of medicinal plants and medical lore. Higher forms of medical practitioners had connections with increasingly higher and more powerful forms of power and thus had more esoteric and specialized knowledge. The possession of this knowledge was protected by institutionalized procedures of schooling and professional rights and privileges.

Disease causation was also placed in a hierarchy, and the cause was treated by the class most competent to deal with it. Since a natural cause was often coterminously explained in relation to supernatural causes, patients would seek knowledge of cause and treatment beginning at the lower levels of power and power possessors and uses and ascend to higher and more specialized forms of diagnosis and treatment if lower-level forms did not adequately solve problems. Thus, from commonly known attempts at curing, they might have gone through increasingly higher levels to diviners, diagnosticians, lower-order shamans, and higher-level shamans. Finally they reached the most skilled specialists in their society (see chart below).

DISEASE CAUSATION AND MEDICAL SPECIALISTS

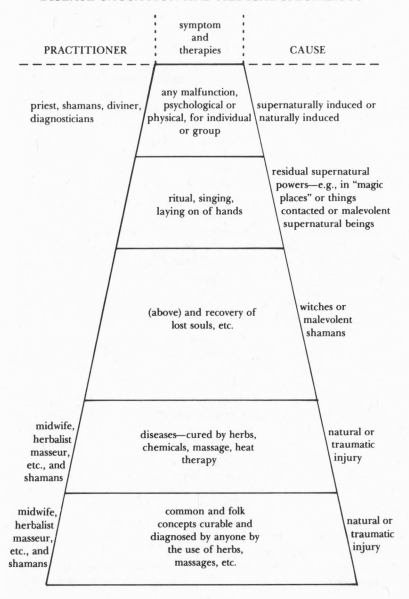

PRACTITIONER	symptom and therapies	CAUSE
priest, shamans, diviner, diagnosticians	any malfunction, psychological or physical, for individual or group	supernaturally induced or naturally induced
	ritual, singing, laying on of hands	residual supernatural powers—e.g., in "magic places" or things contacted or malevolent supernatural beings
	(above) and recovery of lost souls, etc.	witches or malevolent shamans
midwife, herbalist masseur, etc., and shamans	diseases—cured by herbs, chemicals, massage, heat therapy	natural or traumatic injury
midwife, herbalist masseur, etc., and shamans	common and folk concepts curable and diagnosed by anyone by the use of herbs, massages, etc.	natural or traumatic injury

DISEASE CAUSATION AND SOURCES
OF CURATIVE POWER-KNOWLEDGE

Most illnesses and in fact all misfortunes were more likely to be explained ultimately by the absence or presence, use or nonuse, control or lack of control of supernatural forces (power) present in all aspects (persons, objects, intangible forces) of the universe. This power was, according to California Indian cosmology, differentially distributed in both time and space and came from the sacred "dream time" when the universe was created. Through the action of power in the beginning of time, three or more hierarchically ordered worlds were created, each occupied by beings having differing degrees of power. In the upper world lived supernatural beings created at the primordial beginning of the universe. They were beings of very great power who could be utilized by man to control natural circumstances and thus were potential resources for the cause as well as the curing of diseases (Bean 1974a).

In the middle world, the natural world in which man resided, all things contained varying amounts of residual power which could act for or against man. In the lower world were a number of other beings (often associated with particularly malevolent power), some of whom man could communicate with for use of their power. They might, however, act independently against man and cause various disasters as well as fortunate circumstances.

It was from the various supernatural power resources in these various worlds that the inspiration and powers of the shamans ultimately derived. The amount of power one received or was able to control determined the nature and degree of curing and the position of the shaman. Shaman-doctors, for example, who were recipients of power from the highest of power resources, were generally considered the most effective doctors, while the lower-level doctors received most of their abilities, and hence power, from the lesser beings in the middle and lower worlds.

Although ultimate disease causation lay in the realm of supernatural action-forces and most curing forms involved varying degrees of supernatural curing rituals, they were almost always combined with practical medical treatment therapy and posttreatment care. For example, in those cases where there was no apparent natural cause for an illness, herbal remedies were given along with psychic (ritual) healing therapy, as well as with treatments such as massage, heat, bed rest, surgery, and the like.

The theme which ran through either type of curing, supernatural or natural, was, however, one which stressed the restoration of harmony or balance in nature, in interhuman relationships, and in human-supernatural relationships. This theme was more explicitly described for some Native California groups (the World Renewal Cult of the Yurok, Hupa, Tolowa; the Chungichnish among the Luiseño and Gabrielino), but the general principle is found throughout all of California.

The basis of this theme lies in the idea that oppositions and/or conflict could cause disease as easily, and perhaps more readily, as the quixotic nature of the supernatural beings, whether these oppositions-conflicts were disruptive social conditions, taboo violations, selfishness (going against basic community values), or the merging of things or people which were naturally opposed (enemies, tabooed kin, menstrual blood with sacred objects, contact with personages from differing levels of reality).

VARIETIES OF SHAMANIC ROLES

Shamans were ranked according to the amount of power they demonstrated through successful performance of the shamanic arts, such as curing, transformation, divination, and control of natural and supernatural phenomena (heat and cold, the elements); these demonstrations often symbolized their area of occupational specialization.

The greatest shamans tended to be those who could transform themselves into other forms of life, a special class rarely described and somewhat like Eliade's conceptualization of the "White Shaman"—one who had greater powers than others and was crystallized into a purely positive role with an altruistic personality. White shamans could not use their power in any negative way—not even to protect themselves from the malevolence of others if that protection demanded that they act malevolently in turn (Eliade 1964).

Among some groups these doctors (for example, Cahuilla *pavuul*) were recognized aboriginally. Among others (for example, Pomo) they seem to have been the product of the postcontact revelations and an attempt to give shamanism and doctoring new roles in ethnicity-maintenance, which they accomplished by refusing to act negatively against their own people. Their new role demanded that they maintain cultural integration at a time of great cultural stress. If they indulged in negative uses of power, they would lose their potential role as culture heroes who could hold an already culturally ravaged people together as an ethnic unit.

Most shaman-doctors, however, were of the "kill or cure" variety that produced good or bad results. They were morally and professionally capable of either and did in fact secure both. They were expected to perform negative acts toward the group's enemies (more clearly the case in lineage-structured societies than in bilaterally structured ones and were frequently visited for these purposes. However, because they had knowledge of witchcraft, poisoning, and the evil of others, they were in a somewhat dangerous and socially tenuous role. When conditions (medical-behavioral-sociological) became acutely unstable within their community, they were likely to be accused, sometimes placed on trial (where they often confessed and thus relieved the harm they had caused), deprofessionalized by their fellow shamans, or slain.

A lower-level shamanic role, the diviner-diagnostician, found in all Native California societies, was distinguished from that of the shaman on the basis of usability of power. Although these individuals had the power and knowledge to diagnose a disease, discover its cause, and perhaps indicate a cure, they did not have the power or applied skills necessary to proceed with the medical treatment. They were called upon to determine a special course of action, after which a specialist shaman or a lower-order "medicalist" (for example, an herbalist) was called upon to act. These roles were usually reserved for men, but in northern and central California, where power forms were often available to women, persons of either sex might hold this position. The diviner also predicted events and located lost, stolen, or misplaced objects.

In most groups there were those who specialized in the uses of herbs for curative and other nonsacred associated medical procedures (for example, massage, midwifery). These medicalists ranked below other practitioners in status and often assisted other medical practitioners as nurses, acting in postoperative care and carrying out the instructions of higher-order shamans. These roles generally fell to older women who tended to pass the roles on to their daughters. Rarely were these roles filled by men, although many men had considerable medical knowledge and used it situationally in relationship to herbal therapeutics in a nonsacred context. These herbalists, as well as other shamans, charged fees for their services and were usually the first to be called when a family found its home remedies ineffective.

Rattlesnake Shamans

The most frequently mentioned shamanic specialist in California was the rattlesnake shaman. He controlled rattlesnakes, cured their bites, and protected people from possible snakebite. The rattlesnake was often seen as the symbol of a supernatural "dream time" personage, especially those associated with the underworld of the cosmology. Snakebite was apparently a very common malady in

Native California, but the shaman's importance is probably attributable more to the symbolic implications of treatment than to his actual medical functions.

Deer- or Antelope-Shaman

A different type of shaman was associated with animals; the antelope- or deer-shaman usually controlled the large game in his group's territory. Often he had contact with the supernatural guardian of the game. In many groups this role was associated with the ability to transform oneself into another form. This shaman was often an ally of particularly powerful beings (usually masters of the game) and a medical practitioner of considerable skill, as well as a political and economic administrator. Within the category of shamans in the guise of animals, we can place the bear-shaman, a man who could transform himself into a bear in order to utilize the great strength of the bear for various purposes—hunting, traveling rapidly, punishing transgressors of social mores, and so on.

Soul Loss

Since loss of the soul through its capture by supernatural forces, accident, or witchcraft or the like was one of the most common causes of disease and death in Native California, it is to be expected that a class of doctors specializing in soul recovery was recognized. Actually, most shamans were specialists in the care of the soul and in most cultures were likely to have as part of their responsibility the recovery of the soul or the discovery of the circumstances that a soul might encounter following the death of the corporeal body. However, in some groups the soul-loss doctors were specialists whose primary focus of concern was care of the soul. They could send their guardian spirits to restore a soul which had been lost or captured by a malevolent spirit or shaman.

Singing Doctors

Among many groups there was a special type of shaman, the singing doctor. This shaman, usually a male, cured by the power of his songs, obtained from supernatural beings, but was also able to effect cures through the "laying on of hands" and the removal of disease-causing objects. He acquired his original power during visions or dreams or by coming into possession of ritual paraphernalia that once belonged to another singing doctor.

MALEVOLENT USE OF POWER AND WITCHCRAFT

Among all groups malevolent uses of power were available not only to legitimate power brokers—shamans and curers—but also to witches or secret poisoners. Invariably, witches were killed if they were discovered and if their executioners had the courage and political power to accomplish the act. Among many groups there was such fear of these persons, and perhaps such an awareness of their potential usefulness, that only under extreme circumstances, apparently, did execution actually occur. These executions were usually approved by a chief and other political elites; but among some groups—for example, Yokuts—the poisoner practiced his discipline without fear of punishment if the chief of the group had given his permission for the action.

The methods of such poisonings varied but generally involved the intrusion of poisoned arrow points, a mucous substance, or powdered concoctions made of noxious or poisonous substances. Sometimes sheer power sufficed. Both sympathetic and contagious magics were used; people feared the use of feces, hair, clothing, or the like and the making of images or dolls resembling the intended victim. The ritual usually included the singing of esoteric songs and/or the reciting of formulas which facilitated or generated the magical action.

The disease-producing objects were often placed in a person's house or even in a communal house, where they were directed at an individual. The removal or prevention of these objects occupied a considerable amount of the time and attention of the people.

THE SHAMAN AS A PROFESSIONAL AND HIS ACQUISITION OF THE STATUS

The vast majority of shamans came from families of shamans or were individuals who had been observed by shamans and then, on showing the requisite abilities, had been recruited, trained, and "graduated" into professional practice by other shamans. In either case, a divine call or sign was an early indicator of desire (sometimes ambivalently received) to enter the vocation. Upon receiving this call, the candidate was given a series of tests by supernatural beings, usually while he was in trance states. During these trance experiences, the individual obtained power, ritual, medical knowledge, and a set of rules which guided relationships among the shaman, his sacred helpers, and his future clients. The individual was also tested by fellow shamans, often in a "school" situation.

Among many groups secret societies controlled the profession—recruiting, testing, training, and graduating the young men and women to their professional specialties.

Doctors were guided by the ethical and behavioral rules of their various societies. In those societies having formal schools and/or secret societies, professional recruitment, training, and behavior were tightly regulated by established rules of membership and obligations in professional activities.

In groups where formal organizations did not exist, professional behavior was controlled informally by shamans who met on regular occasions to compare notes and discuss their activities vis-à-vis one another and their patients.

Doctors were expected to keep secret from the public not only esoteric knowledge, but also much of their practical work. It was important that their public image be enhanced for the good of the profession. This was accomplished by means of extraordinary, extravagant behavior (magicalists), a high standard of living (several wives, better clothing), and specialized clothing and symbols of office (talismans, shamanic costumes, tattoo marks). They behaved like superior persons, often speaking with one another in esoteric languages, which commoners could not understand. They were not supposed to cure members of their immediate families except in the most extreme conditions. Patients were expected to obey the orders (that is, prescriptions: sweating, bed rest, abstention, ingestion of herbal remedies) of doctors, and the doctors were relieved of responsibility for the consequences if these were broken.

Groups varied in their specific rules that defined the doctor-patient relationship, but some general patterns are indicated below:

Doctors were called by patients to treat particular problems. Some doctors received the call supernaturally—that is, they sensed they were needed by particular individuals. Often they dreamed of a specific problem, informed the patient or patients (if it was a group condition), and then offered to provide diagnosis or cure.

Shamans often felt that someone was about to summon them. They were expected to be available to their clients and thus were necessarily specialists, since they were not active in other economic (subsistence) activities.

When a patient called upon a doctor for treatment, a fee was established or the giving of a gift was implied. In most groups, if the doctor was unsuccessful in the cure, he would return all, or at least a portion, of the fee. This was done in part to protect himself from the accusation that he killed or sickened, rather than cured, the patient for monetary reasons and in part because he had failed in his professional assignment. If he could not cure the patient, he might call upon other specialists to help. For that matter, a patient's family might call in two or more doctors simultaneously to provide care. Fees depended on the type of disease, the length and danger to the doctor of the cure, and the rank and economic status of the patient. Usually a shaman attempted to fit his fee to what the market would bear.

Certain life conditions created special medical problems, particularly in the case of warfare. Since warfare in California was frequent (Bean 1974 ms.) and resulted in considerable numbers of traumatic injuries, it was a time of intense activity on the part of doctors. Much like modern medics, Shamans frequently were active on the battlefront, stemming the flow of blood from wounds, removing arrows, providing psychological support to the more seriously wounded. Often they would supervise emergency first-aid operations until the patients could be removed by litter to their home village, where their wounds could receive more detailed attention, both natural attention and the all-important supernatural. Among several groups there were shamans who specialized in removing arrow points, while others would perform the necessary dressings and postoperative care.

POSTCONTACT PERIOD

It is obvious from early mission period reports that European diseases were making serious inroads into Native California population levels well before Europeans arrived en masse. As a result, there was an increased development of cultic beliefs that emphasized a punishing god (for example, the rise of the southern California Chungichnish Cult) and a general outbreak of witchcraft accusations as new, unexplained, and seriously ravaging diseases struck the indigenous peoples. With the arrival of more and more Europeans came new medical procedures that were often more efficacious and more militantly promoted by whites, with the result that many of the medical functions of the traditional doctors were no longer allowed or needed. Suspicion of the efficiency and efficacy of the native doctors by their own people and persecution of native curers by the whites led to some reduction in their status among their own people and in many cases even their death, although a vigorous underground network of native curers continues today.

Various European religious groups (fundamentalist Protestant, the Shakers) found fertile audiences of people keenly concerned with disease and disease cure. And these religions offered a familiar conceptualization of supernatural curing based upon faith, not an unknown or even unfamiliar concept to most native groups. The difference they allowed was that any member of a cult or religion could receive a spiritual calling, even if for only a short time, and be able to cure with it. Any individual receiving the spirit could become a curer, not just the age-old specialist, the shaman. As these new religious ideas entered California, new concepts replaced old, and the nature of the shaman's relation to the sacred (power sources) changed. In several areas, especially in association with new Indian religious movements (Ghost Dance), the concept of curer changed drastically. A more direct contact with the sacred was allowed to all individuals.

However, it should not be assumed that traditional doctors sat by idly or complacently and allowed themselves to be relegated to oblivion. As the Europeans entered California, they brought with them a new materia medica; and being eclectic and pragmatic in adopting new ideas, California shamans continuously sought to learn these new powers and use them within their medical practices. In fact, the two groups exchanged knowledge of what was useful and comfortably adaptable to each other's cultural pattern.

The more immediate reaction of shamans appears to have been to experiment with old medicines and procedures in treating the new diseases, while at the same time bringing new European medical potentials into the native materia medica. This is a process that still goes on, especially in more recent years, as the number, type, and kind of patent medicines available over the counter have been incorporated into the materia medica of the native curers.

But more important is the fact that the diseases themselves have been redefined into two basic categories: (1) diseases which are the white man's diseases, with their attendant cures; and (2) those which are Indian diseases and have their own proper and efficacious cures and treatments. In addition, native doctors have an edge over their white contemporaries in several ways. They are generally acknowledged to be able to cure diseases which whites cannot or do not often cure or attend to among Indians—for example, cancer, psychic disorders, and alcoholism. Furthermore, Western curative practices have problems that seem insurmountable to some Native Californians: costs, doctors' "negative" attitudes toward patients (that is, impersonal care), inaccessibility to immediate health care, American hospital regimes. Even when facilities and services are available, Native Americans often prefer their own medical treatment. In recent surveys of health conditions and delivery systems among Native Californians, it was discovered that most Indians prefer a doctor who specializes in coming to reservation clinics (a rare occurrence) to those who use off-reservation facilities, even if the degree of care—more medicines, increased technology, immediacy of life-sustaining equipment—is considerably better in such facilities (Bean and Woods 1969).

Moreover, with the increasing concern of the dominant culture about ecological considerations and with what appears to be a renaissance of appreciation for traditional Native American philosophies and life-styles by non-Indians as well as young Native Americans, the status of the native doctor has risen considerably within the past few years. As Myerhoff has pointed out for the Luiseño, the contemporary Indian shaman acts as a culture hero who symbolizes the valuable ethnic background of the Native Californian. He was, and is, the repository of most, if not all, of his people's knowledge of the past, their roots (Myerhoff 1966). But more significantly, shamans still function as the principal creative-active philosophers for their congregation by bridging the oppositions existing between their culture and other cultures. They still cure, direct ritual life, create symbols of ethnicity, draw power from the sacred to the secular world, and act as statesmen advising the secular leaders of Native American peoples.

CONCLUSION

In conclusion I would like to suggest that the term *folk curer* fails to describe the professionalism of medical delivery skills of many medicalists in non-Western societies. The elite medicalists in Native California, as well as in other areas of this continent, as Vogel (1970) has clearly demonstrated, were in fact highly skilled, well-trained professionals, recognized as such by their own peoples. Thus, the term *folk curer* does not apply universally to non-Western curers. The term should, I think, be used exclusively for those practitioners who operate on the level of "common knowledge and concepts of disease." The fact that there are in most societies medical specialists who have control of medically applicable knowledge, are paid for their services, and are so recognized by their constituents sets them apart from a term such as *folk curer*.

We must also remind ourselves that the non-Western medical practitioners do in fact have well-developed medical skills, that they do, despite a symbolic use of "magical" techniques, employ many scientifically validated procedures ranging from surgery, to chemotherapy, to psychiatric skills.

What we know now is but a shadow of what once was. We need more research in the medical functions of Native American peoples. We are still rather ignorant about theories of disease causation as well as curing processes. There is much to be discovered about medical botany, massage, chemotherapy, psychiatric treatment, and the uses of drugs among these peoples.

The failure of Western scholars to appreciate and utilize much of this medical knowledge from other cultures surely stems in part from a combination of sources: our own ethnocentrism and cultural arrogance regarding Western medicine is joined with the need of non-Western medicalists (not unlike our own) to keep valuable knowledge secret and limited to an elite class for profit and prestige.

The persecution that non-Western medicalists have received from westerners has further limited our ability to acquire new knowledge, as has the overemphasis of anthropologists and folklorists on the fascinating "magical" conceptualizations of disease and its curing with which most cultures surround their practical methods. Thus, our concern with the esoteric has obscured the scientific contributions of the people we have pretended to understand.

But the situation is changing slowly, as this conference at UCLA in 1973 demonstrates. Increasingly, medical specialists, anthropologists, and folklorists discover an appreciation of the varieties of medical practice in various cultures. Vigorous debate is beginning. Furthermore, as non-European medicalists become less harassed, as they feel more confident of respectful attention, and as their ethnicity receives greater validation, they will become more open to providing data, so that the exchange of scientific information between cultures will be facilitated.

BIBLIOGRAPHY

Bean, Lowell John
    1974a. "Power and Its Implications in Native California." *Journal of California Anthropology* (Fall, 1974).
    1974b. "Social Organization in Native California." In *Antap: Essays in Socio-economic Organization in Native California*. Ed. Lowell John Bean and Tom King. Ballena Press.
    1974c. "Warfare in Native California." Unpublished MS.
Bean, Lowell John and Corinne Wood
    1969. "The Crisis in Indian Health." *Indian Historian*, 2, 3 (Fall, 1969), 29-33.

Eliade, Mircea
   1964. *Shamanism: Archaic Techniques of Ecstasy.* Princeton: Princeton
      University Press
Myerhoff, Barbara
   1966. "The Doctor as Culture Hero: The Shaman of Rincon." *Anthro-
      pology Quarterly,* 39, 2, 60-72.
Vogel, Virgil J.
   1970. *American Indian Medicine.* Norman: University of Oklahoma Press.

American Indian Foods Used as Medicine

VIRGIL J. VOGEL, *Mayfair College, City Colleges of Chicago*

In the course of investigating the large number of plant products used as medicine by the American Indians, I was interested to discover that a large number of these plants were also used as food. Although not all medical plants were used as food, nearly all important food plants had medical uses. It is sometimes true that the parts used for medicine, such as roots, tubers, stems, leaves, fruits, flowers, seeds, or pollen, were not always the same parts that were used as food. Yet they coincided with sufficient frequency to arouse curiosity about the possibility of mythological foundations for this phenomenon. To take one example: maize, or corn, the most widely cultivated plant among aborigines of the New World, was not only a major part of the food supply for Indians from Peru to the upper Missouri; both the grain and other parts of the plant were also an important element in the pharmacopoeia of these tribes. The maize plant was, moreover, deeply embedded in their mythology and ritual. Maize was generally regarded as either a god or a gift of the gods.

Similar status was found for other cultivated and wild plants that will be mentioned below. This phenomenon gave rise to the question whether Indians made any sharp distinction between substances used for nutrient purposes and those used for cures. A perusal of vocabularies from a dozen languages disclosed that terms for food and medicine were not similar, a sufficient indication that the distinction was not lost. Moreover, the Zuñi had different terms for wormwood (*Artemisia wrightii*) used as food and wormwood used as medicine.[1] But this was, as I think subsequent remarks will show, a distinction without much difference.

To discover the basis of the American Indians' attitude toward these plants, it is necessary to understand their definition of medicine, which was quite different from that ordinarily held in white society. To most Indians, medicine signified a complex of ideas, rather than remedies or treatment alone. George Bird Grinnell, who was intimately acquainted with the northern Plains tribes, has furnished the following explanation of these beliefs:

> All of these things which we speak of as medicine the Indian calls mysterious, and when he calls them mysterious, this only means that they are beyond his power to account for. . . . We say that the Indian calls whisky "medicine water." He really calls it mysterious water—that is, water which acts in a way that he cannot understand. . . . In the same way some tribes call the horse "medicine dog," and gun "medicine iron," meaning mysterious dog and mysterious iron. He whom he calls a medicine man may be a doctor, a healer of diseases, or if he is a juggler, a worker of magic, he is a mystery man. All Indian languages have words which are the equivalent of our word medicine, sometimes with curative properties; but the Indian's translation of "medicine," used in the sense of magical or supernatural, would be mysterious, inexplicable, unaccountable.[2]

A glance at the map, to which the Indians have contributed so many geographical names, reveals their varied application of the term *medicine*: Medicine Bow, Wyoming; Medicine Hat, Alberta; Medicine Lake, Montana; Medicine Lodge, Kansas; and Medicine Mound, Texas. There are also, in Indian parlance, such examples as big medicine, bad medicine, good medicine, love medicine, medicine dance, medicine pipe, medicine drum, and war medicine.

"Whereas we think in terms of drugs, ointments, or cathartics which will benefit the body in a predictable fashion," wrote Robert E. Greenlee, "the Seminole thinks of benefits which one can produce only through the office of the medicine man." This functionary believes that he can surely cure if he can recite the prescribed medicinal formulas, perform the necessary rites, and blow on the brewed medicine in a certain way. His medical theory arises from the reasoning that "he can control the forces of nature and hence make disease yield to his personal efforts."[3] Consequently, curative agents are indeed "medicine," but only one kind of medicine, and that only in association with prescribed rites. The medicine man is entrusted with these rites as well as with ceremonies connected with birth and death, magical ceremonies, and the perpetuation of tribal lore.

Still another instance of the manifold meanings of *medicine* is apparent in the Iroquois practice of soaking seed corn in a liquid in which certain herbs had been boiled. This mixture was called "corn medicine" and was believed to protect the corn from parasites and also to insure healthy growth.[4]

Earlier we quoted Grinnell's definition of Indian medicine as something "mysterious." In another and perhaps more precise sense, it signifies power. Terms for unseen personal power abound in the languages of primitive peoples: the Melanesian *mana*, the Iroquois *orenda*, the Algonquian *manito*, and the Dakota *wakan* are examples. According to one Indian:

> All life is wakan. So also is everything which exhibits power, whether in action . . . or in passive endurance. . . . For even the commonest sticks and stones have a spiritual essence which must be reverenced as a manifestation of the all-pervading mysterious power that fills the universe.[5]

According to the Jesuit priest Father Julien Binneteau, writing in 1699, the Indian "jugglers" claimed that "medicinal herbs are gods, from whom they have life, and that no others must be worshipped. Every day they sing songs in honor of their little manitous, as they call them."[6] Conceivably it is for such reasons that in the Tewa language all nouns denoting plants have their own gender.[7]

Medicine power is often attributed to a fetish or charm adopted to typify a tutelary demon or mystery guardian. These creatures were sometimes animals, but frequently they were plants. Clans named for plants were especially common among the agricultural Pueblo tribes. The Hopi, for example, had twenty-six clans named for plants.[8] Sweet Medicine, the culture hero of the Cheyenne, had a vegetal origin. According to their legend, an all-purpose medicine called Sweet Root was an anthropomorphic spirit who impregnated a Cheyenne virgin, and the subsequent child was named Sweet Medicine.[9]

If medicine means power, it makes no difference whether a plant is consumed as nourishment or as a curative agent or is used for some purpose unrelated to either of these. The power obtained is the same, and the distinction is lost in practice, if not also in theory. As Hoffman has indicated:

> In addition to the alleged medicinal virtues extolled by the preceptors, certain parts of the trees and plants are eaten on account of some mythic reason, or employed in the construction or manufacture of habitations, utensils, and weapons, because of some supposed supernatural origin or property. . . .[10]

An example of the quest for power is the feast which was given by Winnebago chiefs whenever an epidemic threatened. According to Radin's informants, it was given "for stopping the spread of the sickness, whatever it may be, and for repairing the ravages caused thereby."[11]

Evidence of the associations among food, medicine, and the notion of mystic power is to be found in the mythology and ceremonials of many Indian tribes. Of the six festivals or thanks-givings of the Iroquois, according to Morgan, five are related to the food supply. These are called Maple, Planting, Strawberry, Green Corn, and Harvest festivals. The association of food and medicine is shown in their thanksgiving prayer:

> We return thanks for all herbs, which furnish medicines for the cure of our diseases. We return thanks to the corn, and to her sisters, the beans and squashes, which give us life. We return thanks to the bushes and trees, which provide us with fruit.[12]

Of all plants used for food and medicine, none is more widely evident in Indian myth and ritual than maize. Frank Waters informs us,

> It is inconceivable that any Hopi ceremonial could be conducted without corn meal, so varied is its use and so significant is its meaning. It was their belief that corn was a divinely created spirit, the corn mother, so that when corn meal was given in prayers, spiritual thanks was being offered to the creator. . . . We cannot overemphasize the importance of corn in the mythology of the New World. According to the Popol Vuh, the ancestors of the Quiche Mayas of Guatemala were four perfect men made from maize. The Navajos also hold that the prototypes of man were created from corn. Maize was sacred through-out the New World centuries before the first record of it in a European language was made in Columbus's log.[13]

The use of maize in healing and ritual among the Zuni has been described by Matilda C. Stevenson:

> Corn meal wrapped in bits of husk is presented to the theurgist who is asked to visit the sick. Similar presents are made to men and women invited to take part in ceremonies and are used also to notify members of organizations of meetings, etc. The packages are always presented with a prayer and the recipient prays.[14]

One can examine a collection of myths or songs for any tribe or region in which plants were important means of subsistence or healing with the assurance that many of these will deal with plants and their divine origin. Jacobs found that of ten content motifs in Clackamas Chinook myths, food was mentioned more than any other subject except kinship relations.[15]

Doubtlessly we are all familiar with the Ojibwa myth of the origin of corn as it is popularized in Longfellow's *Song of Hiawatha*, which draws upon the exploits of the renamed Ojibwa culture hero, Manabozo. Four times Hiawatha wrestled with Mondamin; and after the last match, when Mondamin was slain and buried, Hiawatha watched the grave for Mondamin's expected resurrection:

> And before the summer ended
> Stood the maize in all its beauty
> With its shining robes about it
> And its long, soft yellow tresses;
> And in rapture Hiawatha
> Cried aloud, "It is Mondamin!
> Yes, the friend of man, Mondamin!"

Such origin myths can be found, in the appropriate culture areas, for wild rice, tobacco, pumpkins, and other plants, as well as for important food animals like the buffalo.

The genesis myth of the Blackfeet tribe tells how Old Man, the creator, introduced the people to food and medicine:

The first people were poor and naked, and did not know how to get a living. Old Man showed them the roots and berries, and told them that they could eat them; that in a certain month of the year they could peel the bark off some trees and eat it, that it was good. . . . The first people that he created he used to take about through the timber and swamps, and over the prairies, and show them the different plants. Of a certain plant he would say, "The root of this plant, if gathered in a certain month of the year, is good for a certain sickness." So they learned the power of all herbs.[16]

With this brief introduction let us examine a few of the more notable examples of wild and cultivated plants which were used by Indians for both food and medicine.

The most outstanding example, of course, is corn (*Zea mays*). Maize is the Haitian aboriginal name for the American Indian's greatest contribution to the world food supply. Indians used it in a variety of food products, including hominy, pemmican, pone or corn bread, popcorn, sagamité, samp, and succotash. Indians also used corn for several medicinal purposes, as we do today. The Inca writer Garcilaso de la Vega (1539-1610) remarked that the Spanish were particularly impressed

with the remarkable curative properties of corn, which is not only the principal article of food in America, but is also of great benefit in the treatment of affections of the kidney and bladder, among which are calculus and retention of the urine. And the best proof I can give of this is that the Indians, whose usual drink is made of corn, are afflicted with none of these diseases.[17]

The *Badianus Manuscript* on Aztec medicine (1552) prescribed a decoction of ground corn in water, called *atole*, for "heat in the heart," dysentery, and the promotion of lactation in women. A poultice of it was also made for infant inflammation.[18] Maya medicinal texts prescribed raw maize soaked in water for blood in the urine, and it was roasted or crushed with the leaves of a species of *Dioscorea* to poultice a sore or swelling.[19]

At Santa Clara Pueblo, New Mexico, the following remedy was used for swollen glands in the neck:

> An ear of corn is laid on the warm hearth near the fire, and the patient is told to set his feet on it and rub it to and fro. . . . In two or three days the swellings are said to subside.

The same people gave blue corn meal mixed with water for "heart sickness," "palpitations, pains near the heart or diaphragm." At San Ildefonso corn pollen was especially recommended for palpitation of the heart. Black corn with red streaking was considered good for a woman at her periods; the remedy is probably an example of the doctrine of signatures.[20]

The Chickasaw Indians treated itching skin and sores produced by scratching by burning old corncobs and holding the affected part over the smoke.[21] Alabama Indians pounded up kernels of corn, mixed the meal with water, and poured the mixture through a sieve over the head of a patient with "slow fever." They also rubbed the body with it.[22] The Catawba used corn grains as sympathetic magic objects in eliminating warts.[23]

Indian uses of corn were quickly adopted by white settlers. In 1672 John Josselyn, the New England herbalist, pronounced "Indian wheat [corn]" to be "excellent in cataplasm, to ripen any swelling or impostume. The decoction of the blew [blue] corn is good to wash sore mouths with. It is light of digestion and the English make a kind of loblooy of it to eat with milk, which they call sampe."[24]

John Brickell of North Carolina told how an Indian doctor "took the rotten Grains of the Maiz, or Indian Corn, well dried and beaten to Powder," and cured an "ulcer" on a white man's leg.[25] This may be an early example of an unknowing application of the principle of antibiotics.

Corn smut (*Ustilago zeae*), a fungus, was used for food by both the Omaha and Pawnee Indians. The spore fruits were gathered as soon as they appeared, while firm and white, and boiled.[26] At San

Ildefonso Pueblo corn smut was stirred in cold water and drunk as a remedy for diarrhea. At Santa Clara Pueblo some women used it in the same way as a remedy for irregular menstruation.[27] The Zuñi Indians used corn smut for a medicine given to women during parturition to hasten childbirth by increasing the severity of labor. It was given also to stop hemorrhage after childbirth and for abnormal lochial discharge. The treatment was the same for all three purposes—a pinch of *Ustilago* was put into a small quantity of warm or cold water and the infusion was taken at intervals.[28]

The virtues attributed to *Ustilago* by the Zuñi were accepted at least in part by white medicine when that substance was made official in the *United States Pharmacopoeia*, 1882-1894, as an aid in childbirth. It served the same purposes as the older drug ergot, although it was considered weaker and of lower toxicity.

Corn silk was also used as a food and medicine. The Missouri River tribes gathered the silks and, after drying them in the sun, stored them for use as food. For this purpose the dried corn silks were ground with parched corn, which was said to give sweetness to the compound.[29] A tea of corn silk was used in pioneer domestic medicine as a remedy for acute bladder infections and as a diuretic.[30] Corn silk was also an officially recognized diuretic in the *USP*, 1894-1906, and the *National Formulary*, 1916-1946. Corn starch and corn oil have also been recognized drugs in the pharmacopoeia.

Generations of rural folk have feasted on the astringent fruits of the persimmon tree (*Diospyros virginiana*), which are considered edible only after the first frost. Persimmons were also an important food and medicine to the Indians, to whom we owe the name. It was a delicacy to the Comanche[31] and to other southerly and southwestern tribes. The Cherokee boiled the persimmon fruit for a medicine taken for bloody bowel discharges,[32] and the Alabama boiled the roots for a tea used in "bowel flux."[33] The Catawba boiled the bark for an infusion used to wash a baby's mouth to cure thrush.[34]

In the mid-eighteenth century Jean Bossu wrote that the southern Indians used this fruit to make a bread which resembled gingerbread and was dried for use on long trips. He considered the persimmon an excellent astringent and a superb remedy for dysentery and bloody flux. The powdered seeds mixed with water and strained through a cloth made a drink which he recommended for kidney stones.[35] A student of Dr. Benjamin Barton at the University of Pennsylvania wrote his dissertation in 1792 on the chemical and medical properties of the persimmon.[36] There is no space here to enumerate the favorable reports on this fruit by early writers on American materia medica, among whom are John Lawson, John Brickell, Peter Kalm, Isaac Bartram, Benjamin Barton, Johann Schoepf, Francis Porcher, and A. Clapp.[37] The unripe persimmon fruit was official in the *USP*, 1820-1882. Because of its tannin content, it was used as an astringent.[38]

In widely separated places, Indians cultivated several species of the gourd family for food, medicine, and utensils. The only one of them to become an official drug was the pumpkin, (*Cucurbita pepo*), the dried ripe seed of which was official in the *USP*, 1863-1936, since it was used for anthelmintic and taeniafuge purposes.

The Maya used pumpkin sap as an application to burns.[39] Pumpkin was the "maycock" of the Virginia Algonquians, and the Swedish botanist Peter Kalm was convinced of its American origin because he was informed by the Indians that they had pumpkins "long before the Europeans discovered America, which seems to be confirmed by the accounts of the first Europeans that came into these parts who mentioned pumpkins as common food among the Indians."[40]

Mrs. Stevenson reported that *C. pepo*, called "squash," was used by the Zuñi for both food and medicine. The seeds and blossoms made an external application used to bring relief from the effects of cactus needles.[41] Yuma medicine men administered an emulsion of pumpkin and watermelon seeds to wounds.[42] The Menomini used the seeds of squash and pumpkin to facilitate the passage of urine. The seeds were pulverized in a mortar and the powder mixed with water.[43] Catawba Indians chewed pumpkin seeds fresh or dried and swallowed them as a kidney medicine.[44]

In a paper prepared for the American Medical Association in 1849, Dr. Francis Porcher said that pumpkin seeds yielded an essential oil which, when mixed with water, furnished a cooling and nutritive milk; when boiled to a jelly, the seeds were said to be a useful diuretic.[45] In the form of an infusion, as well as in a pulpy mass, pumpkin seed was long a favorite home remedy among whites for intestinal parasites and through that use was introduced to the medical profession.[46]

That Indians manufactured maple sugar and syrup (from *Acer* spp.) in precontact times has been well established.[47] In 1771 Bossu wrote that "the French who are settled at the Illinois have learnt from the Indians to make this syrup, which is an exceeding good remedy for colds and rheumatisms."[48] In 1748 Peter Kalm wrote to Cadwallader Colden of New York to ask for seeds of the "Sugar-Maple, and whereof the Indians in some places make a sort of sugar."[49] Three years later Kalm wrote a treatise on maple sugar,[50] in which he held, among other things, that maple sugar cured "scorched wounds." The Louisiana historian Du Pratz held that maple sugar was an excellent remedy for stomach troubles.[51] The same claim was made by Baron de Lahontan, and Dr. Benjamin Rush wrote a laudatory treatise on the nutritional and medical benefits of maple sugar, in which he revealed that Thomas Jefferson planted a maple grove and used no other kind of sugar in his family.[52]

Maple sugar and syrup were used for food and medicine by all tribes which had access to maple trees. References to it are found in writings of Audubon, Barton, Brickell, Joutel, Keating, Henry, Lafitau, Lahontan, Marryat, Pursh, and Schoepf. Samuel Stearns, the herbalist, wrote that "the juice as it runs from the tree is good in the scurvy, and the sugar and molasses for coughs and other diseases of the breast."[53]

The Winnebago mixed maple sugar with sumac leaves and three unidentified substances in a remedy for diarrhea.[54] Both the Potawatomi and the Ojibwa squeezed bloodroot juice on lumps of maple sugar for use as lozenges to relieve sore throat. The Ojibwa also cooked maple sugar with the root bark of the paper birch to make a syrup for alleviation of stomach cramps. The bark of the maple tree was used for a diarrhea remedy, and the pith of the twigs was used in an eye lotion.[55]

Wild rice (*Zizania aquatica*), though not cultivated, was an important cereal to the Indians in the northern Great Lakes region, as well as in scattered places much farther south.[56] Jenks has called it the most nutritious single food that the North American Indians consumed. The Menomini tribe took its name from the native word for this grain, which was one of their main foods.

John Long reported in the 1790s that wild rice was an ingredient (with maple sugar) of a baby food used among northern Indians.[57] John D. Hunter wrote that the Osage made a gruel of wild rice and wild licorice tea, which was given to cholera morbus patients after steam baths and cathartics.[58]

The tuberous roots and bases of the stems of the cattail (*typha latifolia*) have been used as food by the Klamath of Oregon[59] and by Indians of California, Arizona, and the upper Missouri, as well as by the Abnaki of the Northeast.[60] Hunter reported that Plains Indians used the root as a diuretic and that it was a common remedy in "dropsyes, menstrual, and syphilitic diseases."[61] Louisiana Houmas boiled the stalks to make a tea for whooping coughs.[62] The Flambeau Ojibwa used the root fuzz for "war medicine." The Ojibwa and Potawatomi chewed or pounded the root to make a poultice for sores and inflammation.[63] The Omaha and Ponca used pieces of the stem in making a ceremonial object called *niniba weawan*, which was used in the *wawan* ceremony. The down of the cattail was used by them as a dressing for burns and scalds and on infants as a talcum to prevent chafing.

All important varieties of beans (*Phaseolus* spp.) that are used as food in America were cultivated by the Indians.[65] The importance of beans to many tribes is indicated by the prevalence of the bean dance in widely separated places. Beans were used primarily for food, but there were also medical uses. Josselyn declared that "Indian beans [kidney beans] ... are better for physic and chyrurgery than our garden beans."[66] Nicholas Monardes, the physician of Seville, wrote of beans from Cartagena, in South America, which were used for fevers, purges, "diseases of mixte humors, beeyng grosse and in the paines of the Joyntes, and it is a universal purgation."[67] John D. Hunter said that a small red bean growing in Arkansas was used by Indians as an emetic, an abortive, and a narcotic taken in preparation for war and to produce dreams.[68] Safford mentioned red beans as a principal narcotic in ancient America.[69]

Oak acorns (from *Quercus* spp.) were widely used as food both on the East Coast and in California and to a lesser extent in the Plains area. In California especially it was a major food. Generally Indians first removed the bitter-tasting tannin from the acorns by a leeching process and then ground them into a flour used to make bread.[70]

Josselyn wrote that New England Indians boiled acorns in lye from maple ashes to extract the oil, which was then used "to annoint their naked limbs; which corroborates them exceedingly. They eat it likewise with their meat."[71] The Penobscots ate acorns to induce thirst, since it was thought beneficial to drink plenty of water.[72] The Yuki of California used the bark of *Quercus lobata* in a diarrhea remedy, and some northern California tribes used oak galls in a remedy for sore eyes.[73]

The fruit of the manzanita shrub (*Arctostaphylos petula, A. glauca, A. tomentosa,* etc.) was widely used as food, fresh or cooked, by western Indians. The Klamath ate the berries and smoked the leaves for tobacco.[74] The Yuki, the Miwok, and other California tribes also made a cider from the berries. The Miwok chewed the leaves for stomachache and cramps.[75] Palmer said that some Indians ground the dried fruit into a flour to make bread, and the Paiute used the leaves for tobacco and medicine.[76] Some tribes crushed the astringent leaves for a remedy for bronchitis and dropsy. A tea made from the berries was used as a wash for poison oak infection. The Atsugewi used a decoction of the leaves on cuts and burns.[77]

The Jerusalem artichoke (*Helianthus tuberosus*) is one of several members of the sunflower family that were sometimes cultivated by the Indians. Unlike the other sunflowers, which were used for the seeds and the oil extracted from them, this plant was valued for its tubers, which were known to frontiersmen as Indian potatoes. Despite its misleading name, this is a native American plant,[78] and the Siouan name for it, *topeka*, was given to the capital of Kansas.

All the Nebraska tribes used the tubers of the wild plant for food.[79] In recent times it was cultivated for food by some of the Hopi.[80] Susan Scully reports that some Indians (not identified) sought to relieve rheumatic pains by eating the heads or by drinking a tea made from the leaves and stalks.[81]

SUMMARY

Time and space do not permit descriptions of more than the eleven substances listed above, which have been selected for their relative significance and importance in illustrating our theme. In an appendix we briefly list eighteen more, but these are but a small fragment of the number that might be listed as sources of food and medicine among the Indians.

In concluding, we must consider two problems related to the tentative hypothesis here set forth that Indian food and medicine are spiritually and mythologically linked. One, touched upon at the beginning, is the fact that the plant parts used for food were sometimes not the same as those used for medicine. It seems, however, that if the Indians held that spiritual power resided in the whole plant, it was only reasonable that the edible parts be used for food and for internal remedies and that the inedible parts be used for external remedies or for charms and ceremonial purposes.

Another problem is that a plant is sometimes used only as food in one tribe and only as medicine in another, so far as the facts are revealed in the literature. A possible explanation for this discrepancy is that investigations are incomplete. Thorough studies of the ethnobotany of many tribes are yet to be made and, perhaps, can never be made for some of them at this late date. Early observers were seldom scholars, and later investigators have come from different specialties, such as botany, medicine, anthropology, and agricultural science, and the results may reflect the special interests of these investigators. Moreover, it is well known that Indians are often reluctant, for religious and other reasons, to reveal their secrets concerning medicinal plants, so that the more obvious food and economic uses are easier to discover and record.

APPENDIX

SELECTED LIST OF ADDITIONAL INDIAN FOOD AND MEDICINAL PLANTS

Common name	Scientific name	Source: food use	Source: medical use
Butterfly weed	*Asclepias tuberosa*	Report U.S. Commissioner of Agriculture, 1870, p. 405.	Vogel, *American Indian Medicine*, pp. 287-88.
Gooseberry	*Ribes* spp.	Scully, *Treasury of American Indian Herbs*, 1970, p. 47	H. H. Smith, *Ethnobotany, Potawatomi*, p. 82.
Hickory	*Carya ovata*	John Smith, in L. G. Tyler, ed., *Narratives of Early Virginia*, p. 91.	Hu Maxwell, *American Forestry* 24 (April 1918), p. 211
Indian turnip, or Jack-in-the-pulpit	*Arum triphyllum*	Vogel, *op. cit.*, pp. 321-22.	*Ibid.*
Juniper	*Juniperus* spp.	Robbins, *et al.*, *Tewa Ethnobotany*, pp. 39-40.	*Ibid.*
May apple	*Podophyllum peltatum*	Vogel, *op. cit.*, pp. 334-36.	*Ibid.*
Milkweed	*Asclepias syriaca*	Fernald & Kinsey, *Edible Wild Plants*, 1943, pp. 324-25.	Vogel, *op. cit.*, pp. 336-37.
Mushrooms	*Fungi*	Scully, *op. cit.*, pp. 67-68.	Vogel, *op. cit.*, pp. 163-64, 236.

Oregon grape	*Berberis repens*	Scully, *op. cit.*, p. 47.	Vogel, *op. cit.*, pp. 343-44.
Papaya	*Caria papaya*	Oviedo, *Natural History of the West Indies*, Chapel Hill, 1959, pp. 85-86.	Vogel, *op. cit.*, p. 412.
Pecan	*Carya illinoensis*	Carlson and Jones, *Papers Michigan Academy of Sciences*, XXV, 1939, p. 520.	*Ibid.*
Piñon	*Pinus edulis*	Stevenson, *Zuñi Ethnobotany*, 30th Annual Report, BAE, p. 70.	*Ibid.*, p. 53; L. S. M. Curtin, *Healing Herbs* (Los Angeles: Southwest Museum, 1965), pp. 155-56.
Prickly pear	*Opuntia* spp.	Vogel, *op. cit.*, pp. 79-80.	*Ibid.*, pp. 186, 209.
Squash	*Cucurbitae*	Stevenson, *op. cit.*, 66-67.	*Ibid.*, pp. 45-46.
Sunflowers	*Helianthus* spp.	Thomas Hariot, *A Briefe and True Report of the New Found Land of Virginia*, New York, 1903.	H. H. Smith, *Meskwaki Ethnobotany*, 1928, p. 215.
Tuckahoe, Arrowhead, or Wapato	*Sagittaria latifolia*	Gilmore, *Indians of Missouri River Region*, p. 65.	H. H. Smith, *Potawatomi Ethnobotany*, p. 37.
Wild strawberry	*Fragaria* spp.	Coville, *Contributions U.S. National Herbarium*, V, p. 98.	H. H. Smith, *Ojibwe Ethnobotany*, p. 384.

Yellow	*Nelumbo lutea*	Fernald &	H. H. Smith,
pond lily		Kinsey, *op. cit.*,	*Menomini Ethno-*
		p. 200; Gilmore,	*botany*, pp. 42-43.
		op. cit., p. 79.	

NOTES

1. Matilda C. Stevenson, "Ethnobotany of the Zuni Indians," *Thirtieth Annual Report, Bureau of American Ethnology*, 1908-1909 (Washington, D.C.: Government Printing Office, 1915), p. 65.

2. George Bird Grinnell, *The Story of the Indian* (New York: D. Appleton-Century Co., 1935), pp. 180-181.

3. Robert F. Greenlee, "Medicine and Curing Practices of the Modern Florida Seminoles," *American Anthropologist*, n.s. 46 (1944), 317-319.

4. F. W. Waugh, *Iroquois Foods and Food Preparation* (Ottawa, Canada: Government Printing Bureau, 1916; reprint, 1973), pp. 18-19.

5. Ruth Underhill, *Red Man's Religion* (Chicago: University of Chicago Press, 1965), p. 21, citing LaFlesche.

6. Reuben Gold Thwaites, ed., *The Jesuit Relations and Allied Documents*, 75 vols. (Cleveland: The Burrows Bros. Co., 1896-1901), LXV, 65.

7. Wilfred W. Robbins, John P. Harrington, and Barbara Freire-Marreco, *Ethnobotany of the Tewa Indians*, Bureau of American Ethnology Bulletin no. 55 (Washington, D.C.: Government Printing Office, 1916), p. 8.

8. Alfred F. Whiting, *Ethnobotany of the Hopi* (Flagstaff, Ariz.: Museum of Northern Arizona, 1966), p. 57.

9. John Stands in Timber and Margot Liberty, *Cheyenne Memories* (New Haven, Conn.: Yale University Press, 1967), pp. 27-28. There are variations to this story. See also Peter Powell, *Sweet Medicine*, 2 vols. (Norman: University of Oklahoma Press, 1969), pp. 53-54, 460-466.

10. Walter J. Hoffman, "The Midewiwin or 'Grand Medicine Society' of the Ojibwa," *Seventh Annual Report of the Bureau of American Ethnology*, 1885-1886 (Washington, D.C.: Government Printing Office, 1891), p. 197.

11. Paul Radin, *The Winnebago Tribe* (Lincoln: University of Nebraska Press, 1971), pp. 271-272.

12. Lewis H. Morgan, *League of the Ho-de-no-sau-nee or Iroquois* 2 vols. (New Haven, Conn.: Human Relations Area Files, 1954), I, 175-176, 194.

13. Frank Waters, *Book of the Hopi* (New York: Ballantine Books, 1969), pp. 64-67.

14. Stevenson, *op. cit.*, p. 100.

15. Melville Jacobs, *The Content and Style of an Oral Literature: Clackamas Chinook Myths and Tales* (Chicago: University of Chicago Press, 1959), p. 128.

16. George Bird Grinnell, *Blackfoot Lodge Tales* (Lincoln: University of Nebraska Press, 1971), p. 139.

17. Alain Gheerbrant, ed., *The Royal Commentaries of the Inca Garcilaso de la Vega, 1539-1616* (New York: The Orion Press, 1962), p. 53.

18. Emily W. Emmart, ed., *The Badianus Manuscript* (Baltimore: Johns Hopkins Press, 1940), pp. 252, 257, 320-321.

19. Ralph Roys, *The Ethno-Botany of the Maya* (New Orleans: Department of Middle American Research, Tulane University, 1931), p. 249.

20. Robbins et al., *op. cit.*, p. 97. The use of the past tense herein does not necessarily signify that the practice described is no longer current; because the sources, however, are not always recent, prudence requires the use of the verb *was*.

21. John R. Swanton, "Social and Religious Beliefs and Practices of the Chickasaw Indians," *Forty-Fourth Annual Report of the Bureau of American Ethnology*, 1926-1927 (Washington, D.C.: Government Printing Office, 1928), p. 268.

22. John R. Swanton, "Religious Beliefs and Medical Practices of the Creek Indians," *Forty-Second Annual Report of the Bureau of American Ethnology*, 1924-1925 (Washington, D.C.: Government Printing Office, 1928), pp. 473-672.

23. Frank G. Speck, "Catawba Herbals and Curing Practices," *Journal of American Folklore*, 57 (1944), 46.

24. John Josselyn, "New-England's Rarities Discovered," in *Archaeologica Americana: Transactions and Collections of the American Antiquarian Society*, IV (Boston, 1860), 105-238.

25. John Brickell, *The Natural History of North-Carolina* (Raleigh, N.C.: Trustees of the Public Libraries, 1911), p. 396.

26. Melvin R. Gilmore, "Uses of Plants by Indians of the Missouri River Region," *Thirty-Third Annual Report of the Bureau of American Ethnology*, 1911-1912 (Washington, D.C.: Government Printing Office, 1919), p. 62.

27. Robbins et al., *op. cit.*, p. 67.

28. Gilmore, *op. cit.*, p. 68.

29. Stevenson, *op. cit.*, pp. 61-62.

30. John U. Lloyd, *Origin and History of all the Pharmacopeial Vegetable Drugs . . .* (Cincinnati: The Caxton Press, 1921), p. 355.

31. Gustav G. Carlson and Volney H. Jones, "Some Notes on Uses of Plants by the Comanche Indians," *Papers of the Michigan Academy of Science, Arts, and Letters*, 25 (1939), 526.

32. James Mooney and Frans M. Olbrechts, *The Swimmer Manuscript: Cherokee Sacred Formulas and Medicinal Prescriptions* Bureau of American Ethnology Bulletin no. 99 (Washington, D.C., Government Printing Office, 1932), p. 275.

33. W. E. S. Folsom-Dickerson, *The White Path* (San Antonio, Tex.: The Naylor Co., 1965), p. 72.

34. Speck, *op. cit.*, p. 46.

35. Jean-Bernard Bossu, *Travels in the Interior of North America* (Norman: University of Oklahoma Press, 1962), p. 194.

36. James Woodhouse, *An Inaugural Dissertation on the Chemical Properties of the Persimmon Tree* (Philadelphia: the author, 1792).

37. Virgil J. Vogel, *American Indian Medicine* (Norman: University of Oklahoma Press, 1970), pp. 345-346.

38. Edward P. Claus, *Gathercoal and Wirth Pharmacognosy*, 3d. ed. rev. (Philadelphia: Lea and Febiger, 1956), p. 235.

39. Roys, *op. cit.*, p. 258.

40. Peter Kalm, *Peter Kalm's Travels in North America*, 2 vols. (New York: Wilson-Erickson Inc., 1937), II, 517.

41. Stevenson, *op. cit.*, p. 597.

42. Aleš Hrdlička, *Physiological and Medical Observations among the Indians of Southwestern United States and Northern Mexico*, Bureau of American Ethnology Bulletin no. 34 (Washington, D.C.: Government Printing Office, 1908), p. 249.

43. Huron H. Smith, "Ethnobotany of the Menomini Indians," *Bulletin of the Milwaukee Public Museum* 4, 1 (1923), 33.

44. Speck, *op. cit.*, p. 45.

45. Francis P. Porcher, "Report on the Indigenous Medical Plants of South Carolina," *Transactions of the American Medical Association*, 2 (1849), 711.

46. Lloyd, *op. cit.*, p. 236.

47. H. W. Henshaw, "The Indian Origin of Maple Sugar," *American Anthropologist*, 3 (1890), 341-352.

48. Bossu, *Travels*, cited in Henshaw, *op. cit.*, p. 345.

49. Cadwallader Colden, *The Letters and Papers of Cadwallader Colden*, 7 vols. (Collections of the New York State Historical Society, 50-56, 1918-1923), IV, 76.

50. Kalm, *op. cit.*, II, 461, 774.

51. Le Page du Pratz, *Histoire de la Louisiane*, 3 vols. (Paris, 1758), II, 36.

52. Benjamin Rush, "An Account of the Sugar Maple-Tree of the United States . . . ," *Transactions of the American Philosophical Society*, 3 (1793), 64-81.

53. Samuel Stearns, *American Herbal or Materia Medica* . . . (Walpole, N.H., 1801), p. 218.

54. Radin, *op. cit.*, p. 217.

55. Huron H. Smith, "Ethnobotany of the Forest Potawatomi Indians," *Bulletin of the Milwaukee Public Museum*, 7, 1 (1933), 68; *idem*, "Ethnobotany of the Ojibwe Indians," *Bulletin of the Milwaukee Public Museum*, 4, 3 (1932), 357, 377.

56. Charles E. Chambliss, "The Botany and History of *Zizania Aquatica* L. ('Wild Rice')," *Annual Report of the Smithsonian Institution, 1940*, pp. 369-382; Gardner P. Stickney, "Indian Use of Wild Rice," *American Anthropologist*, 9 (1896), 115-121.

57. Albert E. Jenks, "The Wild Rice Gatherers of the Upper Lakes" (extract from *Nineteenth Annual Report of the Bureau of American Ethnology* [Washington, D.C.: Government Printing Office, 1901], pp. 1083, 1086).

58. John D. Hunter, *Manners and Customs*, p. 433, cited by Jenks, *op. cit.*, p. 1086.

59. Frederick Coville, "Notes on the Plants Used by the Klamath Indians of Oregon," in *Contributions from the U.S. National Herbarium*, 5 (Washington, D.C.: Government Printing Office, 1897-1901), 90.

60. V. K. Chesnut, "Plants Used by the Indians of Mendocino County, California," in *Contributions from the U.S. National Herbarium*, 7, 3 (Washington, D.C.: Government Printing Office, 1902), 310; Merrit L. Fernald and Alfred C. Kinsey, *Edible Wild Plants of Eastern North America* (Cornwall-on-Hudson, N.Y.: Idlewild Press, 1943), pp. 82-84; *Food Products of the North American Indians: Report of the U.S. Commissioner of Agriculture, 1870* (Washington, D.C.: Government Printing Office, 1871), p. 408.

61. John D. Hunter, *Manners and Customs of Several Indian Tribes Located West of the Mississippi* (Minneapolis: Ross and Haines, 1957), pp. 384-385.

62. Frank G. Speck, "A List of Plant Curatives Obtained from the Houma Indians of Louisiana," *Primitive Man*, 14 (1941), 60.

63. Smith, "Ethnobotany of the Potawatomi," p. 85; Hoffman, *op. cit.*, pp. 200, 390.

64. Gilmore, *op. cit.*, pp. 64-65.

65. Lawrence Kaplan, "Cultivated Beans of the Prehistoric Southwest," *Annals of the Missouri Botanical Garden*, 43 (1956), 189-251; William W. Tracy, *American Varieties of Garden Beans*, U.S. Department of Agriculture Bulletin no. 109 (Washington, D.C.: Government Printing Office, 1907).

66. Josselyn, *op. cit.*, p. 194.

67. Nicholas Monardes, *Joyfull Newes out of the Newe Founde Worlde*, 2 vols. (New York: Alfred A. Knopf, 1925), I, 52-53.

68. Hunter, *op. cit.*, pp. 376-377.

69. W. E. Safford, "Narcotic Plants and Stimulants of the Ancient Americans," *Annual Report of the Smithsonian Institution, 1916* (Washington, D.C.: Government Printing Office, 1917), p. 424.

70. C. A. Browne, "The Chemical Industries of the American Aborigines," *Isis*, 23 (1935), 408-409; Harold E. Driver, "The Acorn in North American Indian Diet," *Proceedings of the Indiana Academy of Science*, 62 (1952), 56-62; E. W. Gifford, "California Balanophagy," in R. F. Heizer and M. A. Whipple, eds., *The California Indians*, (Berkeley and Los Angeles: University of California Press, 1967), pp. 237-241; Gilmore, *op. cit.*, p. 75.

71. Josselyn, *op. cit.*, p. 182.

72. Frank G. Speck, "Medical Practices of the Northeastern Algonquians," *Proceedings, Nineteenth International Congress of Americanists, Washington, 1915* (published 1917), p. 309.

73. Chesnut, *op. cit.*, pp. 343-344.

74. Coville, *op. cit.*, p. 102.

75. S. A. Barrett and E. W. Gifford, "Miwok Material Culture," *Bulletin of Milwaukee Public Museum*, 2, 4 (1933); reprint Yosemite National Park, Calif.: Yosemite Natural History Association, n.d., pp. 61-62.

76. Edward Palmer, "Plants Used by the Indians of the United States," *American Naturalist*, 12 (1878), 599.

77. Paul E. Schulz, *Indians of Lassen Volcanic National Park and Vicinity* (Mineral, Calif.: Loomis Museum Association, 1954), p. 163.

78. J. H. Trumbull and Asa Gray, "Notes on the History of Helianthus Tuberosus, the So-Called Jerusalem Artichoke," *American Journal of Science and Arts*, 3d ser., no. 3 (1877), 347-352.

79. Gilmore, *op. cit.*, 131.

80. Whiting, *op. cit.*, p. 97.

81. Susan Scully, *A Treasury of American Indian Herbs* (New York: Crown Publishers, 1970), p. 112.

Communication Networks and Information Hierarchies in Native American Folk Medicine: Tewa Pueblos, New Mexico

RICHARD I. FORD, *University of Michigan*

I

No other investigation into aspects of Native American culture can match the depth and range of information about Native American folk medicine. Observed since European contact, indigenous curatives have been recorded by explorers, doctors, and anthropologists alike. Vogel's encyclopedic summary has spared us the task of either recapitulating the history of this inquiry or tabulating the Indians' many significant contributions to our pharmacopoeias.[1] The legacy of their folk medicines has benefited all mankind.

A closer inspection of the original sources from which we obtain this medicinal lore, however, raises some methodological problems. Rarely are we given the number of native informants who provided this invaluable information, nor do we know how representative of a particular culture their knowledge was. The fascination Americans have had for Indian medicine men leads one to wonder how much of our knowledge is derived from the specialist, as opposed to the everyday home herbalist.[2] These caveats can be rephrased as two questions: how differential is knowledge of curing agents in Native American cultures, and how have discrepancies in medicinal lore affected our understanding of Native American folk medicine? If knowledge of folk remedies is indeed unevenly distributed, the next question is, how do people gain access to the information possessed by others so that the well-being of the population is not jeopardized?

These are serious questions that have not been adequately answered in the study of North American folk medicine. To focus attention on the Eastern Pueblos of New Mexico, we know that earlier investigators (Curtis, Laski, Parsons, White) were infatuated by the ceremonialists at the expense of the nonspecialists. At the same time, these sodality members are loath to reveal many of their secrets, the essence of their power and authority. Alfonso Ortiz, to whom much of this study is indebted, aptly records in his significant study of the Tewa that when he, a native speaker, asked probing questions, he received the poignant reply: "Let us give you water and we shall tell you more," that is, you will learn if you are initiated.[3] In my own studies analysis of medicinal practices obtained from several excellent consultants reveals obvious preferences for certain medicines and actual differences in experience with curatives (table 1). These disparities beg for an explanation.

II

In learning about folk medicine certain problems are inherent. Although some forms of information can be derived from errors in unsuccessful trials, this freedom is usually denied a patient. His goal is to regain a balance with nature, to return to a state of well-being, and not to exacerbate an already abnormal condition. Consequently, the acquisition of new medicinal information for most members of a culture occurs during stressful situations and must be affirmative. There is another constraint. Illness or sickness is a culturally recognized state of being that may befall anyone. When one is diagnosed and classified as sick, one has socially sanctioned relief from many obligations. At the same time, however, in small-scale subsistence-level societies, the inability of a member to perform daily chores often creates a burden for others. Therefore trial-and-error learning is potentially dangerous for the patient and too time-consuming, under most circumstances, as long as others must assume the patient's duties. In societies fettered by these rigid constraints, the outside observer would expect general principles for organizing classes of folk medicines to have priority over the learning of specific cures. By this means speed is achieved even though only partial information is known. This leads to the further conclusion that one need not control a great deal of specific information about illness or medicine in order to be cured.

From a practical standpoint sickness is a personal and social inconvenience; the sooner a remedy is prescribed, the happier all will be. Therefore diagnosis requires a code that permits the rapid

Table 1

A LIST OF ILLNESSES AND REMEDIES USED BY FIVE SAN JUAN CONSULTANTS
(in order of preference)

HAY	CONSULTANT A		CONSULTANT B		CONSULTANT C		CONSULTANT D		CONSULTANT E	
	COLD	HOT	COLD	HOT	COLD	HOT	COLD	HOT	COLD	HOT
p'ôn hay (H;C) headache	suts' ę́ę̌gi nanphuu inmortal	yeva wéná osaa púu okáwą̈ phéh tų̈ tobacco stamp steam	nanphuu inmortal	osaa púu tų̈ okáwą̈ phéh	nanphuu suts' ę́ę̌gi	osaa púu yeva wéná tų̈	nanphuu tay kaa suts' ę́ę̌gi poe p'ay hun	osaa púu yeva wéná	nanphuu	phá' wówá tų̈ nwą̈ą̈ tobacco stamp
see hay (H;C) stomach-ache	suts' ę́ę̌gi inmortal khá' póvi	mansu púu yeva wéná osaa púu	suts' ę́ę̌gi khá' póvi	osaa púu yeva wéná pagé	suts' ę́ę̌gi	osaa púu yeva wéná t'óe	suts' ę́ę̌gi inmortal khá' póvi	osaa púu hųų t'óe pagé	suts' ę́ę̌gi	phá' wówá yeva wéná
ts'an wą̈ hay (H) fever	phisaa woe suts' ę́ę̌gi		phisaa woe suts' ę́ę̌gi mentholatum		phisaa woe nanphuu		phisaa woe suts' ę́ę̌gi inmortal		phisaa woe nanphuu	
k'ay foe hay (H) sore throat	suts' ę́ę̌gi khá' póvi		suts' ę́ę̌gi khá' póvi		suts' ę́ę̌gi khá' póvi		khá' póvi suts' ę́ę̌gi		khá póvi	
okhüwa'a (H;C) wind-strike	inmortal	okáwą̈ phéh koyáyi	inmortal	okáwą̈ phéh koyáyi nwą̈ą̈ kanela	inmortal	okáwą̈ phéh koyáyi	inmortal	wą̈ą̈ sáa	inmortal	wą̈ą̈ sáa nwą̈ą̈ kanela

H = hot   C = cold

selection and administration of a curative. However, if information about specific remedies is not universal, then the general rules which make up the code must be rather simple and straightforward and permit a high degree of redundancy so that all can share them without ambiguity. In addition to social and temporal constraints, there is another: the message of illness must be diagnosed in the same terms by the patient and by those closest to him. Once they are in accord, administration of a cure can begin.

From the situation described up to this point, we can deduce two additional features of the information system and communication network that function to prevent ineffectiveness in the initial efforts at curing. First, the rules must be general enough to enable everyone to learn them, and the communication network linking members of the society must be open so that alternative medicines can be found and applied. Second, with time so critical, one cannot go from relative to relative or neighbor to neighbor indefinitely. Therefore a higher authority is required, a specialist who can be appealed to to recheck the diagnosis and prescribe any number of alternative medicines he has at hand. He, too, knows the rules, but his power is derived from, and sanctioned by, still higher authorities governed by more general principles recognized by the community. However, when the society's economic basis is household production and when an "embedded" political organization is present, specialists are only part-time, and therefore they do not have the time to remedy each and every ailment. Specialists, "medicine men," are not part of the open network of communication for obtaining cures and medicines; they can treat only a restricted and finite number of patients.

We would be remiss if we limit an examination of folk medicine to remedies applied under the stress of illness. In fact, one must make sure that illness in the Western sense is not itself a subclass of yet a higher category related to well-being and prosperity. The communities I am discussing are egalitarian, with most activities relating to sustenance conducted by the household (*Kehgee*),[4] and at the same time the individual is deemphasized and submerged in favor of the solidarity and corporateness of larger social groupings. Thus, while new remedies for sickness may be added to one's personal repertoire, for the benefit of the group specific preventatives that avert illness and bad luck must be known to everyone and taught in a variety of situations or unspecified contexts.

To recapituate briefly, three testable propositions emerge from the foregoing discussion. First, general principles of the classification of illness and cures must be highly redundant and have priority over knowledge of specific remedies. In other words, a hierarchy of information about medicine exists in any society, but it is the underspecified, more abstract ideas that must be shared by community members rather than the exact qualities of each known cure, which are almost impossible to teach to everyone without ambiguity. Second, since information about particular medicines is not familiar to every member of a culture, for maximum effectiveness communication networks must be open to alternative sources of diagnosis and remedies. If correct, this proposition predicts that communication networks will mirror the information hierarchy— that is, that persons with differential knowledge will have equal and unimpeded access to each other, but accessibility to those few individuals with specialized training in medicinal lore will be restricted. Third, in a study of medicine, specific prophylactics that affect the maintenance of life and general well-being will receive emphasis over specific cures for sickness.

III

Folk medicines are used in the Tewa Pueblos today, although their importance is dwindling. Initially, when I started my fieldwork, I followed the procedure practiced by most ethnobotanists and obtained from a number of consultants lists of plants used as specific remedies. Table 1 contrasts the medicines used in preferential order by five older women in San Juan Pueblo for curing five common illnesses. Each woman is extremely knowledgeable; yet all have different preferences and even fail to acknowledge some plants favored by others as cures for certain ailments. To reconcile these differences, I had to revamp my procedure and begin my analysis at a higher level of generalization—a very difficult task when one starts, as I had, from the lowest taxonomic level—the specific cures. Thus, to understand Tewa folk medicine, or any other, we must start with general structural principles.

Ortiz has recently provided a detailed study of the Tewa world view.[5] Located along the Rio Grande and its tributaries from Santa Fe northward to the confluence with the Rio Chama, five Tewa-speaking pueblos are active today. The basic overarching principle is a duality that establishes contrastive sets in thinking about man and nature. These communities have a nonexogamous moiety organization that divides its members into a Winter side and a Summer side. Symbolically the Winter group is associated with hunting, maleness, and cold, while the Summer group represents plant foods, femaleness, and warm weather. Colors, geographical areas, and even games are antithetically divided.

The principle of opposition crosscuts the earthly and spiritual orders. All Tewa who have been initiated into their fathers' moieties but have not joined a sodality are termed Weed People or, more formally, Dry Food People.[6] They constitute the lowest earthly level. From their ranks six male *Towa é*, who protect the community, are annually selected, three from each moiety.[7] Adults who have been initiated into sodalities and are thereby members of the highest order are referred to as Made People.[8] Other Dry Food People who have actively participated in rituals can be selected for lifelong lay positions as assistants to their moiety sodality, each of which draws members from only its initiates. The other six associations recruit members from both moieties. These three levels are associated with three spiritual levels from which its members can seek assistance.

The Made People go through a long training period during which they learn their society's rituals, prayers, and symbols. Chartered in the origin myth, each sodality is impowered to assure some aspect of good health and long life. Each Made Person, upon finishing, receives a terraced bowl, called a "lake," within which he prepares medicine water. Combined with the proper ritual, this liquid becomes an elixir. This discussion indicates that ascertaining folk remedies by starting with the simple opposition *hay:woe* (illness:medicine) does not explain Tewa folk medicine and contains only part of the information needed to understand the importance of medicines in the first place.

The Tewa theory of illness is presented in each variant of the origin myth.[9] When the people emerged from the underworld, many became ill. Once again the Winter and Summer headmen decided all should return to their home under the lake. The Hunt headman opened a fetish and found it filled with pebbles and cactus spines; someone was a *chuge⁇i⁇*, a witch. This was the beginning of evil, misfortune, and illness, *t'án*. To counter witchcraft and to cure the people, the Bear (*Kay*) medicine men were created. Once again the people emerged but this time with the knowledge that man was empowered with both good and evil and that the Bear medicine men and other Made People would protect them.

Related to this theory of health and illness is the role of the sun. At the winter solstice the sun reports to the other deities the events of the past year and marks who will die or become seriously ill during the forthcoming year. To avoid this designation people make every effort to assist the sun on its journey from under the lake. They pay their debts, make no new fires, and anoint their joints with piñon pitch "to stay attached to the sun."

As we examine the actual behavior of men and spirits as predicted by the origin myth, the concept of duality again enters: both men and spirits err. The puckish antics of the Yellow Flower Katchina, the same who gives out medicine in Kiva ceremonies, are related in folktales. Nor are the Made People above suspicion. The very nature of their power marks them for public notice, and even a lifetime devoted to good works becomes secondary at death, when for the next twelve days the people watch for auspicious signs in nature indicative of a soul accepted by the Dry Food Who Never Did Become.[10]

From the time of emergence, then, misfortune and well-being, sickness and health were part of the human condition. The Made People were created to protect the people and to sustain good health. Witches cause sickness and jeopardize the proper relations between man and the spirits.

Several levels of misfortune exist, and each is remedied with an appropriate ceremony or medicine. At the most abstract and at the same time most inclusive of these levels, illness, bad luck, and evil are classed as *t'án*. At the next level are two subclasses. Bad luck or misfortune, also labeled *t'án*, is one, and illness or sickness, *hay*, is the other. Beneath these at a third level are specifically named maladies: colds, stomachaches, urinary problems, wind strike, and so on are categories of *hay*, and broken legs, pulled muscles, or lost horses are examples of *t'án*. Each of these is treated by the appropriate *woe*, "medicine." For example, at the level of greatest specificity, *suts'éegi*ʔ (pennyroyal; see the Appendix for the English and Latin equivalents of Tewa plant names) may be chewed and swallowed by some to relieve a sore throat. Likewise, charms to ward off misfortune are categorized as medicinal, as are the ceremonies of the Made People that bring prosperity to the community.

Returning again to the origin of the Tewa and their sodalities, the dual division of Winter and Summer, with their associated symbolic referents, is paramount. It permeates all aspects of Tewa thought and is part of medicinal cures as well. A distinction between "hot" and "cold" is made for both specific illnesses and their remedies (table 2). A few medicines, depending upon preparation, are "of the middle." These are usually mixtures of medicinal agents used to alleviate or prevent forms of bad luck. Following from the principle of opposition, an illness classified as hot must be cured with its opposite, a cold medicine, and vice versa for cold illnesses. Table 1 lists five of these with their more popular cures. Most illnesses (*hay*) are either hot or cold depending upon the time of year or source of the malady. Others are always either hot or cold; for example, fever is only hot. Some afflictions, such as wind strike, are not recognized by Anglos.

In addition to the hot-cold classification, yet another crosscuts medicinal lore and is basic to diagnosis. The sex of the patient is important. Some medicines are only for men and are used particularly as war medicine or during ceremonial participation. Others are prescribed for women. Sexual differences are rarely a

Table 2

SOME ITEMS CLASSIFIED AS HOT—COLD—OF THE MIDDLE BY SAN JUAN PUEBLO

Hot

bear fat	foot racing	spearmint
beans, pinto	jet	sulphur
beef	juniper, one-seeded	tea
buckskin	nutmeg	tobacco
chile, red	okawa phe	Vick's
cinnamon	osha	wormwood
coffee	sagebrush	wool
corn	sheep	yerba mansa
Douglas fir	snakeweed	yucca (baccata)
fetid marigold		

Cold

antelopes	fish	potato
apples	fowl	rabbits
birds	gilia, white	rose petals
cañute	inmortal	silver
chile, green	jacks (game)	tops
contrayerba	lamb's quarters	turquoise
cottonwood leaves	mentholatum	watermelon
deer's blood	mint	
dog bone	pennyroyal	

Of the Middle

bread	dog bone + osha	wheat
pigs		water

problem because the contexts are so precise. The exception may be during childbirth, when the strengths of the medicine must be recognized. However, since a midwife is present, she knows the differences that others may not.

Two distinct information hierarchies are distinguishable in the Tewa pueblos. One is knowledge of the general principles delineated above and some cures for named illnesses. Persons possessing this amount of information are generally Dry Food People, but some are Made People. Within this level, as table 1 demonstrates, knowledge is variable. The second consists of specialists who have training in folk medicine at all levels, although again there are internal differences. These experts are all Made People.

When we examine an actual diagnosis of an illness, *hay*, afflicting a Dry Food Person, we can witness the priority accorded the general classifying principles and concomitantly find support for our first proposition. Ordinarily the senior woman in a household makes the initial diagnosis by her perception of the symptoms and by a description given by the patient. If the patient is a woman perceived as suffering from a cold ailment, she is treated with a medicine classified as hot and thus appropriate for women. A hot medicine administered to relieve internal problems is usually steeped; cold medicine is ground or stirred into water. All medicines are given according to a formula following the sacred numbers: four doses once a day or four, four days. Each illness is treated with one medicine at a time; if the first does not work, a second is tried. But the initial curatives may not work, and the family may not know another cure and/or have an alternative medicine on hand. As long as the condition is not deteriorating, a relative, friend, or neighbor will be *asked* for advice and medicine. This is *always* given without payment, and requests are *never* denied.[12] The crucial point illustrated by table 1 is that one does not have to know or possess these curatives. As long as the suggested remedy fits the proper hot or cold category, it is reliable. Thus, following the communication of a component of a simple binary statement, hot or cold, additional information about the medicine is not needed before it is tried, and one does not have to learn to recognize and to collect every medicine known to the Tewa. The open communication network assures access to the collective information about folk medicine held by individuals in the community, as well as to curatives themselves that are not possessed by every household.

Even though witches are the primary source of misfortune, there is a pragmatic side to folk medicine as well. The evil in the world need not be directed by a witch against a person. Bad spirits exist, but they can be countered through leading the right kind of life, carrying the proper charm, or applying an appropriate medicine. A hot stomachache, for example, that responds to a dose of ground *inmortal* root in water, provokes no further thought; but if it persists after four dosages, then other actions are required, and one does think about *t'án* and *chugeʔiʔ*.

Before the assistance of a specialist is sought, other sources of cures or relief are available. Although the *Towa é* do not cure directly, they are involved in the health of the community in two ways. First, they guard the Made People during their ritual retreats and the pueblo during all ceremonies to assure that each is brought to proper completion. Second, they are associated with the two masked *Tsaveyoh*, one hot and one cold, who are village disciplinarians but at the same time can cure.[13] When they are leaving the village following their annual December visitation, they are empowered to whip people who are not following the Indian way; yet the same whip can touch a person at points of chronic pain to cure it. They also give pieces of wild game meat to bring good health, and, finally, for sick people they will dispense spruce needles to be chewed by a wife or mother and given to the patient.

Catholic saints can also cure through petition and self- or familial dedication. This obviously is an introduced institution, but the underlying premise is indigenous. One will pray to the saints for assistance in the same manner that a Dry Food Person will appeal to ancestral Dry Food People Who Are No Longer at one of the four shrines located near the village. For the saints, dedication may include presentations of new garments, a pilgrimage to Chimayo, or sitting with them during a dance. Household saints are sometimes brought by Spanish to bless homes within a Tewa pueblo in exchange for food.

Since curing by Dry Food People is serial treatment with one remedy at a time, each may prove ineffective; consequently, the patient's condition worsens, and a specialist must be approached. This may be a midwife, a Bear sodality medicine man, or another Made Person.

Midwives are Made People but not necessarily *Kay* members.[14] They *never* refuse assistance but may request payment for services. Furthermore, in contrast to Dry Food People, who treat each illness with a single remedy at a time, they often prepare medicinal mixtures. Likewise, as *Patowa* they can mend fractures and administer massages, which, as we might expect, are called "rubbing on medicine."

A midwife, precisely because of her accessibility, does approach the status of a full-time specialist. She aids in deliveries, helps the mother after delivery, assists the chronically ill, and is available to all in need. She is frequently visited by Indians from other tribes and by Spanish neighbors.

All Made People counteract *t'án*. Each sodality sponsors ceremonies to benefit the people. The Women's society assists the safety of travelers leaving the Tewa world to trade or hunt; the Scalp society provides medicine for warriors; the moiety headmen cure other ailments. Since the head of the Winter side is cold, he can relieve fever and heal burns, both hot sicknesses. His hot Summer counterpart can remedy those suffering from acute coldness. But the most important sodality is the Bear. Laski has given a detailed description of their recruitment, training, and rituals.[15]

With an offering of husk-wrapped cornmeal held in the right hand, one approaches a Bear man for assistance. He can *refuse* a request and *must* receive some payment. To cure minor illnesses, he may act alone or in concert with another member, depending upon the patient's condition. He administers to the patient for four days, giving massages, medicines, perhaps sucking out foreign objects, and dispatching the illness to the west beyond the Tewa land. Acute cases of witchcraft are very serious, requiring the coordinated efforts of most Bear members. Clairvoyance for discovering and disposing of witches is achieved by partaking of an herb. At the conclusion they will leave the patient with medicines to hasten his recovery. However, their role goes beyond curing individuals. They clean the earth navels[16] and keep witches from blocking the blessing of the Dry Food People Who Never Did Become. In addition, they hold communal cleansing rites to expel all witches, and they respond similarly when epidemics threaten the well-being of the community.

The nature of the Tewa communication network supports the second of our propositions. It is always open for easy access to general knowledge and for alternative medicines and thus assures prompt treatment in the absence of detailed information about medicine. On the other hand, the Bears and other Made People are the higher authority who through years of training and experience possess the most information about all medicines and are the only ones empowered to fulfill the general goal of seeking life for the community. Despite this knowledge, they are farmers and herders like everyone else and not full-time specialists. They lack the time to handle every case of *t'án*, and the communication network, including the formality of requests and costs of services, provides that they will be available to treat the most serious cases and to assure protection for the village.

It should be further noted that it is the Made People who introduce new medicines into the pueblo. They have contacts with others with similar knowledge in other pueblos and even with Spanish *curanderos*, and from them they obtain new remedies.

Our third prediction is that information related to the general welfare be learned in specific detail and in a variety of contexts. Again, the hot-cold classification applies. When the Summer headman has ritual authority over the pueblo, children are forbidden to play with bows and arrows and even jacks, cold-producing games; in wintertime these are fine recreation, unlike the warm-associated shinny or kickball. Jet and coral are worn during summer dances, but not the cold turquoise and silver. Anyone can admonish a violator of these edicts, for all in the village will suffer the untoward consequences. Similarly, charms to protect against witchcraft are carried by everyone and placed above the hearth to protect the household. Mothers frequently ask if a child has his root of *Okáwą-phéh* or a husband his *osaa púu* before they leave the house. If it is lost and none is in the house, a neighbor will gladly give it as he would any medicine.

Other actions are practiced by all at times of special ritual or crisis. On All Souls' Day in November the extended family (*matu'i*) joins an elder member of the family who concludes a household ritual of thanking the ancestors by sweeping all the evil spirits away from the relatives and taking them to the west for disposal. In like manner a newborn child is swept clean of bad luck by all visitors. Finally, following a death the smoke of the juniper is used to fumigate against witches and the return of the deceased's spirit. These are specific acts, few in number and witnessed from childhood, that must be followed for the benefit of all.

IV

A comprehensive explication of folk medicine in Native American life has rarely been accomplished. To record only remedies as they are traditionally practiced is insufficient for attaining this goal, since medicinal concepts and practices are embedded in every facet of a culture and consequently are almost impossible to isolate as a separate system. The generalizations deduced and examined in this essay are an attempt to gain a processual understanding of medicinal knowledge in several linguistically related communities, although they undoubtedly apply throughout the continent. We have discovered that knowledge of particular cures is not universal within a pueblo, perhaps cannot be, and need not be as long as underspecified general principles are easy to learn and shared by all residents. From this basis specific medicines can be obtained through an open communication network. However, such a system appears limited to the application of a single remedy at a time for each ailment. Moreover, each person in the hierarchy of accumulated information is approached in increasingly more formal manner, and their information is more costly to secure. Finally, the goal of folk medicinal treatments is maintenance of general well-being, which is also the collective objective of the ceremonialists who occupy the highest human information level. They, however, are unable to act in every case of illness, and thus specific preventatives against misfortune and evil, the most inclusive level of the folk classification, are learned early in life, are few in number, and are continuously reinforced.

Our objective now is to transcend the excellent comparative studies of curatives and to discover the general rules governing folk medicine in all cultures. Time is short, but I suspect that another great legacy from the American Indian awaits us.[17]

APPENDIX

IDENTIFICATION OF PLANTS REFERRED TO IN TEXT

Tewa Name	*Common Name*	*Scientific Name*
huu	one seeded juniper	*Juniperus monosperma* (Engelm.) Sarg.
inmortal (Sp.)	antelope horns	*Asclepias capricornu* Woodson
kanela (Sp.)	cinnamon	*Cinnamomum zeylanicum* L.
khá'póvi	wild rose	*Rosa Fendleri* Crepin
koyáyi	snakeweed	*Gutierrezia sarothrae* (Pursh) Britt. & Rusby
mansu púu	yerba del mansa	*Anemopsis californica* (Nutt.) Hook. & Arn.
nanphuu	potato	*Solanum tuberosum* L.
nwą̂ą̂	nutmeg	*Myristica* sp.
okáwą phéh	blazing star, cachana	*Liatris punctata* Hook.
osaa púu	wild celery, osha	*Ligusticum Porteri* Coult. & Rose
pagé (Sp.)	fetid marigold	*Dyssodia papposa* (Vent.) Hitchc.
phaa	Spanish bayonet	*Yucca baccata* Torr.
phá'wówá	wormwood	*Artemisia ludoviciana* subsp. *ludoviciana*
phisaa woe	white gilia	*Gilia longiflora* (Torr.) G. Don
poe p'ay hun	watermelon vine	*Citrulus vulgaris* L.
suts' éẹgi'	pennyroyal	*Hedeoma nana* (Torr.) Greene
tay kaa	cottonwood leaves	*Populus wislizeni* (Wats.) Sarg.
t'óe	sagebrush	*Artemisia tridentata* Nutt.
tûu	pinto beans	*Phaseolus vulgaris* L.
yeva wéná (Sp.)	spearmint	*Mentha spicata* L.

SOURCE: Richard I. Ford, *An Ecological Analysis Involving the Population of San Juan Pueblo, New Mexico* (Ann Arbor: University Microfilms, 1968), pp. 262-288.

NOTES

1. Virgil J. Vogel, *American Indian Medicine* (Norman: University of Oklahoma Press, 1970). Bibliographic references to historical sources are also available in Ann Katherine Stimson, *Contributions toward a Bibliography of the Medicinal Use of Plants by the Indians of the United States of America* (M.A. thesis, University of Pennsylvania, Philadelphia, 1946) and William C. Sturtevant, *Bibliography on American Indian Medicine and Health* (Washington, D.C.: Bureau of American Ethnology, 1962).

2. William Thomas Corlett, *The Medicine Man of the American Indian and His Cultural Background* (Springfield, Ill.: Charles C. Thomas, 1935) surveys this specialist at great length, and nineteenth-century herbalists in particular express indebtedness to now-forgotten medicine men.

3. Alfonso Ortiz, *The Tewa World* (Chicago: University of Chicago Press, 1969), p. 175.

4. Richard I. Ford, "An Ecological Perspective on the Eastern Pueblos," in *New Perspectives on the Pueblos*, ed. Alfonso Ortiz (Albuquerque: University of New Mexico Press, 1972).

5. Ortiz, *op. cit.*

6. Ortiz, *op. cit.*, p. 17, called *Whe Towa* (Weed or Trash People), *Nayi wha Towa* (Dust-dragging People), *Ph'eʔ yávi Towa* (Weed People), and *Seh t'a* (Dry Food).

7. Ortiz, *op. cit.*, pp. 61-77.

8. Ortiz, *op. cit.* pp. 79, 164. *Patowa* (Made People) called Fish People in earlier anthropological literature. After years of confusion, Ortiz has provided the proper translation.

9. Ortiz, *op. cit.*, 13-16. Elsie Clews Parsons, "The Social Organization of the Tewa of New Mexico," *American Anthropological Association Memoir*, 36 (1929), 142-150 and *Pueblo Indian Religion* (Chicago: University of Chicago Press, 1939), I, 249-253.

10. Ortiz, *op. cit.*, pp. 79-119, 140. The soul of a Dry Food Person takes four days to reach the underworld; a Made Person's requires twelve. If either was a witch, it dissipates into dust.

11. *Súwá* ("hot" or "warm" in a medicinal or spiritual sense), *oetee* "cold" or "cool" in the same sense) and *Teh Pingeh*, "of the middle of the structure."

12. Today many Tewa women are nurses and hospital aides, who, however, are not classified as Made People and therefore are expected to dispense patent medicines without charge.

13. Ortiz, *op. cit.*, pp. 77, 161.

14. Parsons, *Memoir*, p. 119, states that they are female *Kay*, but this is incorrect at least for the three northern Tewa Pueblos.

15. Vera Laski, *Seeking Life*, Memoirs of the American Folklore Society, 50 (Philadelphia, 1959), pp. 96-117.

16. Ortiz, *op. cit.*, p. 21.

17. I am beholden to a long lineage of folklorists, students of folk medicine, and Gregory Bateson, *Steps to an Ecology of Mind* (New York: Ballantine Books, 1972) for many of my ideas. The assistance and insight of Alfonso Ortiz and Karen Ford pervades this essay; their interest is always appreciated. Support for this research came from NSF grant #659 and the Museum of Anthropology, University of Michigan.

Plant Hypnotics among the North American Indians

WILLIAM A. EMBODEN, Jr.,
California State University, Northridge

Hypnotica was established in pharmacological parlance by the German toxicologist Lewis Lewin[1] to designate an induced state of ataraxis, sedation, tranquility, or stupor brought about by organic (natural sources) or inorganic chemicals. It is an empirical decision to have a term encompassing all of these states, since there is no common chemical or genetic affinity that binds them.[2] In the same sense, *medicine* cannot be used in the restrictive definition of American dictionaries to designate any preparation used in treating disease; to the contrary, medicine may be used to indicate *power* or *force*, natural or supernatural. Among the categories of plant medicines, hypnotics may be used to treat a disease or prevent a disease or may be taken by the medicine man to affect a cure by divination. A corollary of the latter is that the concept of disease must be used to designate any ailment, physiological or psychological, real or imagined. Given this latitude, I shall proceed to consider some of those plants that have the capacity to produce hypnotic states and are known to have been used by the Indian of North America. In the broad sense these are all narcotic in that they benumb the sense to varying degrees.

In enumerating species of plants with hypnotic properties, I wish to point out that this compilation is by no means definitive; the magnitude of even this preliminary study suggests that theories of medicine among the "aboriginal" North Americans and their descendants relied heavily upon quiescent states of mind in effecting cures. This form of therapy harks back to the temple healers of ancient Greece, who practiced their medicine in a templelike sanitarium near fresh springs and by a drug-induced hypnosis (accompanied by versotherapy and melanotherapy as adjuncts to their practice) worked their cures. Such precepts have been traced back to 1920 by some psychopharmacologists who ignore this ancient precedent set by the Greeks, as well as that of the North American Indians.[3]

As to the role of the Indian versus the settler in originating uses for the native flora of North America, one may quote Vogel: "So complete in fact was the aboriginal knowledge of their native flora that Indian usage can be demonstrated for all but a bare half dozen, at most, of our indigenous vegetable drugs. In a surprising number of instances, moreover, the aboriginal uses of these drugs corresponded with those approved in the *Dispensatory of the United States*."[4] Such a bold affirmation of the role of Indian medical uses for plants does much to dispel the common belief that these people contributed little of value to colonial and European medicine. The chanting which frequently accompanied treatment bothered the Europeans in America possibly more than the idea that an "aborigine" might effect a cure. Yet did not the disciples of Aesculapius walk among drugged patients and repeat suggestions to them as a form of hypnotherapy? As for the role of plants in this process, Youngken enumerated a list of 450 plant remedies used by natives of North America.[5] No attempt was made to establish a category of hypnotics, and a thorough survey of all of these has yet to appear. Since the nature of this conference calls for brevity, the following discussion is not indicative of the breadth of use of hypnotics throughout the whole of North America.

In northern California the Capella Indians prized the magnificent red delphinium that encrusts a naked stem in late spring. The root of this larkspur was used to induce sleep in children and those who were ill, as well as to stupefy one's foes or to impair the judgment of an opponent. Another European introduction, *Delphinium consolida*, has now become naturalized along the Pacific coast and is similarly employed. In England it was known as King's consound (the specific name from the Latin *consolida*, meaning "to console in time of distress"). The efficacy of this species is evidenced in its popular name, "staggerweed," not to be confused with locoweed, a species of *Astragalus* that may incorporate selenium from the soil.[6]

The "darnel" of the Bible was undoubtedly an ergotized ryegrass (*Lolium* or *Secale*), in which the narcosis was not from the grass, but from displacement of a grain by the fungus *Claviceps purpurea*. This same fungus occasionally attacks *Phalaris* species, a grass seed frequent in birdseed mixtures. Apart from these, there are two species of grass that do intoxicate. One of these is to be found growing around the upper Rio Grande in the Sacramento–White Mountain region. Known by the name *popoton sacaton*, this grass is probably of Aztec origin: the Nahuatl-derived name means "sleepy grass." *Popoton sacaton* is botanically *Stipa vaseyi* and is most common in Guatemala as a medicant for inducing sleep.[7] A related species of grass, *Stipa viridula*, grows as a perennial herb on the eastern ranges of the Coast Mountains; it, too, has a narcotic effect on the spinal cord and the brain. I can find no citation of its use.

In northwestern United States, *Lycopodium selago*, known as wolf's foot and club moss, is common in the temperate forests, where it thrives on the moisture, shade, and rich humus. Three of these stems, which are only a few inches tall, induce a mild hypnotic narcosis, and eight result in a total stupor or even a comatose state. The Potawatomis gathered *L. obscurum* var. *dendroideum*, or tree club moss, which they used for the coagulating properties of the spores, and the Flambeau Ojibwas gathered the entire plant of *L. complanatum*, which they used as a reviver. The Penobscots used the latter species as well.[8] This would seemingly contradict the contention that *L. selago* is a hypnotic, but lycopodine, an excitant, is doubtless not the only active principle in *L. selago*.[9]

Sophora secundaflora was used by the Kickapoo and Comanche for earache and eye diseases. This small shrub-tree grows in South Texas and produces a fruit bearing one to three coral red seeds that are high in cystine and produce a brief exhilaration followed by a deep comatose state. The Arapaho, Iowa, and Tonkawas used this mescal bean as strong medicine. Usually it was roasted by a fire until it turned yellow and was then macerated and made into a liquid infusion. The use of this seed has been traced to A.D. 1000 and doubtless has a ritualistic significance. It is used by peyote cult leaders and as an ornament and may have predated peyote as an intoxicant. Both the ceremony and the intoxication are closely allied to that produced by *Erythrina flabelliformis*, the coral tree of Arizona.[10]

Among the Lower Chinook and the Quinault of the Pacific Northwest Indians, *Arctostaphylos uva-ursi* was the principal smoking mixture, but there is no evidence that the practice included respiring or inhaling the fumes as a regular practice. *Kinnikinnick*, as the leaves were known to these people, was swallowed on occasion and caused a giddy state with loss of motor coordination. Among the Menomini and Thompson Indians, the bear-berry leaves used as a tea both strengthened the bladder and kidneys and provoked an ample flow of urine. When the dried leaves of bear-berry were mixed with tobacco, it was referred to as *sagack-homi*, indicating the distinction between this mixture and the pure leaf. Records of individuals using *kinnikinnick* ("kinikinik") and becoming so intoxicated as to fall into a fire and remain immobile are substantiated by those who still bear the scars of such an experience.[11] Was it an experience of induced ecstasis, a hedonistic venture, or a sort of medication? This question remains undecided.

If one considers the *brujo* a type of shamanic doctor, then his hypnotic brews must be included in the medical lore of North American Indians. Chief Pablo of the Mahuna tribe of southern California related to his nephew, John Bruno Romero (Ha-Ha-St-of Tawee), the insidious use of *Eschscholzia* (*Eschscholtzia*) *californica* to stupefy.[12] This plant, better known as the California poppy, has a root which is high in opiates. The raw root was sometimes scraped and put into the cavity of an aching tooth, but a more pernicious use was prevalent among the Mahunas, who made a brew of the root to stun enemies. Presumably the same brew could be used beneficially.

Both the bark and the root cortex of the wild black cherry, *Prunus serotina*, were potent sedating agents. The Meskwaki Indians preferred the fresh root bark, but other tribes used the bark of the trunk and branches of young trees. This material added to warm water (boiling denatures the medicine) formed a soothing nervine. Fall was the season for gathering *Prunus* bark; it was rarely stored for more than one year because it lost potency with age. Hydrocyanic acid and its precursors are credited with the hypnotic effects, but it would seem that other agents must be responsible.

Another tree important to the Menomini as a sacred hypnotic was the wafer ash, *Ptelea trifoliata*. The root bark was added to a number of medicines to increase their efficacy. Physiological studies indicate that most of the effects are deleterious, but they do include "vertigo and prostration."[13] It is doubtful whether this tree and its products should be included as true hypnotics. This category may be suggested by the similarity of the fruits to those of the true hops (*Humulus lupulus*), not native to North America but adopted by the Mohegans, Meskwaki, Menomini, and Dakotas for their calming, sedating properties. It is doubtful that the female fruits were discovered independent of the Old World traditions, as alleged by some authors. When hops were brought to America, they had such a strong medical tradition associated with them that their soporific effects could not be ignored.[14]

"Bloodroot" is an apt characterization for the rhizomatous *Sanguinaria canadensis* that is common to eastern hardwood forests, for when pulled from the ground, the broken rhizome exudes a bloodlike juice. This juice was used as a dye for body paint as well as for staining implements. The Rappahannocks made a tea of the root which was not altogether pleasant, for it induced vomiting, but it also served to alleviate the pains of rheumatism. It shares many alkaloids possessed by the opium poppy, since they are in the same plant family. As a nervous system depressant (the quality generally attributed to porphyroxin), it was used under the name *puccoon* to calm and sedate. Rhizomes were collected in the fall and utilized before they deteriorated.[15]

Many Indian tribes used species of wormwood, or *Artemisia,* as a tea for stomach ailments and bronchitis. In California the Yokias of Mendocino County used native *Artemisia* species. At an early date, *Artemisia absinthium* was brought from Europe to the gardens of the colonies in the east to provide a similar medicant. The volatile oils containing absinthin and absinthol have the capacity to benumb by breaking neural synapses. Oils of *Artemisia absinthium* combined with anise, coriander, and hyssop formed the narcotic alcoholic beverage absinthe, which was so popular in France at the end of the nineteenth century. Because it causes permanent neural damage, this beverage is now illegal. The leaves and tops of numerous species of wormwood in America, including the escape, *A. absinthium,* found their way into Indian medicine.[16]

Among the Cherokees, *Lobelia cardinalis* was prized as an antispasmodic, as *Lobelia inflata,* known to settlers as Indian tobacco, was among other Indian groups. Although it was smoked for asthma, bronchitis, and similar respiratory disorders, it was also used as a tea. *Lobelia cardinalis,* the common red *Lobelia,* was noted by Millspaugh to have marked properties as an acrid narcotic nervine.[17] The same may be said of the other species insofar as they contain lobeline as the principal active ingredient. The Cherokees believed that the root of this plant could rid the body of syphilis. Although the claim is unsubstantiated, it is certain that all of the North American species of *Lobelia* used by the Indians were debilitating in the sense that they caused giddiness by acting upon the central nervous system.

The use of *Datura* in North America extends between both coasts and throughout the world has a pantemperate and pantropical distribution. Wherever it grows, it is used, and all parts of all species are narcotic. The subject of its use among the North American Indian is worthy of a dissertation. Perhaps the most extreme example of its use is to be found among the Algonquians, who used *Datura stramonium* (jimsonweed) and allied species in coming-of-age rites (much as *D. meteloides* was used in the Southwest). Among the Algonquians, a youth was kept in a semisomnolent state for as long as twenty days so that he might forget the things pertaining to his youth.[18]

Actea alba, or white cohosh, and *Cimicifuga racemosa*, or black cohosh, both grow in rich woodlands of the eastern states; the range of white cohosh extends farther south and west. The two genera, while distinct in the particular, give the appearance of being morphologically similar and were used by the Indians for rheumatism, troubled menses, and difficult parturition. Although a Dr. Williams typified the general opinion of early settler-doctors when he referred to *Cimicifuga* as being useful only by "Indians and Quacks,"[19] it came into common use and entered the *United States Pharmacopoeia* because of its effective action on nerve centers. Millspaugh states that it was a favorite among "all tribes of the aborigines." In the utilization of *Actea alba*, a tincture is made of the whole plant, but only the pulverized root of *Cimicifuga racemosa* is employed. Wheeler noted that this plant relaxed the patient and was a favorite in treating hysteria (which seemed prevalent among settlers in the colonies).[20] An insoluble resin has been called cimicifugin or macrotin, but neither term properly characterizes the chemical, which is simply a precipitate of that which is not soluble in water. Because of its widespread popularity among the Indians of the East, it became known as squaw tea. This epithet has been too broadly applied (for example, to *Ephedra*) to have any validity for botanical nomenclature.

An ancient tradition in China associated the root of *Phytolacca acinosa* with both ginseng (*Panax*) and mandrake (*Mandragora*); thus it became an esteemed root and was used for a host of ailments. In this species, as well as the American species, there is a hypnotic property. It was used in American home remedies for everything from headache to cancer; indeed, one of the popular names for the plant was "cancer-root." An overdose leads to a paralysis of the respiratory system, and death may ensue. Despite the possibility of drastic consequences, the pokeroot continued in many home remedy books as a hypnotic capable of alleviating pain. Since poke was plentiful, it was often used to adulterate belladona.

According to Romero, *Phytolacca americana* (*decandra*), was used by the Indians of the Pacific Southwest for its narcotic properties.[21]

He extols the virtues of the plant and notes that it is to be preferred to morphine, opium, and cocaine. He further notes that it was very important in making Indian formulas. This same genus had long been popular in Asia and western Europe for the narcotic properties of the root. It was to be found in the British *Extra Pharmacopoeia* of 1804.

Garantoquen was a name in common parlance among the Indians of the northeastern states for *Panax quinquefolium*, which, according to Father Jartoux, they regarded as a powerful root. Although much controversy now surrounds the actual effects of this root, it has achieved an unprecedented popularity as a panacea of all sorts and as an aphrodisiac. Russian scientists claim that it serves to stimulate endocrine function while acting in a more general capacity as a tranquilizer. Millspaugh reported the physiological action to induce somnolence, among other things.[22] It is what Soviet scientists term an adaptogen, since it has no toxic principles and is efficacious in relieving stress and combating disease.

Yellow jasmine refers to *Gelsemium sempervirens* of the southeastern states. This yellow-flowered vine is not related to the true jasmine of Europe. There is dispute whether the virtues of the roots and flowers as a narcotic were first discovered by the natives of North Carolina or one of the early physicians among the settlers. John Brickell mentions it as one of the plants useful in a host of diseases, and his writings did not originate with him but are an account of Indian uses of native herbs.[23] This plant was a valuable hypnotic in cases of convulsions, childbirth, and "stitches in the side."

Mysterious is perhaps the best way to describe the species of *Monotropa*, or Indian pipe, that suddenly appear as ghostlike apparitions under beech trees. It has justly earned its name "corpse plant" because of is waxy, translucent, clammy nature; upon the slightest touch, it turns black. In the northeastern states, Native Americans had long known the value of the fresh juice of *Monotropa uniflora* for inflamed eyes and for overcoming nervous irritability, including spasms and epileptiform fits. In the nineteenth century John King recommended it in a dried form as an excellent substitute for opium.[24] No disagreeable side effects are reported for this saprophytic herb, and it seems rather unusual that it never entered any materia medica here or in Europe. Now that the native stands of hardwood forests are disappearing, this herb is becoming increasingly rare.

Orchids have long had a reputation as nervines, sedatives, and antispasmodics; they are especially prized for hysteria. Most notable in the orchid family is the genus *Cypripedium*, or lady's slipper orchid, several species of which were at an earlier time prevalent in eastern bogs and woodland and some of which were found in the western states. Before the arrival of Europeans, the American Indian chewed the fibrous and acrid roots of some of these species, especially during the period of menstruation and during childbirth. *Cypripedium pubescens* (*C. calceolus* var. *pubescens*) is the yellow lady's slipper orchid that was once quite common. Its eradication may be traced to its systematic extinction by herb gathers who prized the roots of the orchid because of information they gleaned from Indian healers. A closely related species, *C. parviflorum*, was especially valued by Cherokee women for labor pains, hysteria, and insomnia. In addition to these two species, the Penobscots employed *C. acaule* as an important nervine. A common practice seems to have been to restrict the use of these orchids to the diseases of women. (Since *hysteria* is derived from the root word denoting *womb*, it is inapplicable to males. The male of the species may suffer madness or instability, but never hysteria). The Pillager Ojibwas seemed to have a preference for *C. pubescens*, but among other tribes *C. luteum* was used for the same purpose.[25]

It would seem that this orchid was usually assigned to the realm of a medicant for female disorders in pre-European times; a notable exception to this rule is the Menomini, who used *C. acaule* in general practice as a nervine.

The use of orchid roots had been common in Europe, but the species used were nonnarcotic, for the most part, and were a foodstuff. Millspaugh tells us that *C. luteum* was regarded by these colonists as the best American substitute for valerian. From the dried roots they made a tincture with two parts alcohol by weight.[26] The decanted mixture has the color of a ruby port and the scent of fecal matter. For this reason, some prefer it as a tea. The resurgent interest in herbs has led to the appearance of fairly large quantities of this root in herb shops in Los Angeles. With the availability of commercial tranquilizers, it seems unnecessary to pillage the few remaining native stands of this beautiful flower that shuns cultivation. A closely related species, *C. parviflorum*, was given to Cherokee women in the throes of childbirth, in cases of hysteria, and in insomnia. In addition to these two species, the Penobscots employed *C. acaule* as an important nervine. Assignation of the female gender to this plant was pre-European, for the Pillager Ojibwas were using *C. pubescens* for female disorders (although the Menomini used *C. acaule* for male problems, this would seem to be somewhat of an exception).[27]

If the notion of nervines, sedatives, and tranquilizers seems to be a contemporary North American obsession, a backward glance will reveal the many hypnotic plants which the Indians of North America used to advantage as important hypnotic medicants.

NOTES

1. Lewis Lewin, *Phantastica, Narcotic and Stimulating Drugs, Their Use and Abuse* (reprint ed. London: Routledge & Kegan Paul, 1964) pp. 27-31.

2. W. G. Clark and J. del Giudice, eds., *Principles of Psychopharmacology* (New York and London: Academic Press, 1970), pp. 251-252.

3. Anthony Horden, "Psychopharmacology: Some Historical Considerations," in *Psychopharmacology: Dimensions and Perspectives*, ed. C. R. B. Joyce, Mind and Medicine Monographs, no. 17 (London: Tavistock Publications, 1968), pp. 104-105.

4. Virgil J. Vogel, *American Indian Medicine* (Norman: University of Oklahoma Press, 1970), p. 6.

5. Herbert W. Youngken, "Drugs of the North American Indians," *American Journal of Pharmacy* 96, 96, 485-502; 97, 97, 158-185; 98, no. 98, 257-271.

6. J. C. Th. Uphof, *Dictionary of Economic Plants*, 2d ed. (New York: Stechert-Hafner Service Agency, Inc., 1968), p. 175.

7. L. S. M. Curtain, *Healing Herbs of the Upper Rio Grande*, Laboratory of Anthropology, Santa Fe, New Mexico (Santa Fe, N.M.: Rydal Press, 1947), pp. 163-164.

8. Vogel, *op. cit.*, pp. 340-341.

9. Charles F. Millspaugh, *American Medicinal Plants: An Illustrated and Descriptive Guide To The American Plants Used As Homeopathic Remedies: Their History, Preparation, Chemistry, and Physiological Effects* (New York: Boericke and Tafel, 1887), pp. 180-184.

10. William A. Emboden, Jr., *Narcotic Plants* (New York: Macmillan Co., 1972), pp. 56-57.

11. James Swan, *The Northeast Coast; or, Three Years' Residence in Washington Territory* (1857; reprint ed., Seattle: University of Washington Press, 1972), pp. 85, 155.

12. John Bruno Romero, *The Botanical Lore of the California Indians with Side Lights on Historical Incidents in California* (New York: Vantage Press Inc., 1954), pp. 34-35.

13. Millspaugh, *op. cit.*, p. 34.

14. Vogel, *op. cit.*, pp. 318-319.

15. Millspaugh, *op. cit.*, pp. 22-23.

16. Vogel, *op. cit.*, p. 396.

17. Millspaugh, *op. cit.*, pp. 97-99.

18. Charles B. Heiser, Jr., *Nightshades: The Paradoxical Plants* (San Francisco: W. H. Freeman and Company, 1969), p. 143.

19. Stephen W. Williams, "Report on the Indigenous Medical Botany of Massachusetts," *Transactions of the American Medical Association* (1849), p. 914.

20. William Wheeler, *Boston Medical and Surgical Journal* (1839), p. 65.

21. Romero, *op. cit.*, p.65.

22. Millspaugh, *op. cit.*, p. 70.

23. John Brickell, *The Natural History of North Carolina, With an Account of the Trade, Manners, and Customs of the Christian and Indian Inhabitants* (Dublin: James Carson, 1737; reprint ed., Raleigh, N.C.: J. Bryan Grimes and Trustees of Public Libraries, Raleigh, 1911), p. 92.

24. John King, *The American Dispensatory* (Cincinnati, 1866), p. 530.

25. Vogel, *op. cit.*, p. 392.

26. Millspaugh, *op. cit.*, pp. 170-171.

27. Vogel, *op. cit.*, p. 330.

Medical Folklore in Spanish America

FRANCISCO GUERRA, M.D., *Madrid, Spain*

INTRODUCTION

Medical folklore in Spanish America has two major components: a magical element that results from the blending of pre-Columbian religions with the Catholic dogma of the conquistadors and another element of botanical lore that combines the aboriginal use of medicinal plants with the Renaissance tradition of herbals, which was prevalent among Spanish physicians during the colonization. These cultural elements are also present in the Philippines; but in Brazil the aboriginal contribution is almost absent because the Tupi-Guarani Indians were progressively overshadowed by a larger population of African Negroes with magic beliefs of their own.

Nowadays social security systems have forced scientific medicine into urban areas, but even there, and above all in rural communities, Spanish America remains fast to traditional folk medicine.

PRE-COLUMBIAN MAGIC

Disease among higher civilizations in pre-Columbian America was conceived as a supernatural phenomenon resulting from sin, rather than from sorcery, foreign-body intrusion, or soul abduction. Besides major deities, both male and female, there was a pantheon of gods specializing in punishing man with certain diseases according to the sin committed.[1] Among the Aztecs, Tlaloc, the god of the waters, punished with rheumatic ailments; Xipetotec, the flayed god, with exanthematic diseases; Macuilxo-

chitl, the god of pleasures, with diseases of the genitals; Xochiquet-
zal, the goddess of love, with incurable buboes, and so on. Among
the Mayas[2] Hunab, the god-creator of the universe, had his son
Itzamma, the lord of heavens, married to Ixchel, the goddess of
pregnancy and medicine. Minor gods controlled different diseases:
Xoquiripat and Chuchumaquic induced hemorrhages; Xix and
Patan, blood vomits; Ahalpuh and Ahalgana, jaundice and ulcers
in the legs. The Incas, too, believed that Viracocha, the sun and
creator of this world, had sent his elder son, Imaimana, to teach
man the use of medicinal plants. Mamacocha, the sea, was worshipped to avoid sickness and to recover health; the Conopas, or
minor gods, and the magical remains, Huacas, were also revered
for the same purpose.

Pre-Columbian religions had outward signs and liturgical ceremonies very similar to the sacraments of the Catholic Church.
Notable among them was confession, used as a medical procedure
to obtain spiritual catharsis in the sick. The *yolmelaua*, or vocal
confession, of the Aztecs was usually preceded by the steam bath at
the *temazcalli* and involved a very active participation by the
physician: if the ailment was of minor importance, he would only
apply drugs; but if the patient was seriously ill, then the physician
would tell the patient to confess his sins and would insist on actively
searching the mind of the sick until he declared everything that
had been troubling his conscience for years. The *ichuri*, or vocal
confession, among the Incas followed a similar procedure; there
were confessors for light and grave sins, and the ritual for the
second kind included the inspection of the entrails of a guinea pig
and the stoning of the back of the patient until all sins had been
declared. The sick completed the cleansing of the body with the
opacuna, or bath in running water. Similar procedures can be
found among other pre-Columbian civilizations.

THE CATHOLIC HAGIOLOGY

The spiritual conquest and the colonization of America by Spain
meant the establishment in the mind of the Indians of a Christian
theology. The Indian gods were replaced by Christ the Healer, his
mother, the Virgin Mary, and hundreds of auxiliary saints with
supernatural powers of healing. For the Spaniards prayer was the
traditional elevation of the soul to God in reverent request,
particularly for health, and in fact was an act of religious virtue to
be used in disease. Furthermore, in the Catholic doctrine it was licit
and worthy to pray to the saints as intermediaries to God. The use
of prayer in the medical folklore of colonial Spanish America can

be accurately assessed by an analysis of the printing in that area up to 1821; this was the date marking the end of Spanish rule in most of the colonies on the mainland. A fairly good idea of the cultural patterns of that period can be derived from a comparison between the total number of books printed and those devoted to medicine or prayer, combined with a tallying of the prayers addressed to Christ, the Virgin Mary, or the saints.

In Mexico City there was a total of 13,023 books known to have been printed between 1539 and 1821; of them there were 730 medical items, mostly graduation theses, 638 prayers to God, 981 to the Virgin Mary, 1,494 to the saints, and even a higher number of sermons. Religious publications, in most cases of prayers asking for health, were five times more numerous and printed in much larger editions than the medical items. While about one hundred copies of a medical item were usually printed, over one thousand were commonly issued in the case of prayers; and sometimes, for example in the case of epidemic diseases, second and third editions of the same item were published in the same year. The advocations of the Virgin Mary were far more frequently used than the prayers to Christ or any saint. Lima had 4,725 printed books, 268 related to medicine, 41 prayers to God, 67 to the Virgin Mary, and 63 to the saints. Guatemala City followed in number of publications with 2,487 imprints, 161 dealing with medicine, 66 prayers to God, 58 to the Virgin Mary, 125 to the saints, and 18 sermons. Manila had 541 imprints, 6 dealing with medicine, 8 prayers to God, 25 to the Virgin Mary, 48 to the saints, and 32 sermons. The issues of the presses in other colonial cities of Spanish America followed very much the same pattern: prayers had a dominant role in therapeutic procedures and the Virgin Mary was the most frequent advocate to God in the request for health.

MAGICAL SYNCRETISM

Pre-Columbian religions, like the Catholic Church, accepted a female supernatural entity as having a major influence in the treatment of disease. It naturally followed that the Aztec Teteoinam, the Maya Ixchel, the Inca Mamacocha, and the like became immediately identified by the Indians with the Virgin Mary of the Spaniards, also the Mother of God. The Aztecs, for instance, called her Tonatzin, "Our Lady," and the shrine of the Virgin Mary, under the advocation of Our Lady of Guadalupe, was indeed built in Mexico on the temple of Teteoinam, the Aztec mother of gods. This syncretism was easily spread throughout Spanish America, and the Indian population continued to worship the old supernatural healing power under a different image and name.

At the same time the medical value of the Catholic prayer for the American Indians was firmly established by the First Mexican Council of the Catholic Church in 1555, which quoted the words of Pope Innocent III that "many times bodily illness is due to spiritual indisposition, and applying a remedy to the ailment of the soul, our Lord sends health to the body...."³ The consequence of this doctrine for the Indian population was the adaptation of their spiritual catharsis, which existed in pre-Columbian civilizations as natural psychotherapy of immense curative power, into the vocal confession of the Catholic Church.⁴ Furthermore, the special minor gods—*tlalocs* of the Aztecs, *conopas* of the Incas, and the like in other American civilizations—which were capable of inducing or curing specific ailments, found their equivalents in the rich hagiology of the Catholic Church. Nowhere else in the world can be found as great a variety of prayers, particularly novenas, for the cure of specific diseases as those printed in Spanish America, mainly in Mexico, and addressed to saints who were considered special patrons for specific ailments. The list of these patron saints reads like the headings of a textbook of pathology: Saint Rocco in epidemics, Saint Sebastian for contagious diseases, Saint Raphael in parturition, Saint Nicholas in throat ailments, Saint Lucy in blindness, Saint Dominic for sterile women, Saint Jerome against lust, Saint Boniface in cases of sodomy, and so on. All these saints had a pre-Columbian ancestor, and even Saint Boniface could trace his ancestry among the Aztecs to Tezcatlipoca, the queer one, one of the most powerful gods. The relevance of this syncretism is felt today, when despite the advances of scientific medicine, these prayers are still printed and used in the treatment of diseases.

THE INDIAN HERBALS

The use of plants in the treatment of diseases was an extended practice among pre-Columbian civilizations. The Aztec *ticitl*, the Maya *ahmen*, or the Inca *callahuala* were native physicians trained in the identification and use of medicinal herbs. Since this knowledge was transmitted by oral tradition, only after the conquest of America did written records of the aboriginal pharmacopoeias begin to be known. The beautifully illustrated *Badianus Codex*, written by Martin de la Cruz in the middle of the sixteenth century, represents the summit of Mexican medical botany. For the Maya the best example is the medical formulary in the *Book of the Chilam Balam of Ixil*, compiled late in the eighteenth century. In South America the riches of medical botany among the Guaranis are exemplified by the *Villodas Codex*, written in the middle of the eighteenth century. America gave some of the most active natural drugs, such as coca, cinchona, and ipecacuahna, but it does not seem that they were used in pre-Columbian America for their anaesthetic, antimalarial, or antidysenteric effects. In this respect two important points must be emphasized: some drugs affecting higher cerebral functions had deep cultural significance and were used in religious experiences for their well-known pharmacological effects. This was the case for the hallucinogens used by the various groups: the Aztecs employed mushroom *teonanacatl*, cactus *peyotl*, vine *ololuihqui*, datura *toluah*; the Incas, *coca* leaves and *yage*; the Arawaks and Caribs, the snuff of *cohoba*. There were, furthermore, brain stimulants consumed daily as infusions, such as maté, cocoa, and certain teas which because of their high content in caffeine are even used today for the same purpose.

But the true nature of the materia medica of the American Indian has been misunderstood for centuries. Their use of drugs in the treatment of diseases was not related to their pharmacological action. For instance, the use of plants, minerals, or animal materials in a gastric ailment had nothing to do with an antacid or sedative effect. The *yoyotl* kernels carried to prevent hemorrhoids in Mexico have no effect on the blood vessels, although they contain thevetin, a very active cardiotonic; on the other hand, *yoloxochitl*, the heart flower, recommended as a heart tonic, lacks this effect. Drugs were used in disease for their alleged magical virtues completely unrelated to pharmacological activity. This, we must remember, was in complete agreement with their concept of disease, which was ascribed to supernatural forces.

THE COLONIAL FORMULARIES

Newly discovered America was hailed as a great repository of drugs by European physicians, who expected to find in the New World the supplies of materia medica which for centuries had been imported from the Orient.[5] Early explorers such as Fernandez de Oviedo (1526, 1535) emphasized the value of the American drugs in his writings, afterward popularized by the books of Monardes (1565), which were translated into several languages. The field research on drugs culminated in the sixteenth century with the work of Francisco Hernandez in Mexico between 1571 and 1578, and his findings were incorporated into the books of Mexican authors like Farfan (1592), Barrios (1607), and Ximenez (1615). It was not until 1778 that Ruiz and Pavón surveyed the native drugs of Peru and Chile and still later, in 1796, that Sessé and Moziño carried out their survey of the drugs of Mexico and California. The official interest of Spain and the heavy expenses of these explorations were well justified by the extensive use of native Indian drugs by the colonial population. However, since the end of the seventeenth century, there began to appear, mainly in Mexico, medical formularies that claimed to have been written by the eremite Gregorio Lopez (1672); they included practically no native drugs and were inspired by the European formularies of the medieval period. In the eighteenth century this type of manual was very popular with the Jesuit missionaries. In Mexico the formulary by J. de Esteyneffer (that is, Steinhoffer [1712]) was reprinted several times and had the unique characteristic of having next to the drugs recommended for each disease marginal notes indicating the special saint to whom one should pray. In the Guarani missions of the Jesuits, these formularies remained unpublished for many years. Those by P. Montenegro and M. Villodas were based on native drugs, but the one with the greatest repute, by Padre Sigismund Asperger (Apergers), was based on European texts of little value. The use of these formularies is deeply rooted in the medical folklore of Spanish America, and next to the native oral tradition in Indian drugs, they are the basis of household therapy.

COROLLARY

In large areas of Spanish America, and Brazil and the Philippines as well, scientific medicine shares a place with botanical remedies and prayers to saints and the Virgin Mary, who specialize in the cure of certain ailments. Folk medicine, with its botanical lore and supernatural elements, has an important place today in the treatment of mental and physical ailments in Spanish America.

NOTES

1. Francisco Guerra, *Acculturation of the Concept of Disease in Ancient Mexico* (Bucharest: XXIIᵉ Congrés International d'Histoire de la Médicine, 1970), pp. 151-152.

2. Francisco Guerra, "La Medicina en la América Precolombina," in *Historia Universal de la Medicina*, ed. Pedro Laín Entralgo (Barcelona: Salvat Editores S.A., 1972), pp. 297-324.

3. Francisco Guerra, *The Role of Religion in Spanish American Medicine* (London: Medicine and Culture, Wellcome Institute of the History of Medicine, 1969), pp. 179-188.

4. Francisco Guerra, *The Pre-Columbian Mind* (New York: Seminar Press, 1971), pp. 274-281.

5. Francisco Guerra, *Historia de la Materia Médica Hispano Americana y Filipina en la Epoca Colonial* (Madrid: Afrodisio Aguado S.A., 1974).

The Role of the *Curandero* in the Mexican American Folk Medicine System in West Texas

JOE S. GRAHAM, *Sul Ross State University, Alpine, Texas*

In spite of the great strides made by scientific medicine in this century, folk medicine is still a viable force in the lives of the Mexican Americans of West Texas. To understand why, one has to consider, first, the fact that the Mexican Americans of West Texas constitute a culture that until recently was almost completely apart from the Anglo culture. They belong to what Américo Paredes identifies as the regional group[1] whose ancestors came to Texas as colonists from Mexico when Texas was still Mexican territory. This group felt their way of life threatened by the English-speaking invaders of their homeland, and "their reaction was inward, in search of greater cohesion and homogeneity within their inherited traditions. This is reflected in their folklore."[2]

So in spite of the long acquaintance between the Anglo and the Mexican American peoples, cultural traits have been slow to merge. This is particularly true of folk medical practices.[3] When the Anglos came with their system of medicine, it was no more readily adopted by the Mexican Americans than other facets of Anglo culture. Lyle Saunders explains why:

> Medicine so interpenetrates and is penetrated by all other areas of organized group life, that it is difficult to separate even conceptually. No medical act has meaning out of its cultural context, and a given act may have quite different meanings in different cultures. It is this close identification of medicine with the whole of culture that makes difficult the transplanting of medical techniques from one culture to another.[4]

In West Texas the term *scientific medicine* became almost synony-
mous with *Anglo medicine*—and still is. To my knowledge, there is
not one licensed Mexican American doctor practicing in the whole
rural region between Del Rio and El Paso, separated by over four
hundred miles—this in spite of the fact that over half of the
population is Mexican American.

Perhaps as important as cultural isolation is another factor which
has kept the Mexican Americans from assimilating the Anglo
medical practices: there was no void of medical theories and cures
to be filled when the Anglos came. Some of the folk medical theory
and practice of these Mexican Americans comes from seventeenth-
century Spain, as George Foster[5] and Ari Kiev[6] have shown. Most
of their medical knowledge, however, comes from the indigenous
peoples of the New World, whose *curanderos* ("folk healers") were
highly respected by the invading Spaniards, who believed that the
native healers were repositories of occult knowledge and curing
magic.[7]

The Mexicans had a folk medicine system long before they
became Americans, and as Lyle Saunders explains about the folk
medicine of all peoples:

> [Folk medicine] is usually not a random collection of beliefs and
> practices; rather, it constitutes a fairly well-organized and fairly
> consistent theory of medicine. The body of "knowledge" on which it is
> based often includes ideas about the nature of man and his relation-
> ships with the natural, supernatural, and human environments. Folk
> medicine flourishes because it is a functional and integrated part of the
> whole culture, and because it enables members of cultural groups to
> meet their health needs, as they define them, in ways that are at least
> minimally acceptable.[8]

Thus, having their own (to them) orderly and logical system of
medicine, they refused to reject it in favor of the medicine of the
invading Anglos. When they did begin to accept Anglo medicine,
they continued to hold on to their own folk medical practices.

Because of the inability of scientific medicine to cope with several
of the Mexican American folk maladies, it is, by itself, inadequate
in serving the needs of that culture, as Martinez and Martin have
pointed out in a 1966 article in the *Journal of the American Medical
Association*. They claim that "medical care is inadequate to the
extent that it ignores [folk illnesses]. . . ."[9] Much of the illness
found among West Texas Mexican Americans is folk illness,
unknown among Anglos and consequently looked upon by most
Anglo doctors as evidence of ignorance and superstition.

There are many in the culture who rely extensively upon

scientific medicine for certain kinds of illness, but many prefer folk medical practices to Anglo medicine; they turn to the doctors only as a last resort. In a study made among the urban Mexican Americans in Dallas, of the seventy-five people interviewed, one-fifth of them reported having never visited a physician, and two-fifths of them had never received service from local health clinics.[10] Because of several factors—among others, the cost and unavailability of medical help—the percentage not utilizing scientific medicine is probably greater in the West Texas area. For example, until recently, when she retired as a *partera* ("midwife"), Mrs. Juan Aguilar delivered an estimated 95 percent of the Mexican American babies born in the town of Marathon, Texas, a town of about one thousand inhabitants, over half of whom are Mexican Americans.

In contrast to this underutilization of scientific medicine, all of my informants (well over thirty in number) had relied on folk medical practices at one time or another. This is especially true for five maladies which the Mexican Americans themselves identify as not afflicting Anglos: *mal de ojo* ("evil eye"), *empacho* ("surfeit"), *susto* ("magical fright"), *caída de la mollera* ("fallen fontanel"), and *mal puesto* ("sorcery"). At one time or another, all of my informants had suffered from one or more of these five ailments, even though almost half of my informants either had a college education or were then in college. The Dallas study revealed that over 97 percent of the seventy-five informants knew about each of the five diseases; 85 percent had specific knowledge about symptoms and etiology for all except mal puesto (only 67 percent knew of this); 85 percent knew of therapeutic measures for all except mal puesto (only one-third knew or would admit knowing about this); and 95 percent claimed that either they or members of their families had suffered from one or more of these ailments.[11] Significantly, there appeared to be no relation between this belief in folk medicine and folk maladies and such characteristics as age, education, or place of birth.[12]

Thus, it is apparent that for whatever reasons, Mexican Americans continue to rely heavily upon the folk medicine system of their culture, even though they may utilize scientific medicine as well. One of the most significant—and in Anglo culture most often overlooked—reasons for this is that many of the folk cures work, and as Saunders points out, "it [folk medicine] requires only occasional success to maintain its vigor."[13]

In their understanding and treatment of illnesses, the Mexican Americans do not distinguish between psychic or emotional illnesses and physical illnesses;[14] rather they distinguish by cause: *mal natural* is illness resulting from natural causes, and mal puesto is illness resulting from supernatural causes, mainly witchcraft. Mal natural is considered to be within the realm of God; mal puesto, within the realm of the devil.[15] The diagnosis of the ailment determines not only what the problem is, but also who is to do the curing. Pragmatically, if one cure does not work, another will be tried. The failure of a cure does not mean that the cure was not efficacious, but rather that the diagnosis was not sound. Sometimes the failure of a cure to work is blamed on the patient's waiting too long before seeking help. Thus a patient may use home remedies, local folk practitioners, physicians, and the curandero—all for the same malady.

When someone in the Mexican American culture becomes ill, there is an attempt to match the cure with the cause. The diagnosis is usually given first by members of his family or by the patient himself. There is little tendency to run to the doctor or curandero with every ailment, as is oftentimes the case in Anglo culture. For minor ailments such as colds, burns, and headaches, the sick depend upon folk remedies shared by the whole culture and known to most adults in that culture. For more serious ailments such as mal de ojo, susto, or empacho, the patient may turn to a neighborhood healer, one who is not a curandero but has accumulated a greater knowledge and understanding of folk medicine than the average mother or grandmother in a family has. Such folk maladies as these and cases of mal puesto are seldom taken to a physician because the physician knows nothing about the proper cures, and besides, he would probably think the patient superstitious. Patients with such serious ailments as pneumonia, appendicitis, broken bones, and serious wounds are taken to the physician, for he understands and can deal with these ailments. In case of childbirth the patient may call on the physician or the partera. The *sobador*, or folk chiropractor, is consulted for bad sprains and bruises and, in some cases, for broken bones.

If an ailment will not respond to home remedies or to the ministrations of a neighborhood healer or a physician, the patient will then be taken to the curandero, who is, to many Mexican Americans, the ultimate source of medical knowledge. If the curandero diagnoses the ailment as mal natural other than the five previously mentioned psychosomatic ailments, he may treat the patient with herbs or, in many cases, if the patient has not already consulted a physician, send him to one. Some curanderos claim to be able to cure all maladies, physical and psychological.

I cite two instances of physical ailments cured by a curandero in Ojinaga, Mexico, just across the Rio Grande from Presidio, Texas. Seventy-eight-year-old Alicia Dominguez of Redford, Texas, suffered a stroke some sixteen months ago and was almost completely paralyzed. Rather than use her Medicare in an Anglo hospital with Anglo doctors, she went to the old curandero—or rather, at her request, he came to her. Using herb baths and massages and occasionally herb teas, the curandero has restored her so that she has full use of both arms and can almost walk unassisted.

The other instance concerns the curing of Oswaldo Ybarra of Alpine, who suffered from some kind of skin disease. As local lore has it, he went to physicians who tried various treatments without success. He was sent to specialists, who also failed to provide relief. At the suggestion of a local physician, he went to a curandero, who, after determining that the ailment was not caused by witchcraft, cured it within a week with herb poultices.

In spite of his abilities in curing physical ailments, the primary focus of the curandero's curative efforts is mal puesto, or witchcraft. Ari Kiev, who sees *curanderismo* primarily as folk psychiatry and mal puesto as psychological responses to societal pressures, claims that the curandero is more effective with psychosomatic and psychiatric illnesses than with physical illnesses because he understands the former better.[16] He further claims that for less serious neurotic disorders, the curandero is probably better equipped to help than the professional psychologist.[17]

The curandero, who has no counterpart in the Anglo culture in west Texas,[18] has antecedents in both the Old and New Worlds. Beltran claims that the curandero is the descendant of the old Aztec *ticitl*.[19] In his book on Aztec medicine, Gordon Schendel refers to the ticitl as belonging to a category of Aztec physicians of the type usually found among Neolithic peoples. He states that the ticitl were "sorcerers who were comparable to the shamans, or 'medicine men,' of the nomadic North American Indians and the 'witch doctors' of African Negro tribes ... [who] ... relied on hypnotism and/or their patient's belief in their supposedly magical powers. They were effective, therefore, where a psychomatic factor was involved."[20]

The curandero has his European counterpart, too, though that counterpart was looked upon as a witch in league with the devil rather than a religious figure in the service of God. This may account for the negative attitude of the Catholic Church and the law toward the curandero in much of South and Central America since the Spanish conquest,[21] and even in the United States to some extent. In their *Malleus Maleficarum* Kramer and Sprenger identify three kinds of witches: "those who injure but cannot cure; those who cure but, through some strange pact with the devil, cannot injure; and those who both injure and cure."[22]

In Peru, unlike West Texas, it is often difficult to distinguish between a *brujo* ("sorcerer") and a curandero, because like the brujo, the curandero sometimes uses black magic to cause injury.[23] Martinez and Martin found a similar problem in Dallas.[24] In West Texas, however, this confusion is seldom the case; almost without exception my informants from West Texas claimed that the curandero uses only white magic to heal patients, though he might use the curse of God to force a brujo to remove a hex from a patient. The curandero of West Texas fits the description of the second kind of witch given in the *Malleus*; in some other areas the curandero belongs to the third class. In all areas, however, the brujo fits into the first class of witches—those who can harm but cannot cure.

In West Texas the curandero sees himself and is seen by others in the culture as primarily a religious figure who has been endowed by God with certain curative and occult powers. Don Pedrito Jaramillo, the best-known curandero in Texas, is a folk religious hero, treated almost as a saint by many of Mexican descent in both Texas and Mexico. A shrine has been built in his memory, and people come hundreds of miles to visit and be cured by his powers, even though he has been dead for many years. His pictures can be found in homes throughout South Texas and in Mexico. Small statues or icons of Don Pedrito are likewise to be found throughout the region. He is called upon in prayers to heal the sick through his spirit. He has become a real folk hero—a folk saint, though not recognized as such by the Catholic Church or priests.

However, many of the folk religious practices, as well as many orthodox Catholic practices, are devoted to warding off the powers of Satan; and the curandero, having received his healing powers as a gift from God,[25] sees himself as a participant in the struggle between good and evil. In this struggle the curandero's principal opponent is the brujo, or witch. In the words of one informant: "The *curandero* has power over the witch. His magic is stronger than the witch's—more potent. It's really his prayers and the cross that he fights with, and the rosary."

In the view of the Mexican Americans of West Texas, the brujo and all spells and hexes are manifestations of the power of Satan. The brujo has made a pact with the devil. He has to pass certain tests to become a full-fledged witch. As one informant explained about a friend who had tried to become a brujo but failed:

He had tests to pass to check his commitment. Among other things, he had to go to where two cattle trails crossed high up in some mountains and call on the devil three times. While doing so the third time, he felt a hot wind blowing and a snake crawled around him. [The symbolism is obvious.] This did not scare him. He was then given a crucifix and told to spit on it and then step on it, thus rejecting all things pertaining to God. He then had to spend the night in a cave in the mountainside. During the night he was awakened by something licking his face. It was a coal-black sheep with silver horns and a gold chain and an amulet around its neck. He couldn't stand this so he called on God, and the sheep disappeared. He feels that Satan is still trying to get him.

I have collected other versions of the initiation of a brujo, all of which include the same symbolic rejection of God through stepping or spitting on the cross or some other gesture.[26]

Belief in witches is almost universal among those whom I have interviewed. There are believed to be several *paninos de brujas,* or witch covens, in the area—all just across the Rio Grande on the Mexican side between Montclova and Juarez. One particularly well-known coven is located across from the Big Bend National Park on a ranch near San Carlos, Mexico. An informant reports an experience her sister witnessed: "While traveling from one ranch to another one time they [the sister and her friends] saw in a wooded area this witches' sabbath thing. They were naked and were having a little dance, like in 'Young Goodman Brown.' The ranch is La Hacienda." The reference to Hawthorne's short story would be surprising, perhaps, except that the informant received her master's degree in American literature last summer.

The witches use their black magic to cast spells and hexes and to make peoples' lives miserable in other ways. The brujo can use homeopathic magic (dolls), or contagious magic (the victim's fingernail clippings, hair, and so on), or even a photograph. The use of photographs in casting spells seems to be a favorite technique in West Texas. Incantations, often prayers said backward, are also common. The witches are usually well paid for these spells. If one individual has a grudge against another or is envious of him, he can go to a witch and for a price have a hex put on that individual. If the victim perceives that he has the symptoms of mal puesto, he then goes to a curandero, who sets about getting the hex removed, often by forcing the brujo to remove it. If the hex goes undetected too long, the damage may already be done before the curandero can act.

A story from one of my informants illustrates the process of unhexing a patient:

> One day one of these witches from La Hacienda, who lived in a house near my sister in San Carlos [Mexico], had something strange happen to her left eye and face. It sort of rotted. She had put a spell on a man there in San Carlos, and his family had taken him to see this old curandero in Ojinaga. In trying to cure him, he found out who had put the hex on the man. He called her and called her, and finally she came, but she was in the form of a turkey. It's a long way from San Carlos. Sure enough, she had the man's picture. The curandero demanded that the bruja remove the spell from the man, but she refused. So he put a curse [of God] on her, and her eye and face rotted. Finally she took the curse off the man and then went out to La Hacienda with some other witches. A week later she came back to San Carlos and she was cured. Later, when she was getting old, she gave all the pictures of people back to them. She said she wanted to do this before she went to live with her son in Ojinaga.

Mexican American brujos can cause mankind the same problems that witches anywhere else can. The *Malleus* gives six different ways that the devil can harm man, and there are stories in my files which indicate that the brujos use all of them. Brujos can cause physical illnesses or diseases, cause death, destroy one's mind, produce impotence, make one jealous of his neighbor, and cause an evil love in a man for a woman or vice versa.

On the other hand, curanderos can cure anything that the brujos can cause, because the power of God is greater than the power of Satan. Like his counterpart in Peru, a curandero in West Texas can deal with problems other than physical illness. He can also "locate lost or stolen property, divine future events, assure success in personal matters, romance, and business, cure insanity and alcoholism, and counteract the effects of witchcraft."[27] People come for hundreds and sometimes thousands of miles to be cured by some of the more famous curanderos, whose reputations have become almost legend.

The folklore in the Mexican American culture about curanderos and their healing powers serves several functions. It validates the folk medicine system by "proving" its effectiveness. It serves to advertise for the more successful healers via oral tradition (although some curanderos, often considered charlatans because they charge for their services, advertise over local radio stations). Most important, however, a curandero's reputation as a successful healer makes him more effective because it increases faith in him among his patients, and faith is the ingredient necessary to all of his cures.

His posture as a religious figure is an important factor in inspiring faith and awe in his followers, who, almost without exception, are devout Roman Catholics and more often than not are poorly educated and underprivileged. This is not to say that the wealthy and educated do not utilize curanderos, for they surely do. His use of the same religious articles (holy water, pictures of saints or of Christ, the crucifix, the Bible, and the rosary) commonly used in worship at home and in church also aids him. He uses prayer extensively—most curanderos can pray eloquently, and these prayers, often read, have a faith-inspiring effect on the patients. Another part of his religious posture is his poverty. Since the curandero never charges (again, those who charge are considered by most in the culture to be charlatans), his home and "office" must be appropriately humble. The successful curanderos do quite well financially, since it is acceptable to take gratuities from grateful patients.

To further enhance the curandero in the eyes of his culture, stories are told to show the superiority of his healing powers over those of the physician. Other stories are told of local physicians' sending patients whom they have been unable to help to a certain curandero, who immediately heals them. True or false, these stories strengthen the healers' reputations and validate the use of curanderismo.

Most studies of Mexican American folk medicine point out the importance of faith in the effectiveness of the cure. This is true in all cultures, especially where psychosomatic and psychological problems are in question. Both the curanderos and their patients recognize the necessity of faith. Every informant that I have interviewed about curanderismo has emphasized the importance of faith in the healing powers of any given curandero. During the process of effecting the cure, the curandero frequently reminds his patients of the necessity of faith. Don Pedrito Jaramillo repeatedly told his patients, "I have no healing power. It is the power of God released through your faith which heals you."[28]

Kiev shows the relationship between faith and the healing of psychosomatic and psychic disorders: "The curandero's approach would appear to be better suited [than that of the professional psychologist] for the depressed patient, providing as it does reassurance, support, and the promise of help. Most crucial, the patient

can hope for improvement by virtue of the faith he sets in the curandero."[29] Curanderismo works because of the faith that the
patient has in the healer and his cures.

Because faith is essential, much of the curandero's efforts are
focused on inspiring faith in his patients. The methods of accom-
plishing this differ, but the goals are the same. Most successful
healers learn early how to manipulate the fears and guilt feelings of
their patients to this end. The most common method of gaining the
faith of a patient consists of convincing him that the curandero has
clairvoyant or divining powers. In the first session with a patient
the healer invariably demonstrates these powers by telling him
facts about his life which the curandero could know only through
clairvoyance. Some healers give vague, general facts about the
patient, facts which could fit almost anyone. These attempts are
often successful, especially when the patient is uneducated and
easily frightened. Some healers, on the other hand, combine their
charismatic personalities with what seem to be real powers of
divination.

As a part of an assignment in a folklore class, a Mexican
American graduate student visited two curanderos to see how they
work. She came away feeling that one was a quack and that the
other was truly a gifted man. The first had attempted to frighten
her into believing in the healer's powers by warning her in a very
sinister manner that someone was out to get her through witchcraft. This, coupled with a very crude attempt at reading her past,
convinced this student that this particular curandera was indeed a
charlatan.

The informant came away from the second healer feeling that he
had real magical powers. She gave this description of the encounter:

> When I got there I went into his little office. The front room is very
> small and there are a few chairs for patients, and a counter with neat
> packages of labeled herbs. I waited my turn and when it came, I was
> ushered into a small back room containing a small table covered with a
> white cloth. On the table was a burning candle, a cross, a rosary, and
> some holy pictures.
>
> As I came in I asked him if there was anything wrong with me—if
> someone had hexed me. He took my hand and looked me in the eyes.
> He closed his eyes—it scared hell out of me—and started slowly drawing
> a circle in the air with his finger, all the while holding my hand. Then he
> told me some things about myself.

The things he told her about herself were specific and true and
therefore convincing. He told her where she was born, that she had

had asthma as a child, that she had a peptic ulcer, that her husband had been killed in Vietnam, and other specific facts about her life. She was convinced that he had no way of finding this out other than through divination. He went on to assure her that she had not been hexed, saying: "If anybody has tried to harm you with witchcraft, I'll know just by looking at you, but I won't know who did it until I hold your hand and do all of this stuff [close his eyes and make circles with his fingers]." His was a convincing performance.

Within the past month I had the opportunity to visit with two curanderos of considerable reputation; both live in South Texas. The first, whom we will call Pancho, lives in San Sebastian, and the other, whom we will call Señor Luna, lives in Laredo, Texas. Although they used different techniques, both attempted to convince me of their magical or divining powers. Pancho is evidently of Italian extraction and spoke some Italian, which impresses some of his patients. He works on Tuesdays, Fridays, and Sundays, and both he and some of his patients whom I interviewed claimed that during the healing sessions, which last from eight A.M. to the early hours of the next morning, he treats as many as five hundred patients. While I was there, over thirty patients were sitting on benches provided for them, patiently awaiting their turn.

When we entered his "office"—a small, poorly lighted, cluttered room added to the back of his house—he attempted to impress us (my contact and two friends were with me) with his knowledge of the occult. When I asked if we could tape the interview, he indicated that he preferred that we did not. Then, showing us a small magnet, he told us that he would wipe the tape clean by passing this small "stone" over the tape, as if the "stone" had magical properties.

He then attempted to impress us with his knowledge of the occult by showing us two books on witchcraft, which he would not let me touch. Since he could not read English, he showed us pictures from the books, commenting upon each. He used a crystal ball and some colored lights for effect as he attempted to demonstrate his powers of divination by reading the past and future of one of my companions. His facts were vague at best, one of the observations being "You are not looking for another job, but you would take a better opportunity if one came along," which was a pretty safe bet. We attempted to look impressed, and he performed the same operation for the other companion.

He showed us several examples of witches' efforts to hex some of his patients. Again, he would not allow me to touch any of the items he showed us, which included a small wax doll in a glass jar, some rather grotesque concoctions in small vials, and some pictures used to hex a patient. He was counteracting the hex by placing the picture of the hexed individual face-to-face with a picture of Christ, rolling them up together, and then wrapping them in a clean white denim cloth. He attempted to convey to us that the cloth had special magical properties.

All in all, the performance was unsuccessful from our critical point of view. My contact, on the contrary, was quite impressed with the healer's efforts. Since he already believed in Pancho's powers, he tended to overlook the weaknesses in the performance and accentuate the good parts. It is evident that similar performances had an inspiring and faith-building effect on many of his less critical patients.

Señor Luna, the curandero in Laredo, also attempted to persuade me to believe in him. His approach was much different from Pancho's—much more dignified. First, his "office" was clean and well lighted, in direct contrast to Pancho's. He began our interview by graciously telling me to record the conversation if I wished. He then gave me a lengthy sermon explaining his theories of sickness and health: we are sick when we are out of tune with God; we get well by getting back in tune with him.[30] Luna's task, as he saw it, was to help his patients get into harmony with the Almighty.

He read a few passages from the Bible and a few paragraphs from a bilingual edition of Mary Baker Eddy's *Science and Health with Key to the Scriptures.* His readings were very dramatic, and he pounded his points home by thumping vigorously on the table and eliciting positive responses from my contact, who had accompanied me.

At the urging of my contact, he attempted to tell me things about my past. The effort required having me hold a crucifix in my right hand while he held my left hand in his own. He, too, dealt in generalities; he made good guesses at times and poor ones at others.

On the way to Laredo my contact had told me that Señor Luna had made him see Christ. Toward the end of our interview, he asked Señor Luna to make me see Christ, too. I was anticipating a dramatic show of some sort, but that did not materialize. Instead, Señor Luna set up a fairly ordinary trick of optical illusion. I was instructed to stare intently at a black and white picture of the face of Christ while he said a prayer—a duration of about thirty seconds. He emphasized that I was to focus on the nose and not move my eyes. Then on his command I was to stare at a spot on a lighted wall. Sure enough, the image appeared there, just as I had expected. He was very happy that I had seen it and asked me to "testify that I had seen Christ" to some skeptics in my contact's family. We repeated the act outside; this time the image appeared in the sky. This simple trick has been a very useful tool in inspiring faith in many of his patients, which is what it is designed to do.

Both of these curanderos seemed honest and sincere. It is easy to see how one less critical than I could be impressed by their performances, and that is what is important. Because of their faith in themselves and their patients' faith in them, both curanderos were effective. Both were able to relieve the distresses of those in their culture who believed in them.

In some cases the patients are motivated by fear as much as by faith in the healers. This is particularly true of those often considered charlatans. Through fear they keep their patients from seeking medical assistance elsewhere, and at the same time they charge exhorbitant fees. An example of this intimidation occurred in Marathon, Texas, about five years ago. My informant's mother-in-law was making weekly trips to Quemado, Texas, to see a curandera, Hermana Juana, about a skin affliction. The healer was charging her forty or fifty dollars a session. Finally my informant, a schoolteacher, went with his in-laws to see what was going on. He detected some trickery and said so to one of the healer's patients. The patient then told Hermana Juana, and the next day she called the mother-in-law and told her that my informant was a very wicked man and that he was going to die by Christmas. She then called his wife and tried to intimidate her, but his wife called him to the phone. He cursed the curandera soundly and threatened her with a lawsuit. She became very conciliatory and said that she would pray for him and that he wouldn't die by Christmas. His parents-in-law were badly frightened; and when he insisted that the mother-in-law be taken to a physician, they told him that the curandera had said that if she went to a doctor, she would die immediately. He persuaded them to take her to a doctor, and she was soon healed. Consequently, they no longer live in fear of Hermana Juana.

These and other examples serve to substantiate the findings of Kiev about the healer-patient relationship. He found that "the substantive psychology and the faith of the native healer in his system might be as important for successful treatment as the scientific accuracy of his methods."[31] Equally as important as his faith in himself is the faith of the patients in the curandero and his system of cures.

This study has presented five generalizations about the folk medicine system of the Mexican Americans in West Texas. First, folk medicine and curanderismo is still an important force in their lives, not only because of cultural isolation, but also because the system works in many instances. Second, the curandero, primarily a religious figure, is highly respected for his curative powers and occult knowledge. Third, belief in witchcraft is common among these people, and much of the curandero's efforts consists of overcoming spells and hexes. Fourth, faith is the essential ingredient in the cures he performs. And fifth, much of the curandero's efforts are designed to inspire faith in his patients and, in some cases, fear. Although these generalizations may not be accurate for all Spanish-speaking peoples in the Southwest, or even for all of the individuals in the Mexican American culture of West Texas, there is much evidence to indicate that they are accurate for the majority in that culture.

NOTES

1. Américo Paredes, "Tributaries to the Mainstream: The Ethnic Groups," in *Our Living Traditions*, ed. Tristram P. Coffin (New York: Basic Books, 1968), pp. 70-80.

2. *Ibid.*

3. In a recent survey I conducted in October 1973 among the seventh and eighth graders in the Marfa, Texas, Independent School District, not one Mexican American child knew of a cure for warts, probably one of the most common folk cures among Anglos. This proved true for other cures. The Anglo children were much more aware of Mexican American folk cures.

4. Lyle Saunders, *Cultural Difference and Medical Care* (New York: Russel Sage Foundation, 1954), p. 229.

5. George M. Foster, "Relationships between Spanish and Spanish-American Folk Medicine," *Journal of American Folklore*, 66 (July, 1953), 201-217.

6. Ari Kiev, *Curanderismo: Mexican-American Folk Psychiatry*, (1968; reprint ed., New York: The Free Press, 1972), pp. 22-32.

7. Foster, *op cit.*, p. 204.

8. Saunders, *op cit.*, p. 146.

9. Cervando Martinez and Harry W. Martin, "Folk Diseases Among Urban Mexican-Americans," *Journal of the American Medical Association*, 196 (April 11, 1966), 147-164.

10. *Ibid.*, p. 162.

11. *Ibid.*

12. *Ibid.*

13. Saunders, *op cit.*, p. 146.

14. Arthur J. Rubel, "Concepts of Disease in Mexican-American Culture," *American Anthropologist*, 62 (October, 1960), 795-814.

15. Arthur J. Rubel, *Across the Tracks*, 2d ed. (1966; reprint ed., Austin: University of Texas Press, 1971), p. 157.

16. Kiev, *op. cit.*, p. 127.

17. *Ibid.*, p. 186.

18. It could be argued that the Christian Science reader is a fairly close counterpart for the curandero in the Anglo culture of this region.

19. Gonzalo Aguirre Beltran, *Medicina y Magia* (1963; reprint ed., Mexico 20, D.F.: Instituto Nacional Indigenista, 1973), p. 81.

20. Gordon Schendel, *Medicine in Mexico* (Austin: University of Texas Press, 1968), p. 47.

21. Douglas G. Sharon, "Eduardo the Healer," *Natural History,* 81 (November 1972), 32, 37, 40-45.

22. Heinrich Kramer and James Sprenger, *Malleus Maleficarum,* trans. Montague Summers (London: John Rodker, 1928; reprint ed., New York: Dover Publications, Inc., 1971), p. 99.

23. Sharon, *op. cit.,* p. 32.

24. Martinez and Martin, *op. cit.,* p. 163.

25. Compare to Beltran, *op. cit.,* p. 82; Sharon, *op. cit.,* p. 41; and Rubel, *Tracks,* pp. 184-185.

26. Cf. Kramer and Sprenger, *op. cit.,* pp. 99-100.

27. Sharon, *op. cit.,* p. 32.

28. Wilson M. Hudson, ed., *The Healer of Los Olmos and Other Mexican Lore* (Dallas: Texas Folklore Society, XXIV, 1951), p. 17.

29. Kiev, *op. cit.,* p. 186.

30. Cf. Sharon, *op. cit.,* pp. 42-43.

31. Kiev, *op. cit.,* p. 4.

Some Aspects of Folk Medicine among Spanish-speaking People in Southern Arizona

BYRD HOWELL GRANGER, *University of Arizona*

The discussion of folk medicine among Spanish-speaking people in southern Arizona will here be limited to that of Mexican Americans. The Mexican American population in Arizona derives largely from Sonora, across the border, a fact that despite one study to the contrary[1] has apparently had little effect on differentiating folk medicine in southern Arizona from that known to Mexican Americans elsewhere. The same folk illnesses are known from South America to northern New Mexico, and in Arizona they do not differ markedly from those known to southwestern American Indians and to Mexican Indians. As a White Mountain Apache recently said, "The Mexican is Spanish and Indian to start with, so there's not really any difference. They still cure the same with the Spirit of God."[2]

Historical references disclose that the Spaniards encountered Indians who, like the rest of mankind, suffered bodily ailments, among other things "devilish stomach disorders"[3] unknown to missionaries. Contemporary Mexican Americans rank stomach troubles among the handful of illnesses which may be termed cultural afflictions.

Mexican Americans classify folk disorders[4] as being brought on by (1) emotion, (2) dislocation of organs, (3) magic, or (4) hot/cold imbalance. Two additional categories are (5) other folk diseases not specified, and (6) Anglo diseases[5] (such as pneumonia or appendicitis). In southern Arizona informants speak in terms of cause, but cause is defined simply as natural (controlled by God) or unnatural (brought on by bewitchment).[6]

Historically, the most interesting cultural affliction may be *empacho*, a digestive ailment, which was noted by early missionaries as native to the Indians. In 1763 Ignaz Pfefferkorn said it was "a dangerous and frequent ailment caused by overeating, chilling and drinking bad water" and that indigo dissolved in urine was a helpful remedy.[7] Today Mexican Americans say *empacho* is food adhering in a mass in the stomach; its symptoms are stomachache, nausea, and weakness. Remedy calls for stomach massage. Massage was also applied in Pfefferkorn's day.[8] As for the prevalence of empacho, a registered Tucson pharmacist reports that every day he sees a half-dozen sufferers requesting remedies for empacho.[9] On his shelves are at least five patent medicines called *desempacho*. Another remedy, widely used in the Southwest, is *tequesquite*, a sodium bicarbonate substance usually found at mineral springs.[10]

A first step in diagnosis is to brew mint tea, which the patient drinks. If it does not help, then the patient has empacho.[11] Further diagnosis requires that the patient lie face down while a female relative or a *curandera* pinches skin near the waist and listens for a snapping noise from the abdomen. If it is heard, empacho is confirmed. Treatment will attempt to reestablish the proper balance of "hot" and "cold" in the stomach,[12] a factor to be discussed later. Empacho, incidentally, may be chronic, attributable to a digestive system which is constitutionally weak, a characteristic which is called *debiles de la estomica*, a term applied to whole families with such a weakness.[13]

Although lead protoxite, known as *la greta*, is used to break up the mass of lodged food, it is not desirable because it has a "cold" quality which may hinder restoring the proper balance of hot/cold.[14] *Asogue* ("quicksilver") with white lead was a remedy widely used in Mexico in 1887 for "empeche."[15] Quicksilver is still a remedy.[16]

Only glancing mention can be made of the hot/cold theory of diseases, which came to the New World with doctors trained in the Hippocratic doctrine of attributing disease to imbalance of the four humors. "Hot" and "cold" do not apply to actual temperatures, but rather to qualities of disorders. Some disorders are viewed as being very cold, others as conversely hot; and foods and medicines must be prescribed to fit the diagnosis so that they will not aggravate an existing imbalance. Emotional upset can lead to hot/cold imbalance. Given that premise, it is interesting to note that some say *empacho* may be brought on by one's being forced to eat something one really does not want;[17] thus empacho, which has a hot/cold imbalance, may stem from an emotional cause.[18]

Foster, investigating Hispanic American folk medicine, conjectures that some popular illnesses may be attributed to characteristics of native temperament not shared by the Old World Spaniard: the latter is "an essentially stable, well-integrated individual with few inner doubts and fears," whereas the Mexican American maintains an outer aspect of assurance which "often masks inner doubts, uncertainties, worries and apprehensions."[19] The assumption may help explain the presence of empacho, not only among Mexican Americans, but among Papago Indians as well.[20] Some assert, however, that it may be brought on by eating heavy foods like rice, potatoes, and bananas.[21]

No such ambiguity as to cause exists with *susto,* a second Mexican American folk illness, sometimes also called *espanto.*[22] Claudia Madsen says that espanto is brought on by meeting a ghost, an experience that frightens the soul out of the person's body. Symptoms include a loss of speech and of appetite, the presence of fever and chills, and dreams about the dead.[23] Susto can eventuate in death. Fright sickness was known to the Aztecs,[24] who believed that it might be caused by a hopping skull, a dwarf woman walking like a duck, an apparition in a shroud, or a footless and headless moaning ghost.[25] It should be noted that separation of body and spirit is devastating, for Mexican Americans believe that the spirit is more important than the body and, therefore, that the spirit *must* be forced back into the body.[26]

Currently, espanto[27] appears to be undergoing a gradual inclusion under susto, which is also brought on by sudden fright, such as a fall or seeing or experiencing a bad accident. In Mexico it bears a wholly descriptive name: *Se le fue la tripa,* "He lost his guts."[28]

Susto in southern Arizona has the same causes as it does elsewhere. Sharp and immediate anger will not cause it, but slow-burning malevolence may.[29] It is also induced by shame, a feeling of not measuring up to one's nuclear family or group. It strikes young and old, rich and poor. In Tucson it struck the son of a Mexican American doctor. The boy became so ill he had to drop out of school. An Anglo psychiatrist was at first unable to help. The barrier which lay between them was one any Mexican American would acknowledge: the man was outside the nuclear family with whom the illness should have been investigated initially. Over many months the psychiatrist broke down the role of "outsider"—a slow process for which medical doctors have no time, but a necessary one with Mexican Americans. Ultimately the boy said that his physical education class had been required to use a trampoline, that he had been deadly afraid to do so, and that he had fainted as he had stepped forward to carry out the teacher's order. His failure led to a feeling of deep shame and to a desperate case of susto. Speaking of the cause made it possible for him to begin to mend.[30]

Susto is dangerous. In a pregnant woman it can cause the birth of a sickly baby.[31] Susto requires speedy and adequate treatment. Usually a Mexican American who falls ill will first consult with his immediate family to delve into the cause of disability. For minor ailments, a female relative who has learned medical lore from her own mother or grandmother is qualified to diagnose and to treat illness. Serious disorders, however, call for the services of a curer, male or female. For minor susto, such as occurs when a child falls and cuts his lip, an immediate step is to give him plain sugar.[32] The victim may also be given sugar and water[33] or orange-leaf tea.[34] Fright illness in southern Arizona and in Mexico is sometimes called *tiricia,* which means "the blues," a name reflecting the mental state and deep fatigue of the person experiencing it. A treatment for tiricia is ordinary bluing,[35] a cure reminiscent of Pfefferkorn's noting in 1763 that Indians used indigo for their "devilish stomach disorders."[36]

For susto too serious for home treatment, a curandero may have the patient lie on the floor or on a bed and sweep over him from the chest laterally upward and downward with the herb *pirul,*[37] with *palo blanco,* or with a household broom.[38] Treatment, in part dependent on the magic of numbers, may take nine days.[39] The treatment is common in southern Arizona.

It is noteworthy that susto is endemic among Mexican Indians to such an extent that it may be considered of Indian, rather than Spanish, origin.[40] Foster notes that susto functions by permitting a person under stress to escape within an illness his own culture sympathizes with and thus to avoid ridicule for personal behavior which may have been unsuitable.[41] Susto in this light may be viewed as an aid to *machismo,* the essential masculinity of Mexican American culture: if a male doesn't measure up, it's not his fault, but the fault of susto.

A bad case of susto can be fatal. One informant's reaction to it is revealing: "Susto is hard to cure—it's better not to get it in the first place."[42]

In a second category, that of dislocated organs, the chief offender appears to be *caída de la mollera,* or "fallen fontanel," referred to in border communities simply as *mollera caída.* Since the fontanel is soft only during infancy, the disorder is confined to young children. Parents, however, believe the fontanel to be near the apex of the head rather than in the location known to doctors.[43] When it falls, the palate also drops, cutting off the child's ability to ingest food.[44] The condition can be induced by a fall or by carrying an infant in a "vertical position before it is eight months old." Symptoms include green or white stools and inability to suck.[45]

To prevent mollera caída, some advocate keeping a tight cap on an infant's head to help the soft bones to set, and mothers should of course avoid pulling the nipple abruptly from the baby's mouth.[46] In southern Arizona, mothers fear mollera caída so much that if the infant develops "cradle cap" (a kind of scalp encrustation), they will do nothing about it for fear of causing the fontanel to drop.[47]

Treatment is relatively simple. Either the mother or the grandmother may fill her mouth with water and suck on the fontanel to bring it back into position. Alternatively, a finger may be forced into the baby's mouth and gentle upward pressure exerted on the palate to raise it and with it the fontanel. The fontanel may also be shaken back into position by holding the infant upside down by the ankles and shaking it gently a specified number of times.[48]

Mollera caída, however, is not confined to Mexican Americans. When it occurs among San Carlos Apaches, they cut the hair over the fontanel and apply a kind of dough which as it dries pulls the fontanel into correct position.[49] Pima and Papago Indians place a finger in the child's mouth to raise the displaced fontanel.[50] Apparently the same concept is—or was—believed in the American South, where blacks gather a child's hair into a tight topknot to hold in place the "thread" that connects the palate and the fontanel, for any possible looseness in the thread would permit the fontanel to sag.[51]

Treatment for mollera caída among Mexican Americans may be done at home, but it requires skill. If the mollera caída resists home treatment, the child may be taken to a curandero.[52]

One way to cure the dislocation is to rub olive[53] oil on the child's head and then dip the head in water while saying prayers.[54] Another treatment, used by a Papago medicine man, is to apply a mixture of sugar, salt, and old fat—or anything sticky—to the fontanel. He also pushes on the roof of the child's mouth.[55]

Among diseases of magical origin may be included *mal aire,* or "being hit by air," another ailment known to both Mexican Americans and Mexicans.[56] In Mexico, to guard against attacks by evil spirits, people may carry amulets. The so-called petrified deer's eye (*ojo de venado*) is a favorite.[57] It is a large brown seed with a dark "eye," something like a buckeye. "Bad air" causes a kind of paralysis or paralytic twitching, often brought on by exposure to sudden changes of air temperature, such as when one steps from a hot tub into a cold room. It may also strike when one is in a fit of anger and hence overheated.[58]

In Tucson, bad air may be induced by blows or very strong sneezing, which causes "swellings, sore eyes and nervous tremblings."[59] It may also cause severe headache or neck pain. Mal aire frequently hits the back between the shoulder blades. The treatment for bad air which hits the back is to have the patient lie face down, place a sanctuary candle between the shoulder blades, light the candle, and press an inverted glass, any size, over the candle until the flame is extinguished. In using up the oxygen, the candle creates a vacuum. The glass is then pulled off, with a loud pop. Says the informant, "Its hurts, but it does the job." The treatment was also used by Aztecs.[60]

Historically, mal aire is linked in another way to the Aztecs, who believed that illness came through the witchcraft of evil air-spirits.[61] On the other hand, *aire de los muertos* ("air of the dead") is known in Galicia, Spain.[62] However, the concept of evil-filled air is not unique. Night air with its powers of darkness has been long and widely feared.

Aside from cupping, a remedy for aching neck calls for heating a dirty pair of men's shorts and laying them on the painful area.[63]

In Mexico a cure for mal aire caused by evil spirits[64] requires cleansing the patient's body with an egg, which is then broken in a saucer and "read." The treatment is identical to that used in the American Southwest for still another folk illness, *mal de ojo*, or "evil eye" sickness.[65] In both Spain and Spanish America exists the belief that some people quite involuntarily and without malice impose illness merely by gazing fixedly at another person. Children are especially susceptible. In addition, some say that jealousy or covetousness may bring on the malady,[66] causing the patient to develop severe temple pains. Symptoms may resemble those of a terrible cold with high fever.[67] Sometimes hysterical behavior results.[68] Failure to diagnose mal de ojo, or mal ojo, or mal puesto at its onset can turn it into a terminal illness. It is therefore imperative that the disorder be correctly diagnosed as soon as possible.[69]

Among Mexican Americans, low mentality is attributable to mal ojo.[70] In such cases mal ojo may be said to serve a social function, as susto does in connection with a deficiency in machismo, for the low mentality is not the fault of the parents any more than the lack of manliness is the fault of the susto victim.

In neither Mexico nor Arizona are doctors believed capable of curing cultural ailments. Diagnosis and cure for mal ojo lie solely within the skill of a curandero. Diagnosis, as for mal aire, is achieved by means of the "egg cure."[71] An informant reports that when a child was extremely ill with cold and fever (an illness called *los ojos*), old-timers used to take a freshly laid egg and, while repeating *el credo* and *Padre nuestro*, rub the child with it from head to toe and then place the egg under the bed overnight. If the egg cooked, the child would recover.[72] The treatment parallels the egg cure elsewhere except that an egg might be broken into half a glass of water, its shape examined to yield a diagnosis: if the egg resembled a sunny-side up fried egg with a clear "eye," the patient had mal ojo. The egg and water mixture rested under the bed to draw out the evil power during the ensuing night.[73]

Only a curandero can handle mal ojo, and the cure can be effected only in private. The curandero takes the patient into the curer's home, makes everyone else in the home leave, and goes to work for a period which may last days, weeks, or even months.[74]

When illness hits a member of a Mexican American family, the first step is family consultation to find an explanation for why the illness struck. Until the answer comes, diagnosis cannot. It is sometimes hard for Anglos to understand that a Mexican American will do nothing to correct illness—not even consent to an essential and immediate operation—before consulting with family members. As for treatment once diagnosis is achieved, in southern Arizona, as elsewhere, home remedies suggested in family council will be administered by the mother or grandmother before the help of a doctor or nurse is sought. Families recognize and treat disorders which doctors scorn, and if a close relative is incapable of helping the sick one, a curer in the neighborhood will be sought for diagnosis and treatment. This system, however, is not applied to "gringo" illnesses, which may be said to have been "introduced" into Mexican American culture and hence have adhering to them no cultural diagnosis or treatment.

As a matter of fact, in all folk illnesses and ailments among Mexican Americans, ethnic attitude is significant. To a large extent the cultural attitude may derive from native roots, for in the mid-1700s Jesuit Joseph Och noted that Indians had stoical patience, never rolling about, moaning, or complaining.[75] Mexican Americans are Spartan. In 1972 a Chicano said that a man is not macho—rough and tough—if he admits to illness; he admires endurance and disdains sickliness, which reflects, to him, moral weakness. But, he added, some illnesses point up that the patient has been mistreated and so provide an escape by giving a rationale for otherwise unsanctioned behavior, or illness may dramatize the evil consequences of cultural change, which causes the victim to fall ill because he has abandoned the old accepted ways. However, doctors are wrong to think that Mexican Americans do not suffer deeply.[76]

According to the same Chicano, health is thought of as a gift from God, a concept wholly accepted by Mexican Americans in southern Arizona. If one becomes ill, he is thought of as "the passive and innocent victim of malevolent forces in his environment." He is not held responsible for becoming sick unless he is being punished for sins.[77] Therefore he must endure the illness as only what he should expect.

The macho attitude toward sickness helps explain why Mexican Americans consider their health adequate even when by Anglo standards they should be seeking medical help for a hacking cough, obvious anemia, the sniffles and fever of a cold. Such minor matters do not interfere with a man's work. One is not ill, furthermore, if pain is absent.

There is one final point, and it is significant in the treatment of ills which may have brought on by sins as well as in the treatment of other stubborn cases. One may always seek the help of God, either by addressing special prayers to saints, such as Saint Apollonia in case of toothache, or one may make a vow to a saint to carry out a special mission if the saint can induce God or the Virgin Mary to save or cure the patient. Too little attention has been paid to pilgrimages to shrines. Mexicans and Mexican Americans are like Chaucer's Canterbury pilgrims in that they embark on pilgrimages for succor and fiesta. One of the most significant annual pilgrimages occurs in early October to Magdalena, some sixty miles south of the Arizona border, some one hundred thirty from Tucson. Pilgrims, some carrying a staff, walk that distance. Their families establish camps along the route for rest, nourishment, and bathing tired feet. On October 4 pilgrims stand for hours waiting their turn to visit the holy image of Saint Francis Xavier—and when they have finally inched their way into the small chapel where his life-size image lies in state, they ask for forgiveness of sins, for cure from doleful illness. If a pilgrim attempts to raise the saint's head from its pillow and fails, the sin is not forgiven. The stricken look on the face of one so condemned is heartrending.

I have stood by silently and watched an apparent grandfather, a young girl with a sickly baby in her arms beside him, pass long slender ribbons of red, yellow, blue, and green over the saint's body; touch the ribbons to the image's forehead, lips, chest, and stomach; then, lips moving all the while, turn and touch the blessed ribbons to the girl and then her child. The ribbons, I know, will be taken home. There they will hang to bring or maintain health.

Votive offerings are a commonplace in cures. In Tucson the image of Saint Francis at the Mission of San Xavier has a coverlet to which is always pinned an ever-fresh batch of tiny silver hearts, limbs, heads, torsos—in thanksfulness for ills cured. From time to time the brothers of the mission detach the votive offerings and place them in jars beside the figure.

In conclusion, it can be stated that in southern Arizona folk medicine is alive and well, believed in and practiced, for an array of ailments for which medical doctors have no cure. As Mexican Americans say, "A doctor charges you, but God cures you."

NOTES

1. Ingrid Poschmann O'Grady, "Childbearing Practices of Mexican-American Women of Tucson, Arizona" (M.A. thesis, University of Arizona, Tucson, 1973).

2. Margie F. McCurry, ed., *Viva la Diferencia . . . a Chicano Cultural Awareness Conference with Emphasis on Health: A Compact Review of the Conference Held at Ghost Ranch, Abiquiu, N.M., May 14-17, 1972.* "Interview with Mike Cruz, 28 Year Old Whiteriver Apache Curandero, and Mr. Fuentes" (Albuquerque; University of New Mexico, n.d.), p. 145.

3. Frances E. Quebbeman, *Medicine in Territorial Arizona* (Phoenix: Arizona Historical Foundation, 1966), p. 9.

4. Arthur J. Rubel, "The Epidemiology of a Folk Illness: 'Susto' in Hispanic America," *Ethnology*, 3 (1964), 268, states that a folk illness refers "to syndromes which members of a particular group claim to suffer and for which their culture provides an etiology, diagnosis, preventive measure, and regimens of healing," illnesses which doctors in the dominant culture do not understand and cannot easily cure.

5. McCurry, *op. cit.*, p. 124. Margaret Clark, *Health in the Mexican-American Culture: A Community Study* (Berkeley and Los Angeles: University of California Press, 1959), p. 164, gives an identical classification. Arthur J. Rubel, in "Concepts of Disease in Mexican-American Culture," *American Anthropologist*, 62 (1960), 797, categorizes under *males naturales* natural causes "within the domain of God", under *mal artificial* those caused by the devil, and under mal puesto "one of the others"; none of these diseases is understood by Anglo doctors and none afflicts Anglos. Claudia Madsen, in *A Study of Change in Mexican Folk Medicine* (New Orleans: Tulane University Press, 1965), p. 100, separates folk illnesses into those with natural and those with supernatural causation but notes that sufferers do not so classify their disorders. (Study accomplished for the Middle America Institute.)

6. Evelyn Siqueiros, "Folk Medicine in the Mexican-American Culture" (Paper prepared for Dr. Frances Gillmor, University of Arizona, c. 1970), p. 2; Margarita Artschwager Kay, "Health and Illness in the Barrio: Women's Point of View" (Ph.D. diss., University of Arizona, Tucson, 1972)), p. 201, agrees. Dr. Kay has devised a system according to levels: "Level I: illness contrasted with health; Level II: illnesses of the physical body and those caused by emotion; Level III: course of illnesses contrasted as being self-limited, mild, or severe; Level IV: generic, grouped by symptoms." On p. 202 Kay says that women sometimes based classification on prognosis or on etiology (caused by germs or by deformity). Each informant in Kay's study interpreted names for disorders as she saw them, without group agreement. It

should be noted that Kay's study was based on interviews with women living in a very small barrio of Tucson. In my experience, although to all surface appearances belief in cultural disorders is fading, in actuality this is not the case, as my fieldwork throughout Arizona for more than a decade reflects: under stress, the cultural illnesses surface strongly.

7. Ignaz Pfefferkorn, *Sonora: A Description of the Province* (Albuquerque: University of New Mexico Press, 1949), p. 214.

8. *Ibid.*, p. 215. Currently, one who knows how to massage properly is known as a *sobanda*; she is not, however, a curandera, for she is not so trained. Massage is used to diagnose where the food mass is lodged.

9. Roy Laos, Interview, November 28, 1973. Mr. Laos is the owner of the Arizona Drug Store in Tucson.

10. Madsen, *op. cit.*, p. 123. L. S. M. Curtin, *Healing Herbs of the Upper Rio Grande* (Los Angeles: Southwest Museum, 1965), p. 182.

11. Mrs. Margarita Hughes, Interview, December 11, 1973. Mrs. Hughes, a secondary-school teacher of cultural awareness, is an active and respected member of the barrio communities in Tucson. Her family, originally from Sonora, are longtime residents of the city. My gratitude goes to Mrs. Hughes for reading and strengthening the present paper by authenticating and adding to its accuracy from a Mexican American's point of view.

12. Rubel, "Concepts," p. 799. Kay, *op. cit.*, p. 151, notes that in one small barrio of Tucson, women believe that if neglected, empacho may lead to severe constipation (*obstipation*, which Kay equates with peritonitis) and death.

13. Hughes, Interview.

14. Rubel, "Concepts," p. 799.

15. Fanny Chambers Gooch, *Face to Face with the Mexicans* (New York: Ford, Howard and Hulbert, 1887), p. 439.

16. Hughes, Interview.

17. Arthur J. Rubel, *Across the Tracks: Mexican-Americans in a Texas City* (Austin: University of Texas Press, 1966), p. 166. William Madsen, *Mexican-Americans of South Texas* (New York: Holt, Rinehart and Winston, 1964), p. 75, agrees.

18. During the interview, Mrs. Hughes had occasion to rub Ben Gay on her hands. She volunteered the information that she so believed in the hot/cold theory that she would wait for her hands "to cool off" before washing them.

19. George M. Foster, "Relationships Between Spanish and Spanish-American Folk Medicine," *JAF*, 66 (1953), 216.

20. Fr. Kieran McCarty, Interview, December 5, 1973. Fr. McCarty is resident priest at the San Xavier Papago Reservation and mission near Tucson.

21. William Madsen, *op. cit.*, p. 75.

22. Rubel, "Epidemiology," p. 270, lists the following names for the disorder: *pasmo, jano, perdida de la sombra.* Foster, *op. cit.*, p. 211, says *espanto* ("fright") has these names: *colerina* ("anger": Peru), *pispelo* ("shame or embarrassment": El Salvador), *chucaque* ("shame or embarrassment": Peru), *tiricia* ("disillusion": Peru), *sipe* ("sibling jealousy," "rejection": Mexico), *peche* ("sibling jealousy," "rejection": El Salvador), *caisa* ("sibling jealousy," "rejection": Peru), *pension* ("sadness").

23. Claudia Madsen, *op. cit.*, p. 105.

24. Virgil J. Vogel, *American Indian Medicine* (Norman: University of Oklahoma Press, 1970), p. 19, says that American Indians suffer from soul loss due to fright or to the soul leaving the body in a dream and not returning. It is also caused by violating taboos or by having unfulfilled dreams or desires.

25. Claudia Madsen, *op. cit.*, p. 105.

26. Hughes, Interview.

27. William Madsen, *op. cit.*, p. 77, says that ghost fright can be treated by giving the sufferer "water mixed with dirt taken from the center of a crossroad."

28. Gordon Schendel, *Medicine in Mexico: From Aztec Herbs to Betatrons* (Austin: University of Texas Press, 1968), p. 143.

29. Hughes, Interview.

30. The information came from an Anglo doctor who prefers to remain anonymous. November, 1972.

31. Hughes, Interview.

32. Informant: Mrs. Lupe Bailon; Collector: Susan Madrid Bailon; Globe, 1953; University of Arizona Folklore Archives. (Hereafter to be noted as follows: Inf.:————; Col.:————; UAFA.)

33. Inf.: Maggie Valencia; Col.: Janice Templin; Douglas, 1962; UAFA. William R. Holland, "Mexican-American Medical Beliefs: Science or Magic?" *Arizona Medicine* (1963), p. 93, says that a Tucson treatment is the insertion of a piece of garlic into the anus on nine nights; if the garlic absorbs, the patient has susto from which he will experience relief after the ninth night. Prayers and candle burning at saints' images are often part of the cure.

34. Claudia Madsen, *op. cit.*, p. 106.

35. Hughes, Interview.

36. Pfefferkorn, *op. cit.*, p. 214.

37. Rubel, *Tracks*, p. 165. A danger of susto is that the patient may become so ill that undiagnosed tuberculosis may result from his decline. According to Rubel, "Concept," p. 805, susto may in fact be confused with tuberculosis.

38. Rubel, "Epidemiology," p. 270. It may originate in the concept that a person has one body but two or more spirits which may leave his body.

39. Foster, *op. cit.*, p. 217.

40. Holland, *op. cit.*, p. 143.

41. Foster, *op. cit.*, p. 211. Foster says that in parts of Spain it is believed that if part of the body is displaced, such as the stomach "falling" because of violent coughing, the condition can be cured only by restoring the organ to its normal position. Foster also notes the occurrence of fallen fontanel in Mexico, El Salvador, and Guatemala.

42. Clark, *op. cit.*, p. 170. An informant said that a baby so afflicted cannot nurse well but "just sucks and smacks his lips all the time."

43. Hughes, Interview.

44. William Madsen, *Mexican-Americans*, p. 74.

45. Claudia Madsen, *op. cit.*, p. 123.

46. William Madsen, *Mexican-Americans*, p. 74.

47. Hughes, Interview. Peter Wild, whose wife is a Mexican American, says that before bathing one must pat his own fontanel to avoid catching cold. Tucson, December 10, 1973.

48. These are methods used generally throughout Mexican American communities, including those in southern Arizona.

49. Aleš Hrdlička, *Physiological and Medical Observations among the Indians of Southwestern United States and Northern Mexico*, Bureau of American Ethnology Bulletin no. 34 (Washington, D.C.: Government Printing Office, 1908), p. 223.

50. *Ibid.*, p. 243.

51. I heard this from my mother, a native of Virginia, c. 1933. My mother in turn had heard it from my grandmother, a native of New Orleans. The belief has also been reported in Tucson in 1965 by Judy O'Kelley, learned from Hal O'Kelley. UAFA.

52. Inf.: Dr. P. Drew; Col.: Gail S. Hood; Tucson, 1963; Inf.: Mrs. G. Barrientos; Col.: M. Cabrera; Yuma, 1964; UAFA. Mrs. Barrientos said that the baby should hang upside down by its heels, and "you jerk three times, simultaneously hitting his heels soundly. You can see immediately the change in the head and eyes."

53. Hughes, Interview.

54. Inf.: Bill Yellowhammer; Col.: Harry Reynolds; Tucson, 1972; UAFA. Both men are half-Indian and half-Mexican American.

55. Inf.: Alice Narcho and Lucy Pablo (Papago); Col.: Loretta Herbst; Tucson, 1962; UAFA.

56. Carleton Beals, *Mexican Maze* (Philadelphia: J. B. Lippincott Company, 1931), p. 26. Kay, *op. cit.*, says a deer eye is dried seaweed seed. A deer eye (*ojo de*

venado) in my collection bears no resemblance to seaweed seed, but Kay may refer to a variety unknown to me.

57. Foster, *op. cit.*, p. 209.

58. Foster, *op. cit.*, p. 209. Foster says the disorder is "perhaps the most frequent Spanish-American explanation for illness." He believes some forms of mal aire are native to Spanish America.

59. Kay, *op. cit.*, p. 222.

60. Hughes, Interview. Mrs. Hughes is of Aztec descent. She reports that cupping is fairly common for such back pain.

61. Frances Toor, "Cures and Medicine Women" *Mexican Folkways*, 1 (1925), 18.

62. Foster, *op. cit.*, p. 210.

63. Inf.: Mr. A. Perez; Col.: M. Cansler; Yuma, 1964; UAFA.

64. It is only recently that I have pieced together from various informants why Mexican American children fear and yet will dance excitedly near a dust devil. It appears that they believe evil spirits are in the dust devil and if they are caught in one, they will become ill, but the temptation to play and tempt fate is too much for them.

65. Rubel, "Concepts," p. 801.

66. William Madsen, *Mexican-Americans*, p. 158.

67. Hughes, Interview.

68. Rubel, *Tracks*, p. 169.

69. Rubel, *Tracks*, p. 158.

70. Hughes, Interview.

71. Claudia Madsen, *op. cit.*, p. 98, says that the egg cure came to the New World from Spain. Foster, *op. cit.*, p. 209, believes that the "only Spanish cure in any way related has to do with defective vision, for which one passes a freshly laid egg across the eyes," but adds that a warm egg rub continues to be used in Spain for many forms of mal de ojo in the clinical sense, so that the magical mal de ojo perhaps came to be cured in the same way in the Western Hemisphere. He also says that chicken eggs were unknown in the New World prior to the coming of the Spaniards.

72. Inf.: Cuca Flores; Col.: Kathleen B. Gilmer; Morenci, 1962; UAFA.

73. Charles August Arnold, "The Folk-Lore, Manners, and Customs of the Mexicans in San Antonio, Texas" (M.A. thesis, University of Texas, Austin, 1928), p. 26.

74. Hughes, Interview. Mrs. Hughes says, "When everyone gets thrown out, it's rough when you have only one room."

75. *Missionary in Sonora: The Travel Reports of Joseph Och, S.J., 1755-1767* (San Francisco, Calif,: California Historical Society, 1965), p. 173.

76. McCurry, *op. cit.*, p. 125. Clark, *op. cit.*, pp. 198-199 and 201, sets forth the same concepts. Mrs. Hughes agrees, saying that when she took twenty-two children on their first visit to a roller-skating rink, one boy made the mistake of admitting to weakness, saying, "I'm sweating and I took a cold drink of water. I'm going to get sick." The others jeered and ridiculed him. As for departing from the old ways, Mrs. Hughes says such action is a recognized cause of illness. "We say, 'You've become too gringo, so you get sick all the time.' How many times have I heard that!"

77. McCurry, *op. cit.*, p. 124. Mrs. Hughes says, "If one is punished for sins, he simply has to put up with it until he atones. That's why Mexican-Americans go to the doctor so seldom—sometimes too late." Kay, *op. cit.*, p. 213, relates that in the section of Tucson she investigated, women believe that colds should run their course, rashes erupt to the full, diarrhea be left untreated, and ulcers drain constantly. She does not, however, delve into ethnic concepts underlying the Mexican American attitude toward such ills.

A Survey of Folk Medicine in French Canada from Early Times to the Present

LUC LACOURCIÈRE, *Laval University*

To present even in its general outlines a panorama of folk medicine in French Canada seemed to me, after I had accepted the invitation to do so, a rash undertaking, as much from a historical as from an ethnomedical point of view.

Although the subject has always fascinated me, because of the family environment in which I grew up (as the son, brother, and brother-in-law of country doctors), as well as because of semi-professional circumstances, such as my participation as an ethnographer in the founding of the Canadian Society of the History of Medicine in 1950, I must humbly assert that my research on empirical or folk medicine and those who practice it has remained somewhat marginal to my major fields of study. My work on this subject has been confined to compiling bibliographical data and to collecting remedies and treatments, verbal devices, anecdotes, folk beliefs, and traditions whenever the occasion has presented itself during field trips over the years.

I will not attempt to present here a complete picture of folk medicine from the early beginnings of New France in the sixteenth century to the present day, since such an undertaking also would entail, to some extent, the outlining of the main stages of the establishment of a formal system of medicine and its evolution into scientific medicine as we know it today. Consequently, I will limit my discussion of the early period to the mere mention of a few dates and references which will serve as historical background to certain observations and material based directly on fieldwork.

The oldest folk remedy noted in the New World was given by the Indians to Jacques Cartier during his stay in Stadacona (now Quebec) during the winter of 1535-1536, when an epidemic of scurvy (*la grosse maladie*) decimated his crew. An infusion made from the bark of the *Annedda* tree proved to have "miraculous" healing powers:

> No sooner had they drunk than they improved in a manner truly and obviously miraculous. For, after drinking of it twice or thrice they recovered their health and were healed of all the disorders afflicting them. So much so that one of the men who had been suffering from the pox for five or six years was completely cured of it by the remedy. When this was seen and known, there was such a rush on the medicine that they almost murdered one another in their eagerness to be first served. So that in six days a whole tree as large and tall as any oak in France was used up. And in those six days it worked more wonders than all the physicians of Louvain and Montpellier using all the drugs in Alexandria could have done in a year.[1]

This tree, identified as the white cedar (*Thuja occidentalis*), was called *l'arbre de vie*, or "the tree of life," by Cartier's contemporaries. However, the incident took place before the permanent settling of New France, and by the time Quebec was founded, the secret and the identity of this panacea were lost, a fact which Champlain was to deplore.

It was between the years 1608 and 1760 that French medical traditions, official or otherwise, were implanted in New France. The annals mention a good number of doctors, surgeons, barbers, and apothecaries established mainly in the cities and frequently in hospitals, notably the Hôtel-Dieu of Quebec and the Hôtel-Dieu of Montreal, which have been in existence since 1639 and 1644, respectively. There numbered among these practitioners many worthy men, such as Michel Sarrasin (1659-1734) and Jean-François Gauthier (1708-1756), botanists and physicians of the king and both celebrated for having given their names to native plants, the pitcher plant (*Sarracenia purpurea*) and the wintergreen (*Gautheria procumbens*), which are currently used in folk medicine.

A medical historian of French Canada notes that besides these scholars, there appeared in rapidly increasing numbers healers and charlatans ("des guérisseurs, des charlatans, des 'fratres' "), as they were called, who traveled about the countryside setting bones and selling herbs and panaceas.[2] Some of these folk practitioners have passed into history, but usually because of their unpleasant dealings with the authorities rather than their exceptional healing powers.

This is notably the case of the Breton Yves Phlem from la

Pérade, a small village on the Saint Lawrence River. He signed a written agreement before witnesses and the parish priest to heal a certain Jean Bilodeau of a very advanced canker on his lower lip. However, Bilodeau died on May 10, 1736, in spite of eight months of treatment. His widow later refused to pay for her husband's treatments; hence the law proceedings in which she was sentenced to pay Phlem for the lodging and food given to her late husband but not for the treatment and care administered by the healer. The latter continued none the less to exercise his art among those people who still had faith in his healing powers.[3]

After 1763, under English rule, the position of official medicine gradually changed. It was not until 1788 that the law specified under the Medical Act that every candidate who wished to practice medicine, surgery, or obstetrics had to be examined by a board whose members were appointed by the governments of either Quebec or Montreal.

For those who were unable to go out of the country to study medicine, an apprenticeship took the place of academic studies. It was only in 1819 that medical instruction was officially offered by a group of doctors, and with the establishment at a later date of the universities, academic medicine continued to evolve. It is not necessary to follow its evolution here, but it should be noted that it would be erroneous to believe that scientific medicine completely supplanted empirical or folk medicine.

We will limit our remaining remarks to folk medicine and a consideration of the different types of healers and their arsenal of cures and treatments. First, what were and what are these healers to whom a clientele, much larger and more credulous than one would suppose, still turns?

There are healing saints who are solicited on certain occasions or to heal specific diseases over which they have a sort of monopoly: Saint Blaise for a sore throat; Saint Apolline for a toothache; and Saint Geneviève, on whose feast day there is a distribution of miniature loaves of bread, to which the power of protecting pregnant women is ascribed. There are those of whom cures or even miracles are solicited in healing shrines: Saint Anne, Saint Joseph, and the Virgin Mary.

Mingled with an ardent faith, a kind of bargaining is done with Saint Expedit and Saint Jude, intercessors of urgent or desperate causes. Every day the local newspapers carry images of these saints or photographs of Pope John XXIII or less universally known benefactors as ex-votos for the fulfillment of promises made to them in return for the granting of favors, generally healing.

Next on our list of healers we would mention (in view of their religious nature) certain priests to whom extensive powers have been attributed. Placed at the head of parishes often lacking doctors, many priests gave medical advice which in the minds of their parishioners made them veritable healers. Their fame often extended far and wide, especially if they gave themselves up to the study of plants or herbs. The names of a few of these priests are found in history. For instance, Father Pierre-Joseph Compain (1740-1806) wrote down for the nuns of the Hôtel-Dieu of Quebec in 1799 his cure for cancer and a remedy for cankers in which spider webs played an important role.[4] People still cite as an effective cure "courvaline," a depurative decoction of different herbs attributed to Father Joseph-Claude Poulin de Courval, as well as the "holy water" of François-Xavier Côté, a preparation, primarily of colcothar, which is used in the treatment of wounds and inflammation of the eyes. Both of these remedies were considered so efficacious that they were included in a manual of therapeutics which was used at Victoria University in Montreal.[5] (It was at this university, no longer in existence, that my father studied medicine.)

As for the traditional healers whose gift is supposed to be hereditary—the seventh consecutive son having, like the kings of France, the mark of a fleur-de-lis under his tongue and *marcous* or posthumous children—they can be divided into two groups, bonesetters (or lay chiropractors) and faith healers.

Bonesetters generally limit themselves to setting fractures and dislocations. Many of them are well known, and people come from great distances to consult them, even from points outside of Canada, such as New England. They generally practice their art as a sideline to render service to the community. As a rule they do not accept money, that is, they do not set a fixed price, but they do not refuse gratuities.

Each region has its own bonesetter, and he is often a member of the third or fourth generation in his family to practice his occupation. This is the case for the Lessard family and the Lamberts of Beauce County, as well as the Boilys of the Saguenay region, whose reputations extend far beyond the area in which they live. For instance, a descendant of a certain Fabien Boily, who was a famous healer, has his picture published regularly in the Montreal newspapers with the brief notice "Still at the same address"; evidently this address is well known and has been for some time.

There is an anecdote frequently told in many areas to demonstrate the great skill of these bonesetters; Marius Barbeau has included it in his portrait of Fabien Boily:

More than once Fabien Boily dared to measure his skill with that of a professional doctor. According to Brigitte Desbiens, Boily had a bone to pick with the doctor of the Escoumains parish. The young practitioner had called him a charlatan.

Greatly provoked, the healer defiantly asked the young doctor, "Do you know cats?"

"Certainly I know them."

"If you do, then prove it."

Boily caught the black cat in the kitchen and dislocated its bones except for those in the neck and spine and placed the cat as an inert mass on the carpet in front of his adversary.

"You killed him, the poor beast!"

"Killed him? Go and look. If you know cats so well, revive him."

"But you're mad!" cried the bewildered doctor.

"Watch this," said the bone-setter.

He took the cat in his hands and while humming "Marie Calumet" [a folksong] he began to work his fingers. In a short time, as if by magic the cat regained its form, shook itself on the carpet, meowed plaintively and got up and hid behind the stove, sending all healers, professional doctors as well as charlatans, to the devil.[6]

The same story is told of the bonesetter Noel Lessard of Beauce County, with the difference that the dislocation and setting of the cat's bones take place before a magistrate in a court of law. Lessard, who was without benefit of counsel, is reported to have said that the cat would be his lawyer; and it was in fact the cat that proved his case.

Faith healers who cure only by touching with the hands or include incantation or prayer in their treatment are more difficult to locate or interview since they dislike having fieldworkers inquire into their affairs. They become known, however, through their numerous legal contentions with the College of Physicians. Since 1939, I have collected at random newspaper clippings of lawsuits which made the headlines of daily newspapers in Quebec and Montreal. The majority of these healers were fined for illegal practice or for extorting money from naive individuals. Those who have been duped have often revealed the unusual practices of the healer, such as those of a man (who shall remain nameless) whose healing power was to be found at the end of his penis and who sent the unsuspecting husband to collect herbs on a distant mountain while he administered his cure to the ailing wife.

However, many of these healers are too cunning to be caught. One such healer has practiced for forty years and has had many lawsuits with the College of Physicians which have gone as far as the court of appeal, but he has always been acquitted. He has allowed himself the luxury of having a large volume of 427 pages edited with all of the testimony presented before the court, as well as a series of photographs and letters from individuals whom he has supposedly cured.[7]

Like other healers who exploit the public, he has a large personnel at his service, and he holds consultation in many cities, where his visits are announced months in advance. Apparently he merely tells his patients that he will think about them, and they have so much faith in him that they go away happy, although lightened of remunerations collected by his assistants. Since he is beginning to feel his age, this healer has recently announced in the newspapers his intention to retire, but he states that one of his nephews will succeed him, since he too has received at birth the gift of healing. This and similar cases leave one skeptical about the sincerity of such commercialism.

This type of faith healer contrasts with another category of individuals who were forced by necessity, at least in the beginning, to intervene in the isolated surroundings in which they lived. These are *sages-femmes*, midwives or wisewomen of the rural milieus, many of whom have already confided their experiences to folklorists. They have existed since the beginning of New France, but they are beginning to disappear now that women generally have their children in hospitals.

Under the French regime, wisewomen were the object of rather strict regulations. We read in the ritual of the Quebec diocese published in 1704 that the priest must "make sure that no one undertakes this responsibility [that is, of being a wisewoman] within the entire parish without his having first examined her faith, good living and her ability to administer the sacrament of baptism in cases of necessity, and having then exacted from her an oath that she will duly carry out her duty." It is not known if these instructions were always carried out to the letter.[8]

From one of my notebooks used in field collecting, I excerpt a few of the reminiscences of a eighty-eight-year-old sage-femme, Mrs. Elzéar Gagnon, who lived in the mountain region of Charlevoix County.

> I began to attend patients in 1893 at the age of thirty-three. I went right up until last year [1945], when I delivered three sets of twins. I've never counted the number of children I've delivered. Over fifty-two years, that must make more than a thousand. I've never had any mishaps.
>
> When you go to a patient, you never know if it's going to be a boy or a a girl. That's up to the good Lord.
>
> I never gave any remedies before labor. I prayed to the Holy Virgin.

There were those who took remedies, though; a growth which grows in the ears of rye is scalded and drunk as a tea. You take a soupspoonful in a cup of hot water before giving birth. [Mrs. Gagnon uses the popular term *acheter*, or "buying," the child.] It prevents bleeding. When the woman lost a lot of blood, I taught quietness and prudence. Nothing unexpected. When there is something unexpected, children falling or a husband who talks too loud, well, the blood flows."

Mrs. Gagnon goes on to enumerate different remedies and foods which she recommends for the churching of the mother: "teas which you make from seven types of herbs: juniper-berry, boxtree, white pine, white fir, red spruce. . . . You mix all that together. It's better when you add a little drop of liquor."[9]

I will not take the time to present interviews with other wise-women or healers who have a special gift, such as blood-stoppers and those who "put out fire" (fever), cure toothaches, and remove warts. Nor will I discuss one of the most important folk practitioners, the blacksmith, since this topic would require a lengthy development. The blacksmith played an important role in the community, where he was recognized as having great healing powers. The curative uses of the *eau ferrée*, or chalybeate water, of the blacksmith are well known.

I will close these few remarks on folk medicine with a brief consideration of the treatments and remedies most commonly practiced.

First, it should be noted that the same remedies are often applied to both humans and animals, especially in the rural areas. This is documented in an old manuscript by a shoeing smith dated 1780 and entitled "Collection of remedies to safeguard horses from diseases and accidents which can befall them, enlarged by several remedies for the human body, prepared by me, Nicolas Joseph Neris, master farrier at Paris, residing . . ." (the bottom of the title page is torn, but the date 1780 is legible).[10] It is a manuscript of 295 pages; unfortunately, I have not had time to inventory it in its entirety. As a sample of its contents, the fourth section is presented as follows: "In which is contained various good ointments, poultices, plasters, essences, waters, powders, nostrums, as much for man as for horses; there is also contained herein remedies for different human diseases and mishaps."

This French manuscript, which contains many parallels with material found in French Canada, deserves special study and could easily be the object of an annotated edition. Similar works have been prepared in Canada. There is, for instance, a manuscript prepared in 1857 by Augustin Stanislas De Lisle, a notary and

RECUEIL

DE REMEDES, POUR GARENTIR

LES CHEVAUX,

des maladies & accidents, qui
peuvent leurs Survenir !

AUGMENTÉ

De plusieurs remedes, pour le

CORPS HUMAIN.

fait par moy, Nicolas Joseph

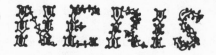

NERIS

Maitre marechal a paris; y
demeurant ... e la bucherie, pres
La p

a pa ...quillet

1780

botanist of Montreal, entitled *Petite pharmacie végétale* ..., which is a family guide to plants and their medicinal properties.

Our richest source of ethnomedical information is still, of course, oral tradition. An inventory of bibliographical sources for French Canada since 1900 reveals that folklorists and students of folklore have collected more than five thousand different folk remedies from Nova Scotia to northern Ontario. About two-fifths of these have been published; the rest are on file at the Archives de Folklore. That means that a lot of work in the areas of both classification and collecting still remains to be done in folk medicine.

Those remedies which have been published to date have been presented simply as alphabetical lists under the name of the disease.[11] This is a cursory classification which is certainly not the most satisfactory. Other systems of classification now under consideration may give more information about the ingredients used, borrowings from the vegetable, mineral, or animal kingdoms, and so on. Even more satisfactory is the method which separates wherever possible remedies of a purely empirical nature from those based on magic and yet reserves an intermediate category dependent on both empiricism and magic.

I will not enumerate examples of medicines made of plants or certain animal or mineral substances. I would mention, however, that in the eighteenth century the correspondence of a nun of the Hôtel-Dieu of Quebec contains about ten remedies, autochthonous to Canada, which she sent to an apothecary in Dieppe, France; some of the ingredients used in their preparation were maidenhair fern, maple syrup, ginseng, spruce gum, pine sap, the foot of a moose, and the musk glands of a beaver. All of these are still used today in folk medicine and even, at times, in official therapeutics.

The survival of remedies based on magic is still remarkably strong. It is only necessary to consider the frequency in remedies of odd numbers, especially three and seven; or the importance attached to colors—red flannel, white wool, and the dung of a black cow to prevent or cure sore throats, and so on; or the importance of gestures made with the left hand or foot; or movement in a certain direction, often in opposition to the orbit of the sun; or removing the bark from a tree in an upward or at times downward movement; or the days of the week and the months of the year which recall the fasti and the days of mourning of antiquity; or the many different kinds of amulets worn arond the neck or carried in a pocket to ward off toothache or whooping cough.

Perhaps the most remarkable magic cures are those which

propose the transference of disease to an animal, a tree, or another object. They are often accompanied by rituals or formulas owing as much to incantation as to prayer.

The belief in transference in folk cures is based on a simplistic conception of disease as a foreign element which has penetrated the body and can be extirpated by transmitting it to someone or something else. The removal of warts, for example, is accomplished by selling them for the low price of one cent; or if the sufferer encounters a funeral procession, they may be taken down under the ground by the dead person; or they may be thrown behind one's back along with peas or a piece of potato or pork with which the warts have been wiped.

The same thing applies to the removal of unwanted hairs. I quote a passage from a manuscript notebook written by a school teacher in 1939: "Have someone give you a piece of fresh pork and rub it on the part where the hairs are to be removed and bury it in the ground [where it is left to rot] and say, 'Cursed hair, remove yourself, just as the devil removes himself from the sight of God and never come back again, never, never, never!' "

The transference of an internal disorder is somewhat more complicated. One can fasten a pain, such as a toothache, to the bark of a tree with the aid of pins or get rid of a pain in the foot by stepping in peat moss and outlining the form of the foot with an object. But it is mainly in cures for rheumatism and similar disorders that this transference to a tree is most widespread.

To get rid of rheumatism, you must follow a path in the woods where no one is likely to pass; when you reach the foot of a tree, any tree at all, dig up the root with your left hand and, holding the tree root between your teeth, say, "Rheumatism, I leave you here and I will take you back when I pass this way again." Then bury the root with your left hand. If you take care to avoid this spot in the future, a complete cure is guaranteed.

Transference to trees has been recorded with fewer and greater numbers of variants by almost every folklorist who has studied folk medicine. However, transference to an animal seems to be less prevalent, at least in its sanguinary form, where the animal must be sacrificed. Two examples of this practice are the application to the body of a skinned cat to cure shingles (zona) or pulmonary disease and the strangling of a mole or mouse to prevent certain disorders.

I have been mainly concerned in this paper with folk medicine in French Canada, but certainly many of the treatments and beliefs outlined here have parallels in other parts of the country, although not all of these folk practices are currently carried out in every area. For instance, Helen Creighton has found a considerable amount of folk medical material in English in the province of Nova Scotia;[12] and J. Frederick Doering has collected ethnomedical practices from the Pennsylvania German settlers of Ontario.[13] Parallels to the Canadian material and the principles on which it is based can be found, of course, throughout the world. But French Canada is rich in folk medical practices, and much important work remains to be done in this field.

To close, I will relate a short anecdote which illustrates, to my way of thinking, how people still respond to folk practices and are spontaneously filled with confidence.

One evening I was recording tales and folksongs in a family in a rural area of Bellechasse County. During a break, I noticed a delightful little girl, six or seven years of age, and wanted to ask her a few simple questions, but she clung to her mother and was visibly embarrassed by the presence of a stranger. Parents always respond when one takes an interest in their children. Noticing that the little girl had warts on her hands, I said, without thinking, "Come and see me. I can make your warts disappear." I had no sooner pronounced those words than the mother literally pushed the child into my arms, saying, "That man can get rid of warts. Go and see him." Not knowing just what to do, I blew on the little girl's fingers.

Well, the next time I went back to see those people, the little girl's warts were gone, and they brought me more children to have their warts removed! That happened twenty years ago, and whenever I go back to that area, people still mention that I have a gift for removing warts. That shows what great faith people have.

NOTES

1. [Jacques Rousseau and Jean L. Launay], *Jacques Cartier et "La Grosse Maladie"* ("Reproduction photographique de son Brief Recit et Succincte Narration suivie d'une traduction en langue anglaise du chapitre traitant des aventures de Cartier aux prises avec le scorbut et d'une nouvelle analyse du Mystere de l'Annedda" [Montreal: XIXe Congres International de Physiologie, 1953], p. [102]).

2. Sylvio Leblond, "Histoire de la médecine au Canada français," *Cahiers d'histoire de la Société historique de Québec*, no. 22 (1970), p. 18.

3. Michel and Georges Ahern, *Notes pour servir à l'Histoire de la Médecine dans le Bas-Canada depuis la fondation de Québec jusqu'au commencement du XIXe siècle* (Quebec, 1923), pp. 435-441.

4. René Bélanger, "L'abbé Pierre-Joseph Compain, prêtre et médecin, 1740-1806," *Saguenayensia: Revue de la Société historique du Saguenay* (Chicoutimi), 13, no. 4 (1971), pp. 106-108.

5. *Traité élémentaire de matière médicale et guide pratique des Soeurs de Charité de l'asile de la Providence* (Publié sous le patronage des Professeurs de l'Ecole de Médecine et de Chirurgie, Faculté de Médecine de l'Université Victoria" [Montreal, Sénécal, 1870], p. 376 and p. 587).

6. Marius Barbeau, "Boily, le remancheur," *Liaison*, no. 13 (March, 1948), pp. 152-153.

7. *Il faut le mettre en prison* ("Le procès intenté à J.-A. Desfosses en Cour criminelle" (Sherbrooke, 1939).

8. [Mgr. Jean-Baptiste de la Croix Chevrières de] Saint-Vallier, *Rituel du diocèse de Québec- par l'ordre de Monseigneur de Saint-Valier, évêque de Québec* (Paris: Simon Langlois, 1703).

9. Luc Lacourcière, manuscript collection at the Archives de Folklore, nos. 190 to 193, collected at Saint-Hilarion, Charlevoix County, in September, 1946.

10. Nicolas Joseph Neris, "Recueil de remedes, pour garentir les chevaux, des maladies et accidents, qui peuvent leurs survenir, augmente de plusieurs remedes, pour le corps humain, fait par moy, Nicolas Joseph Neris, Maitre marechal a paris; y demeurant . . ." (Paris, 1780).

11. More than thirty lists of remedies, well localized and dated, have been published. Among those which have appeared in publications readily accessible, I would mention by way of example the following: E.-Z. Massicotte, "Les remèdes d'autrefois," *Journal of American Folklore*, 32, (1919), pp. 176-178; Horace Miner, *St. Denis, A French-Canadian Parish* (Chicago: University of Chicago Press, 1939), pp. 256-259; Soeur Marie-Ursule, *Civilisation traditionnelle des Lavalois* (*Les Archives de Folklore*, 5-6 [Quebec: Presses de l'Université Laval, 1951]), pp. 170-184; Carmen Roy, *Littérature orale en Gaspésie*, (Musée National du Canada, Bulletin no. 134 (Ottawa, 1955), pp. 61-88; Anselme Chiasson, *Chéticamp* (Moncton, N.B., 1961), pp. 179-188; Catherine Jolicoeur, "Traditional Use of Herbs in Quebec," *The Potomac Herb Journal*, 7, (Winter, 1971), pp. 3-5.

12. Helen Creighton, *Bluenose Magic* (Toronto: The Ryerson Press, 1968).

13. J. Frederick Doering, "Pennsylvania-German Folk Medicine in Waterloo, Ontario," *Journal of American Folklore* (1936), pp. 194-198.

Folk Medicine in French Louisiana

ELIZABETH BRANDON, *University of Houston*

In 1958 a psychiatrist, working at that time in the Department of Psychiatry of the Louisiana State University, stated: "We see that there is an active ongoing movement of folk medicine in this area. . . . Our area, Louisiana, seems to be one of the most fertile fields for research on this type of movement as well as upon herbalists, witch doctors, and black magic practitioners."[1]

A Louisiana public health nurse, working toward a doctorate in public health at the Tulane University School of Public Health and Tropical Medicine, made a similar observation in 1971: "Superstitious beliefs and practices, including voodoo, persist in Louisiana and affect the health practices of these people."[2]

That life in southwestern French Louisiana was conducive to the implantation and continuation of folk practices in medicine is not surprising, for until the second quarter of our century, it was an isolated rural area with low economic and educational standards and little or no communication with the outside world, conditions which did not invite doctors to settle. In antebellum times, plantation medicine, which was better developed in this state than in other states of the Union, did not reach the needy white patients in the region. The casual visits of a plantation doctor in this vicinity hardly provided for the wants of the slaves on the plantation, and the doctor's services were not available to outsiders. Thus, people not supplied with trained physicians' help had to depend on their own treatments or resort to lay healers. The emancipation of the slaves brought the French Louisianian into closer contact with the healing procedures of the black people, who in turn exerted their influence on the practices of the whites.

The advancement of education has diminished perceptibly the popularity of folk practitioners, but it has not obliterated it completely. The healers' existence is justified by their success in treating the sick; the demand of the public has created the supply of nonscientific practitioners. In Louisiana, as elsewhere, the patients seeking the services of these folk doctors do not necessarily belong to the group of population on a lower level of education; many educated people patronize them. To the question as to why patients consult laymen instead of trained physicians, the answer is almost always the same: because there is much that is inconclusive in modern medicine; because hospitals and doctors do not fulfill the needs of the patients; because in a given case the doctor did not cure the illness, especially when it was chronic; and finally, because the healers always demonstrate empathy for their patients and exude optimism, which doctors are incapable or unwilling to do.

In former times a native stock of remedies was available in every household. The materia medica of each family consisted of native herbs, animal substances, and common chemicals and minerals. In herbal medicine the plant—its roots, leaves, stems, buds, flowers, and fruit—could be used; trees furnished bark in addition to the other elements. And always every mother of a French Louisianian family has planted herbs in her garden. "*Mamou*, sassafras, *laurier*, citronella—I have all of these in my garden," reports an informant.[3]

The animal substances sought would be milk, flesh, fat, viscera, bones, and excrements. The list of various chemical and mineral ingredients used includes vinegar, camphor, sulphur, vaseline, soap, turpentine, epsom salts, chalk dust, ashes, charcoal, sand, kerosene (coal oil), baking soda, gasoline, sugar, salt, and ammonia. In every home several of these items were on hand so that poultices, brews, decoctions, teas, infusions, tonics, and ointments could be prepared in case of necessity. If the ingredient necessary to prepare a remedy could not be found, it was replaced by another which could be just as efficient. In folk medicine the practitioner seeks a cure of the symptoms rather than of the disease or the sick organ. And since the symptoms of various diseases are identical or similar, the same concoction may serve many purposes. On the other hand, one illness may respond to many different kinds of treatment.

There are, for instance, innumerable cures for a cold: a tea of leaves of the coral tree, a brew of leaves of *guimauve* (crimson-eye rosemallow, *Hibiscus oculeroseus* Britton); a tea of *chardron* (thistle, *Cirsium horridulum*); an infusion of *herbe à malot* (lizard's tail, *Saururus cernuus*); a tea of leaves of magnolia, sassafras, or citronella; a brew of the bark of a peach tree turned toward the east, a beverage made of sheep's tallow mixed with crushed dried hocks of a pig; an infusion of flowers of the elderberry (*sireau, Sambucus canadensis*); a syrup made of crushed grains of the coral tree mixed with honey, soda, and olive oil. Besides taking remedies internally, a patient suffering from a common cold can also apply remedies externally. There are several rubs that are recommended. Rubbing the body with a salve made of sheep's tallow mixed with turpentine or with a combination of turpentine and olive oil is claimed to be helpful. A rub with *whiskey camphré* seems to be infallible. *Whiskey camphré* is a well-known medication considered beneficial, not only for a cold, but also for other ailments. It is prepared in the following way: "Buy camphor, crush it, pour whiskey over it, keep the liquid in a bottle. It is . . . good to drink a little spoon of it for all sorts of ailments."[4]

There are many ways of treating sores. One can soak the painful place in coal oil, or one can put on it a piece of lard or sheep's tallow. A poultice made of brown sugar and soap may bring the desired result. The same remedy is effective in healing sores caused by a nail scratch or perforation. An additional treatment for this affliction is a poultice of very hot milk. One of my informants explained that he saved his daughter from sure blood poisoning after she perforated her foot with rusty barbed wire. He prepared a poultice with sugar and corn husks and applied it for the duration of the night. This treatment caused such an improvement that on the next day the child could walk again.[5]

Remedies for a sore throat are plentiful. The patient has a choice of gargling with a decoction made of roots of *éronce* (blackberry-bush, *Rubus cuneifolius*) or of blossoms of the *plaqueminier* (persimmon tree, *Diospyros virginiana*). It is also good to gargle with a mixture of honey, salt, and baking soda dissolved in water. An aching throat can be helped by drinking melted tallow or a tea made of elderberry flowers. Rubs of the neck with kerosene, *whiskey camphré*, or turpentine to which sugar and sulphur have been added are other possibilities.

A child that throws up will find relief after drinking an infusion of boiled flies or a bouillon of the inner lining of a chicken gizzard. Other remedies recommended are teas prepared with flowers of pumpkin, red geranium, or *févi* (okra, *Hisbus esculentus*).

Several illnesses can be treated by one remedy. Thus, a tea of leaves of the coral tree cures colds, fevers, inflammations, bronchitis, and stomach cramps. A brew made of magnolia leaves alleviates colic, indigestion, stomach pains, colds, chest congestions, and inflammations. The decoction of sassafras roots brings out spots in eruptive diseases, makes the patient perspire, helps anemia, prevents infections, and cleans blood. A drink prepared with boiled lizard's-tail leaves is used to treat colds, fevers, and colic and to relieve aching gums of teething babies. Sheep's tallow is recommended for problems with kidneys, stomach disorders, abscesses, chafed hands, and rheumatic pains. Whiskey camphré taken internally or applied externally helps stomach cramps, aching bones, headaches, earaches, cricks in the neck, and painful muscles. The juice or an infusion of roaches is good for colds, throat aches, and lockjaw.

Some of the old-time remedies are known by everybody and widely praised. Among them are the following: spider webs to stop bleeding; baking soda and vinegar for a wasp bite; quid of tobacco for insect bites; sassafras tea used as a tonic; whiskey camphré for sprains and cricks in the neck; garlic for worms; dew water for skin; grease of toads, rattlesnakes, or alligators for rheumatic pains; a little bag made of red flannel and filled with camphor or asafetida to ward off disease, brass or copper rings and bracelets to relieve rheumatism; a key on a string around a person's neck to stop a nosebleed.

The French settler brought with him from France and Nova Scotia quantities of domestic remedies transmitted to him from generation to generation. When he settled in Louisiana and became known as the Cajun,[6] he became acquainted with the local flora already used with great success in medical practice by the Indians, from whom he doubtlessly learned many a recipe. Literature reports that the Canadian French *voyageurs* and *coureurs de bois* who visited and often settled in Louisiana valued greatly the Indian's skills in the healing of wounds and chronic sores with poultices and herbs and considered their methods superior to those of the whites.[7] French travelers in Louisiana commented on the success of the Indians' medical treatments. Among them are Jean Bernard Bossu, who recorded his impressions in his *Travels in the Interior of North America, 1751-1762*, and Le Page du Pratz, author of the *History of Louisiana*, who spent several years in the colony in the first half of the eighteenth century. Both of these historians discussed the Indians' curing powers, of which they themselves were often the objects. It would be logical to suppose that a number of the medicines made of herbs and trees native to Louisiana were transmitted to the newcomers by the Indians. Parallels are easy to establish between the two groups, although no documented claims of Indian influences on the Frenchmen can be made at this time. "Louisiana Choctaws boiled the bark of Magnolia grandiflora in water and used the liquid to bathe the body to lessen or prevent itching due to prickly heat."[8] The Cajun uses the leaves of the same plant to apply to itching skin caused by poison oak. The Houmas[9] and the Cajuns found that a tea of magnolia leaves relieved cramps. Both of the groups knew how to make remedies for fevers from the ingredients of the willow: the Houmas made a brew of the roots and bark;[10] the Cajuns prepared a tea from the leaves. Sassafras tea was recommended by the Cajuns to clean the blood. The Choctaws "thinned their blood" by drinking the extract of the boiled roots of the same plant.[11] One of the most prevalent cures for earaches in both cultures was blowing tobacco smoke into the ear of the patient. To cure an abscess the Cajun applied a poultice of *gombo filé*, which is unquestionably an Indian contribution. From the dried leaves of sassafras the Louisiana Choctaws had learned to prepare a powder which became a part of the French cuisine in Louisiana. The powder, called gombo filé, is used to add flavor and give consistency to the famous Louisiana gumbo soup.[12]

The Indians were known to use steam and vapor as therapeutic means. By boiling leaves of the Carolina poplar, the Louisiana Choctaw created a steam for treating snakebites.[13] Reminiscent of these practices is a Louisiana method of healing a wound with the help of steam. An informant reports the following: "When you stick a nail into your foot, put red burning charcoal in a can, then put some tallow and sugar on this charcoal. This makes a steam and when it is hot enough, you have to put the sore foot above the can and leave it there as long as you can stand. The steam pulls out the poison of the sore."[14]

Some of the Indian remedies were passed on to the local population by the white "Indian doctor" who emerged thanks to the popularity of the Indian as a healer.[15] Some of these "Indian doctors" claimed to have learned their nostrums from their contacts with the natives; others maintained that they had absorbed the knowledge and practiced their art during Indian captivity. The popularity of these practitioners all over the United States can be attributed to their frequent advertising in the press, which saw the height of its development in the nineteenth century. Louisiana had several French newspapers in that period, and the notices of these self-proclaimed healers were often featured in them. In one of the issues of the *Courrier de la Louisiane* of 1826, a certain William W. Williams, "Indian doctor," claimed that after "a long intercourse with many different tribes of savages, and much practice . . . [he] gives relief in desperate cases, and when given up by other physicians."[16]

Supernatural elements figure prominently in Louisiana folk therapy. Magical formulas, occult symbolism, and protective amulets are used in preventive and healing traditional medicine. The sign of the cross made with a cat's tail over a sty will make the sty disappear. A toothache can be stopped by wearing a necklace of amber beads or touching the aching tooth with a nail that has not been used. Strings with three, five, or nine knots tied around any part of the body will protect the wearer and relieve his aches and pains. A string, preferably red, wrapped around the little finger will stop a nosebleed. Another remedy for the same affliction is to bury a butcher knife in the ground or wear a key on a string around one's neck. The hemorrhage can also be checked by putting an axe or a saw under the bed of the patient. A black chicken, cut into pieces, can be used with good effect on a snakebite. Two matches crossed on a person's head will rid him of a headache. A child's aching back can be cured in the following manner: an adult should lie down on the floor and have the child walk over his healthy back. If a child suffers from impetigo, somebody left-handed should be asked to hold the child in front of a cupboard door. The door should be opened and closed three times in front of the child. This will cure him.

Some illnesses can be cured by magic transferences. A toad put on one's head is supposed to heal a headache. When the toad dies, the head should stop hurting. In order to get rid of a fever, one should lie down on a heap of cool willow leaves. When the leaves become warm from the patient's fever, they should be thrown out. The fever is to pass on to the discarded leaves. A good remedy for a wound in the foot caused by a nail is to dip the nail in kerosene and then put it above the door; the foot will then stop hurting. The following method of transferring and plugging is suggested for the cure of a child's croup or asthma: "You measure the child next to a tree that grows. Make a hole with a drill just above the child's head and plug the hole with a lock of his hair. As soon as he grows higher than the hole the illness goes away."[17]

In Louisiana, like everywhere else, there is an abundance of supernatural cures for warts. They are supposed to disappear if one rubs them with a stolen dishrag. One can also get rid of them by taking grains of corn, sprinkling them with drops of blood extracted from the warts, and throwing them behind one's back without looking. Rubbing the warts with willow leaves, potatoes, meat, or peas and then burying these substances will make the warts disappear. If you want to transfer warts to someone else, take the string that was tied around the warts or one of the substances with which the warts were rubbed or cut off a piece of wart and then put one of these elements in a box or in a bag and throw it on the road. The warts will settle on the person who picks up the container.

Amulets of all kinds are worn by those who believe in their power. They are made of pecan nuts, alligator teeth, hog teeth, rattles of rattlesnakes, coins, beads of elderberries or chinaberries. These fetishes have the power to heal, protect, or ward off illness. Golden earrings worn in pierced ears cure sick eyes. A sty rubbed with a golden wedding ring will disappear. A red flannel bag filled with garlic or asafetida worn around the neck protects one from many diseases. A penny, dime, or other coin, as well as other charmed objects carried in a pocket or worn, will be an effective protection for the wearer.

A close survey of the field of folk medicine in lower Louisiana reveals three kinds of nonscientific practitioners who cure "natural" and "unnatural" illnesses. An unnatural illness is a disease that was inflicted by somebody claiming to possess magic powers, by a witch doctor or a conjurer, often called a "hoodoo-man" in Louisiana.

The first of the three groups of Louisiana practitioners is the *remède-man*, who treats natural ailments by means of herbs, domestic remedies, and patent medicines available in drugstores without prescription. The second category comprises the sympathy, spiritual, or faith healers, called *traiteurs*, who profess to have God-given powers to heal natural diseases by prayers and charms. To the third group belong practitioners who are supposed to have supernatural means of exercising their profession. They are the ones who inflict and treat unnatural diseases by casting spells and selling hoodoo bags, *gris-gris*,[18] and magic powders.

It is not always possible for an outsider or even a local inhabitant—or, for that matter, the patient himself—to distinguish clearly among these three categories because often a practitioner in one group may combine the methods and elements of treating used by the other two groups. Thus, the herb doctor may borrow from the occult and add to his ointment a charmed alligator tooth to wear, encroaching in this way on the domain of the conjurer. He may at times compete with a traiteur and say prayers while dispensing his botanical remedy. Here are two examples of this lack of delimitation of function of each group:

To cure a boil, he made with a knife a circle around it, said some words and gave the patient a black salve.[19]

I had a sister who suffered from headaches. She suffered all the time. The "traiteur" came and treated my sister. For headaches or for sunstroke he uses leaves of "lilas." He takes these leaves, crushes them and puts some salt, lots of salt, and then some crushed ice. He puts all that on the head. Then he touched the head and said the Lord's Prayer and the Hail Mary.[20]

A faith healer does not use any medicine at all. He treats ailments by magico-religious means. The only things he dispenses are sympathetic-magic objects that he has "treated" by himself, such as handkerchiefs; *cordons,* strings with three or nine knots; nails; or coins. The figure of this white Roman Catholic Cajun traiteur does not differ from the "powwow" healer in the Pennsylvania German communities, the "power doctor" in the Ozarks, or any other faith healer so often described in literature. A more detailed discussion of the Louisiana traiteur can be found elsewhere.[21] In this paper only one aspect of his activities will be considered: his charms.

The treating incantations of the faith healers are shrouded in secrecy and not easy to record. Through the graciousness of an informant, I was lucky to obtain a manuscript with thirteen charms, which were written down in 1907 by my informant's uncle, a known traiteur in Vermilion Parish. A study comparing the Louisiana charms with those of other areas shows striking parallelism. The formulas used in the study were recorded by various collectors in different periods in Britain;[22] in 1850 and circa 1910 in Berry, France;[23] and in the first quarter of the nineteenth century in Pennsylvania.[24]

Religion and magic mingle freely in the charms. Hand in hand go prayers, christological symbols, anointing and laying on of the hands, the presence of Christ, the Virgin Mary, and saints, together with cabalistic numbers and colors, the magic of alliteration, and circles.

The symbol of the cross is often encountered. This symbolism is found in a Pennsylvania charm as well as in some of the Louisiana magic formulas:

Pennsylvania: ". . . make three crosses over the place with the thumbs."

Louisiana: ". . . say this treatment with the thumbs folded in a cross."

Louisiana: "Say from the throat coming down with the hands in a cross."[25]

CURES FOR WORMS

The incantations are directed at the disease itself. Only the adjurations are cited.

1. Pennsylvania: "Worm I conjure thee by the living God that thou avoid this blood and this flesh."[26]
2. A Middle English charm: "I conjure thee little worm, by the Father and Son and Holy Spirit. . . ."[27]
3. A thirteenth-century English charm: "I adjure you, worms, in the name. . . ."[28]
4. Louisiana: "Worm of the heart of Nestor Guidry, I conjure you in the name of God of Jesus Christ and by the force of tears."[29]

The following group of charms has the use of cabalistic colors in common.

1. Berry, 1910, for ulcers in the mouth: "White ulcer, red ulcer, black ulcer, ulcer of all kinds, I summon you to come out of the mouth [name the person] as pure and as neat as our Lord Jesus Christ was born." Say five Lord's Prayers and five Hail Marys.[30]
2. An English cure for ringworm:

   > Ringworm white,
   > Ringworm red,
   > I command thou wilt not spread.
   > I divide thee to the east and west
   > Or the north and to the south.
   > Arise in the name of the Father, Son, and Holy Ghost.[31]

3. Louisiana, for a boil or carbuncle: Circle the boil nine times with a bit of fresh dirt and say: "Black carbuncle, red carbuncle, I conjure you to get out of the body of this person just like Jesus Christ came down from the Cross to go away to the Garden of Olives and not go away to rot in the ground."[32]

The first and the third charms use the mystic comparison between Christ and the sick which is one of the oldest types of parellelisms. All three charms are good illustrations of the practice of exorcism; there is animistic personification of the sickness, which is considered a malevolent entity, addressed by name, and implored to disappear by invoking the benevolent force, alone capable of conquering the evil.

CURES FOR BURNS

1. Berry, 1850: Saint Peter and Saint Paul are crossing a field of "garets." Saint Peter says to Saint Paul: "Whom do I hear crying?" Saint Paul says to Saint Peter: "It is your breath." Then blow three times.[33]

2. Berry, 1910: While passing on St. Blaise Street, Saint John said to our Savior: "Here is a child that is getting burned. Saint John, blow on this child three times." Say: "In the name of the Father and the Son and the Holy Ghost" and the child will get well.[34]

The reference to Saint Blaise is symbolic since this saint's name is often invoked on behalf of the sick, particularly those suffering from afflictions of the throat.

3. Sussex, England: One makes a sign of the cross over the wound and says:

> There came two angels from the north,
> One was Fire and one was Frost.
> Out Fire, in Frost,
> In the name of Father, Son, and Holy Ghost.[35]

4. England:

An angel came from the north,
And he brought cold and frost;
An angel came from the south,
And he brought heat and fire;
The angel came from the north
Put out the fire
In the name of the Father, and of the Son, and of the Holy Ghost.[36]

These two charms have been very popular all over Great Britain.

5. England:

> As I passed over the river Jordan, I met with Christ,
> He said, what aileth thee? Oh Lord, my flesh doth burn.
> The Lord said unto me, Two angels, etc.[37]

6. Pennsylvania: Our dear Lord Jesus went over the land; there he saw a burning brand . . .[38]

7. Pennsylvania: One lovely Sara goes through the land, with a fiery burning brand in her hand . . .[39]

8. Louisiana: Pass your hand over the burn and say nine times: "When Jacquot was crossing the sea someone told him: it kills fire, it kills frost, in the name of the Father and Son and the Holy Ghost."[40]

The Louisiana version combines the main elements which link the eight charms quoted. The Louisiana Jacquot is probably a substitution for Saint John. There is dynamism common to all the versions. In all of them biblical figures are in movement: going, coming, passing, crossing. There is either the idea of cooling off by blowing or the symbols of hot and cold, which are related to the ancient belief of the system of human humors. In his article on English charms, Thomas R. Forbes suggests that some of the charms for burns "give the impression that they were intended more to relieve the pain than heal."[41] The concept of cooling off by blowing seems to bear out this statement.

In the five charms that follow there is analogy of alliteration patter. The prayers are not quoted in the illustrations.

1. Berry, 1850, for a sprain: Say: "Ante, superante te."[42]
2. Berry, 1910, for a sprain: Say: "Pérantéranté, pérantéranté, antournis, antournas."[43]
3. Berry, 1850, for a cut: "Je t'ente, je te désente, je te rente."[44]
4. A Louisiana charm for a sprained back ends with the words: "Parenté, Fusenté."[45]
5. Louisiana, for a scratch: Say: "Je suis parent, parent, parent"; then say: "Je suis parenté, parenté, parenté."[46]

And, finally, I give examples of gibberish pertaining to dangerous bites, in Europe by rabid dogs, in America by snakes.

1. Berry, 1850: "Iram, quiram, caffram, caffrantem, fronsque, secretum, securit, securisit, securtït, seduit,"[47]
2. Yorkshire, England: To be written on an apple or a piece of fine white bread:

> O King of Glory, come in peace,
> Pax, Max, and Max,
> Hax, Max, Adinax, opera chudor.

To be swallowed three mornings fasting.[48]
3. England: Write upon a peece of bread, "Irioni, khiriora, esser, khuder, feres," and let it be eaten by the partie bitten.[49]
4. Herefordshire, England:

> Fuary, gary, nary,
> Gary, nary, fuary,
> Nary, fuary, gary.

Write this on a piece of cheese and give it to the Dog.[50]
5. A Pennsylvania charm ends with the expression "tzing, tzing, tzing," which may be interpreted as an onomatopoeic representation of the hissing of a snake.[51]

6. Louisiana: "Jom see jom jom jerat coq mah jom."[52]
7. Louisiana: "Tiame bomont, tiame faure, mon tiame mon seuron tiame."[53]

The gibberish included in the last group of charms results from mangled Latin words or phrases. This deformation is due to the faulty memory of some informants or to the misunderstanding or mispronouncing of others, while the process of oral transmission was going on. The examples suggest that in the case of a serious illness, such as a bite of a mad dog or a snake, Latin prayers were used to make the charm more effective. Many prayers and incantations are survivals of medieval times, when the church not only permitted but actually sponsored healing practices.

The most notorious of Louisiana practitioners is the group that deals in black magic. Most conjurers, apparently, are black, although some white ones are also known in the area. Many practices of the hoodoo-men stem from medieval European witchcraft, but to those were added voodoo elements brought to Louisiana by the slaves from Africa, as well as by the slaves and freemen of color from the West Indies, particularly from Haiti. For geographical, historical, economic, and cultural reasons, this voodoo influence has been felt more in Louisiana than anywhere else in the United States. The history of Louisiana records many dispensers of black magic, not only among men, but also among women, famous "voodoo queens." The best known among the latter was Marie Leveau, a free New Orleans mulatto who was a descendant of a long line of voodoo practitioners in Haiti. The hoodoo-men and the queens used to distribute for a price various fetishes, potions, and powders. The many powers attributed to these gris-gris included inflicting an illness or eradicating an enemy, as well as preventing and curing "unnatural" illnesses caused by a hex. The clients who used to avail themselves of the services of these practitioners were not all black; many adherents of this cult were white.

The conjurers are still around today, and voodoo activities in Louisiana, instead of dying out, have actually in recent years experienced a renaissance, which is attributed to the influence of hippie culture, with its obsession with fortune telling, astrology, candles, and incense burning. Voodoo rituals continue to exist and to influence the psyche as the health practices of those who believe in it. As in the past, many blacks as well as whites continue to fear the workings of magic and the gris-gris placed on their doorsteps, in the shrubs near their homes, or under their pillows. They believe that by casting a spell, a conjurer can cause a person a dreadful illness, can stop him from growing, can drive him insane or cause his death. The use of malevolent charms in the form of powders, amulets, or hoodoo bags is a daily occurrence in the life of the Louisianians who are addicted to it. The hoodoo bags, often called "sachets," are usually filled with various evil-emanating substances, such as graveyard dust; feathers; hairs from a cat or a horse; bones, nerves, or pieces of dried skin of vultures, lizards, or snakes; scrapings from fingernails; brick dust; dried weeds; teeth or fangs of a snake; a tail of a rat; dead flies; rusty nails, and so on. Fortunately for those who fear a hex, some of the practitioners are involved in fabricating benevolent gris-gris, which have the power of counteracting the evil and restoring the victim to health. Voodoo deaths still occur not only in Louisiana, but in other states as well.[54]

Many people live in constant fear of being conjured. In 1890 Louis Pendleton commented in his *Notes of Folk-lore and Witchcraft* on the condition of Negroes who became despondent and ill when they feared that they had been bewitched.[55] In an article on North Louisiana voodooism published in 1965, Hugh Brown describes the testimony of a sheriff who investigated the case of a Negro accused of the voodoo murder of his wife. During the interrogation the defendant conducted himself normally and was relaxed and coherent until the subject of voodoo came up; "then a coat of fear gripped him and he became too ill to answer the question."[56] Another case of existing fear is related by Bernice Webb in her 1973 study of voodoo mail-order advertising in Louisiana. A high school teacher of English in southwestern Louisiana brought to his class a black candle, which is believed by some to emanate an evil influence. He lit the candle and left it burning. As the candle burned, he observed that many of the students in his class displayed unusual nervousness.[57]

Preparations with underlying supernatural powers are dispensed not only by witch doctors, but also by drugstores and mail-order houses. Drugstores in major cities and smaller towns of Lower Louisiana are popular suppliers of voodoo items. In Houston, where many Louisianians settled, Bichon's Drugs, 412 Travis, is one of the outlets for these goods. An informant in Lafayette stated "that certain local stores have been advised by their headquarters to push voodoo products because of the readymade market waiting for them."[58] Mail-order houses list several categories of goods and preparations. One of the important groups is the "Botanical," which includes all parts of herbs used for voodoo products, although no claim is made for supernatural powers in any of the products featured. "Candle and Incense" is another important category, very popular today. "The Human Image" products play the most prominent role in the voodoo practices in Louisiana. Candles in the form of male and female human figures are one example of this group. Another important aspect are voodoo dolls that can be used for benevolent or malevolent practices. These dolls, handmade in Haiti and retailing from $2.50 up, can be had with pins and a sheet of instructions included. The pins are used to pierce the doll's body in the place where the sender wishes to inflict a wound on the enemy for whom the doll is a surrogate. The catalogs are mailed to Louisiana from such major cities as New York, Chicago, Philadelphia, Minneapolis, Houston, and Los Angeles.[59]

The attitude of doctors toward the traditional practitioners has been variably hostile, indifferent, or interested. Dr. E. LeRoy Hatch reports that his critical attitude and his zeal in presenting folk medicine to his patients as fallacious and inconsistent brought only negative results, while his associate was much more successful with his positive attitude: "With a straight face and apparent attention he would listen to their explanations of cause and cure. Complimenting them for their sagacity, he would then prescribe the necessary treatment, allowing them to continue with their superstitions and nostrums when these were not detrimental to the patient."[60]

The statement of Dr. Hewitt L. Ballowe, author of *Creole Folktales*, who practiced medicine all his life among the Delta Louisianians, is worth repeating: "There are plenty of things I can't understand. One is the power of these people. I've seen them bring about what looked like cures in cases I thought doomed. According to the test-tube analysis, the patients could not live. But they did."[61] Harnett Kane reports how Dr. Ballowe solved the problems of competition with the folk doctors: "He always got along with the remède people, he observes. 'I'm not narrowminded. I told 'em to do their work, I'd do mine; and let the best man win.' Finding a voodoo bag under a pillow, he did not harangue. 'Let's try my stuff, too,' he suggested. The workers with prayers and strings appreciated his viewpoint."[62] Many physicians have manifested their hostile attitude toward the practices of nonscientific healers and have been fighting them openly. "Doctors give lots of trouble to 'traiteurs,' said an informant. "Often the doctors will get together with the State to accuse the 'traiteurs' of practicing medicine illegally."[63]

In recent years there has been a surge of interest in the activities of folk healers and a desire to learn more about folk medicine. Don Yoder points out in his 1971 study that traditional medicine is no longer viewed as a sideshow at a country fair and no longer considered a mere superstition by the educated public. Scholars have started to take traditional medicine more seriously and to view it as a part of the whole cultural background of a people. The function of folk medicine and its relation to the culture of an ethnic group have been recognized. The psychological value in psychosomatic medicine, in community medicine, and in psychiatry is being surveyed presently on national and international levels.[64]

Studies published recently by medical personnel in Louisiana point in the same direction. These studies lead to a better understanding of what causes patients to seek help from folk practitioners and of the psychology of patients who ultimately come to physicians for help. Dr. Wiedorn states that a field investigation, such as he has completed, is of great interest to the doctor, since "it allows for the study of active and widely supported folk medicine as well as the basic emergent processes of a primitive psychotherapy and psychiatric technique." His clinical experience with psychotic healers reveals some techniques of psychological healing which "may throw some light on the problems and processes in modern psychotherapy" and primitive folk therapy.[65]

Considering the fact that folk medicine as practiced in Louisiana influences the population and has implications in public nursing, Julie Yvonne Webb, having done field research, feels strongly that future nurses and health workers should get acquainted with the folk medicine of the region in which they intend to practice. She calls for a study of local traditional health practices to evaluate which ones are helpful or harmless and which ones are damaging. Since the influence of voodoo on peoples' attitudes toward their diseases persists, workers in the health field should know what the practices of voodoo are in order to understand the patients better. Doctors should be more lenient in accepting harmless practices in order to be in a position to counteract the dangerous ones and to introduce modern health ideas and methods. If superstitions and unsafe voodoo practices found in each locality were described and explained to various health workers during their in-service programs, the health education and public health services of the state would be greatly improved.[66]

The same intentions underlie the modern attitudes of certain churchmen. Yoder comments on it as follows:

> Since World War II, also, there has been significant growth of "faith healing" under the aegis of the established, organized religions of the United States. . . .[67]

At the same time, seminary education is including studies of the relation of religion to medicine, and offering widened programs in pastoral counseling, the native ecclesiastical form of psychotherapy. The significance of these movements is that they are attempting to return religious healing, for those who want it, to organized religion.[68]

The desire to understand better the workings of voodoo is also a part of this renewed interest of the Church in folk practices. In a recent article entitled "Brazil's Voodoo Religions Prompt Study by Catholics" in the *Houston Post* of October 19, 1973, this attitude is clearly stated. It is calculated that some 60 million Brazilians actively practice African-based voodoo religions. Father Raimundo Cintra, a Roman Catholic priest who teaches religious history at Rio de Janeiro's Catholic University thinks that the Catholic Church should study voodoo and says: "We're interested in utilizing voodoo's positive aspects so our church can take better care of the people's needs."

It is hoped that this interest of scientific and religious scholars will grow and bear fruit. Fieldwork and a better insight into the positive and negative aspects of folk medicine and voodoo should contribute to the increased ability of doctors to understand and treat their patients. As a result, the confidence of the sick in the organized medical profession will be strengthened and will help to stamp out the harmful practices of witchcraft, which are still dominating the lives of a large segment of our population.

APPENDIX

Ce livre appartient à Nestor Guidry et acheté le 25 avril in 1907

1. *Le traitement de charbon*

Le cerner neuf fois avec un morceau de terre fraîche et dire: "Charbon noir, charbon rouge, je te conjure de sortir du corps de cette personne tel que Jésus Christ a descendu de l'arbre de la Croix pour s'en aller au jardin des Oliviers et *ni au dame* [?] s'en aller pourir en terre."

2. *Le traitement d'érysipèle*

Le cerner trois fois et dire: "A nom du Père et du Fils et du Saint (Esprit)" et faire six croix dessur et dire les mêmes choses.

3. *Le traitement du poireau*

Pointer le poireau neuf fois avec le doigt et dire: "Pique poireau."

4. *Le traitement de mal d'oreille*

Mettre le doigt dans l'oreille jusque l'avoir conjurée et dire cinq fois le Notre Père et le Salue Marie et dire trois fois: "Saint Nestor Guidry, Grand Dieu vivant, mon Patron, chassez ce cruel mal que Saint un tel *sens* [?] a occasionné par le froid ou par le vent ou par l'air, je te conjure par la parole de Jésus Christ, je te conjure par la parole de Jésus Christ, je te conjure par la parole de Jésus Christ" et redire cinq fois le Notre Père et le Salue Marie.

5. *Le traitement de brulûre*

Passer la main sur la brûlure et dire neuf fois: "Jacquot en traversant la mer on lui dit elle tue le tison ou la gelée au nom du Père et du Fils et du Saint Esprit."

6. *Le traitement de sang*

Dire cinq fois le Notre Père et le Salue Marie et dire: "Sang de Saint Nestor Guidry, arrête comme tu étais auparavant et je te conjure par la parole de Jésus Christ" trois fois et redire cinq fois le Notre Père et le Salue Marie et dire le traitement avec les pouces en croix.

7. *Le traitement de ver*

Dire de la gorge en descendant avec les mains en croix de trois à neuf fois: "Ver de coeur de Nestor Guidry, je vous conjure au nom de Dieu de Jésus Christ et par la force de larmes." Le Notre Père après et dire les mêmes choses avec le Salue Marie après.

8. *Le traitement de serpent*

Dire en croix: "Tiame bomont tiame faure mon tiame mon seuron tiame" et faire le traitement neuf fois sur le mal.

9. *Le traitement de repoulure*
[*éraflure, chaboulure?*]

Faire neuf croix sur le mal et dire: "Je suis parent, je suis parent, je suis parent" et dire: "Je suis parenté, je suis parenté, je suis parenté" et faire neuf croix sur le mal.

10. *Le traitement de mal d'oreille*

Mettre les mains sur les oreilles et dire: "Douleur inconnue de Nestor Guidry, je te conjure au nom de Dieu de Jésus Christ et par la force de larmes," après le Notre Père et dire les mêmes choses avec le Salue Marie et faire le traitement de trois à neuf fois.

11. *Le traitement de fontanelle*

"Fontanelle de Nestor Guidry, sois comme tu étais, je te conjure au nom de Dieu de Jésus Christ" et dire à travers de la tête au nom du Père et du Fils et du Saint [Esprit] et faire le traitement de trois à neuf fois.

12. *Le traitement de boureille*
[*bourrier?*]

Passer la main dessus neuf fois et dire: "Notre Seigneur Jésus Christ, passez y la main avant que j'y passe la mienne."

13. *La prière pour rêver*

Dire trois fois: "Je tire la raison du Saint Antoine pour voir qui a tracassé Nestor Guidry" et dire une fois: "Je demande de me faire rêver à mon désir" et dire cinq fois le Notre Père et le Salue Marie.[69]

NOTES

1. William S. Wiedorn, Jr., "Psychotherapeutic-like Technique in Folk Medicine," *Louisiana Folklore Miscellany*, 3 (1958), 20.

2. Julie Yvonne Webb, "Louisiana Voodoo and Superstitions Related to Health," *HSMHA Health Reports*, 4 (1971), 300.

3. Mrs. Gaston Hebert. "Mamou": coral tree (Erythrina Herbacea); "laurier": magnolia (Magnolia Grandiflora).

4. Mrs. Henry Saltzman.

5. Mr. Edgar Boudreaux.

6. *Cajun*: deformation of the word *Acadien*, pertaining to the French people who settled in Louisiana in the years 1764-1785, after their dispersion from Nova Scotia, then called "Acadie."

7. Virgil J. Vogel, *American Indian Medicine* (Norman: University of Oklahoma Press, 1970), p. 116.

8. *Ibid.*, p. 334.

9. *Ibid.*

10. *Ibid.*, p. 393.

11. *Ibid.*, p. 365.

12. *Ibid.*, pp. 364-365.

13. *Ibid.*, p. 255, pp. 351-352.

14. Mrs. Edna Solomon quoting her grandmother's cure.

15. Vogel, *op. cit.*, p. 123.

16. *The Rudolph Matas History of Medicine in Louisiana*, ed. John Duffy (Baton Rouge: Louisiana State University Press, 1962), II, 40.

17. Mrs. Edna Solomon.

18. *Gris-gris*: French word of West African origin meaning fetish or magic charm. In Louisiana it also means a hex or a spell. *Gris-gris* is often used as a synonym for "hoodoo" bag or malevolent charm.

19. Mr. Alphonse Moore, describing a folk doctor's treatment.

20. Mrs. Henry Saltzman. "Lilas": chinaberry tree (Melia azedarach).

21. Elizabeth Brandon, "'Traiteurs' or Folk Doctors in Southwest Louisiana," in *Buying the Wind*, ed. Richard M. Dorson (Chicago: University of Chicago Press, 1964), pp. 261-266.

22. William Henderson, *Notes on the Folk-Lore of the Northern Counties of England and the Borders* (Nendeln, Liechtenstein: Kraus Reprint Limited, 1967). Thomas R. Forbes, "Verbal Charms in British Folk Medicine," *Proceedings of the American Philosophical Society*, 4 (1971), 293-316.

23. Léonard Saint-Michel, "Un petit Formulaire de Médecine occulte découvert en Berry est toujours en usage," *Connaître* (Cahiers de l'Humanisme médical, Folklore et Médecine), 11 (1948), 21-24.

24. John George Hohman, "The Long Hidden Friend," ed. Carleton F. Brown, *Journal of American Folklore*, 17 (1904), 89-152.

25. *Ibid.*, p. 110, no. 23. Louisiana, nos. 6 and 7. The items of the Louisiana collection of charms, included in the Appendix, will be identified by number.

26. *Ibid.*, p. 116, no. 63.

27. Forbes, *op. cit.*, p. 312, no. 170.

28. *Ibid.*, no. 172.

29. Louisiana, no. 7.

30. Saint-Michel, *op. cit.*, p. 23.

31. Forbes, *op. cit.*, p. 308, no. 131.

32. Louisiana, no. 1.

33. Saint-Michel, *op. cit.*, pp. 21-22.

34. *Ibid.*, p. 23.

35. Henderson, *op. cit.*, p. 171.

36. Forbes, *op. cit.*, p. 301, no. 70.

37. *Ibid.*, no. 71.

38. Hohman, *op. cit.*, p. 131, no. 144.

39. *Ibid.*, p. 121, no. 122.

40. Louisiana, no. 5.

41. Forbes, *op. cit.*, p. 301.

42. Saint-Michel, *op. cit.*, p. 21.

43. *Ibid.*, p. 23.

44. *Ibid.*, p. 21.

45. Edward J. Kammer, *A Socio-economic Survey of the Marsh-Dwellers of Four Southeastern Louisiana Parishes* (Washington, D.C.: The Catholic University of America Press, 1941), p. 142.

46. Louisiana, no. 9.

47. Saint-Michel, *op. cit.*, p. 21.

48. Henderson, *op. cit.*, p. 179.

49. Forbes, *op. cit.*, p. 299, no. 38.

50. *Ibid.*, no. 41.

51. Hohman, *op. cit.*, p. 116.

52. Kammer, *op. cit.*, p. 143.

53. Louisiana, no. 8.

54. Webb, *op. cit.*, p. 293.

55. Louis Pendleton, "Notes of Negro Folk-lore and Witchcraft in the South," *Journal of American Folklore*, 3 (1890), 204.

56. Hugh S. Brown, "Voodooism in Northwest Louisiana," *Louisiana Folklore Miscellany*, 2 (1965), 86.

57. Bernice Larson Webb, "A Study of Voodoo Mail-Order Advertising in Louisiana," *Louisiana Review*, 2 (1973), 68.

58. *Ibid.*, p. 65.

59. *Ibid.*, pp. 65, 67, 68, 70, 71.

60. E. LeRoy Hatch, M.D., "Home Remedies Mexican Style," *Western Folklore*, 3 (1969), 163.

61. Harnett T. Kane, *Deep Delta Country* (New York: Duell, Sloan and Pearce, 1944), p. 246.

62. *Ibid.*, p. 245.

63. Mr. Alphonse Moore.

64. Don Yoder, "Folk Medicine," in *Folklore and Folklife*, ed. Richard Dorson (Chicago: University of Chicago Press, 1972), p. 211.

65. William S. Wiedorn, Jr., *op. cit.*, p. 13.

66. Julie Yvonne Webb, *op. cit.*, p. 300.

67. Yoder, *op. cit.*, p. 210.

68. *Ibid.*, p. 211.

69. These thirteen charms in the Appendix are transcribed in correct French from a photocopy of a handwritten collection of charms made in 1907. The copy was too indistinct to reproduce. For more information see p. 222.

Hohman and Romanus: Origins and Diffusion of the Pennsylvania German Powwow Manual

DON YODER, *University of Pennsylvania*

Occult folk medicine is the type that makes use of charms, formulas, spells, conjurations, and blessings in the attempt to heal the ills of man and of beast.[1] In the European and American practice of folk medicine, the formulas used are in most cases ancient in origin and are related to the word-magic of primitive as well as complex cultures in all parts of the world. The formulas have been transmitted to the present generation of healers by traditional means, by the direct channel of oral tradition passed from one practitioner to another, by the side channel of printed as well as manuscript charm books, or by the combined method of written word plus oral instruction as techniques are passed from one generation to the next.

The problem with which this paper deals is that of determining the immediate European sources of the standard printed American charm collection. It is not our purpose to review the European scholarship on the remote origins of individual charms nor to trace their transit in European cultures.[2] Our material is derived from the Pennsylvania German culture, where occult folk medicine—called in Pennsylvania German dialect *Brauche* or *Braucherei*[3] and in English "powwowing"[4]—has existed widely since the seventeenth- and eighteenth-century emigration from the German-language areas of central Europe to colonial Pennsylvania. Powwowing, as it is commonly known today, has existed in urban as well as rural contexts down to the present time.[5]

Since 1820 a standard printed corpus of magical charms has

existed for the Pennsylvania Germans, a book entitled *Der lang verborgene Freund*, published in Reading, Pennsylvania, by a German emigrant named John George Hohman. This book has been reprinted in numerous German editions, in toto, and in pirated collections under slightly varying titles. It has been twice translated into English, and a double chain of English versions has come down to the present time from the two independent translations. These were (1) *The Long Lost Friend* (Harrisburg, 1856), and (2) *The Long Hidden Friend* (Carlisle, 1863).

The commonly "received" edition today, published in cheap paperback and sold along with dream books and horoscopic literature under or over the counter at many bookstores (even at the University of Pennsylvania bookstore for my own students) is the Harrisburg English translation. The Carlisle edition went through several later printings. It was also spotlighted by its use in two scholarly articles: (1) Carleton F. Brown, ed., "The Long Hidden Friend by John George Hohman," *The Journal of American Folk-Lore* 17 (1904), 89-152, and (2) Robert Byington, "Powwowing in Pennsylvania," *Keystone Folklore Quarterly* 9 (1964), 111-117. The Harrisburg edition has been reprinted not only in Pennsylvania, but also in Maryland, New York, Illinois, and elsewhere; it is, as I have stated, still in print and, obviously, still in use.

Hohman is in several ways, intentionally or unintentionally, a mystery man, one of the most influential and yet most elusive figures in Pennsylvania German history.[6] He appeared in Pennsylvania in 1802, when he landed at Philadelphia on October 12 on a Hamburg vessel with his wife and son Philip. According to nineteenth-century documentation, he and his wife served for several years as redemptioners to pay their passage. Soon, however, Hohman's name began to appear on broadsides of both an occult and literary nature. For the rest of his life, until 1846, when he disappeared from the scene, we have a stream of print—books, pamphlets, chapbooks, and broadsides—issuing from his pen. These include the first printed American version of the *Himmelsbrief*, or "Letter from Heaven";[7] an extensive book on household medicine (1818);[8] the most complete edition of New Testament apocrypha published for the Pennsylvania Germans (1819);[9] the powwow book (1820); and various ballads and spiritual songs, some of which he himself composed or amended.[10] During the time of his broadside peddling, he seems to have lived near Reading, in Rosenthal (Rose Valley) in Alsace Township, where he presumably farmed on a small plot and eked out a meager existence with his publications. In his expansive foreword to the book, he underlines his "compassion for my suffering fellow-men" which led him to publish and asks the reader rhetorically "Do I not deserve the rewards of God for it? . . . Besides I am a poor man in needy circumstances, and it is a help to me if I can make a little money with the sale of my books."

Hohman himself was a practitioner of occult folk healing, as witnessed by the twelve testimonials from individuals, named and in some cases with addresses, from Bucks and Berks counties, Pennsylvania, whom he claims to have cured from "wheal in the eye," ulcer, sore mouth, burns, "wild fire," headache, convulsions, and other ailments. His preface also gives a lengthy defense of his book and similar books on the grounds that they provide cures for many ailments which medical doctors have failed to help. His defense emphasizes the religious underpinnings of occult healing—the healing is "done by the Lord."[11] He also rejects the common tendency of compilers of occult literature to remain anonymous or to indulge in pseudepigraphic subterfuge: "I sell my books publicly, and not secretly, as other mystical works are sold. I am willing that my books should be seen by everybody, and I shall not secrete or hide myself from any preacher. I, Hohman, too, have some knowledge of the Scriptures, and I know when to call and pray unto the Lord for assistance."[12] And finally he places himself "upon the broad platform of the liberty of the press and of conscience, in regard to this useful book, and it shall ever be my most heartfelt desire that all men might have an opportunity of using it to their good, in the name of Jesus."

After his final book was published in 1846,[13] Hohman disappeared from the Pennsylvania scene; so we know neither where he came from in Europe before his emigration in 1802 nor where he died in America after the publication of the final book in 1846. But between these dates he published more influential printed materials for the folk religion and folk medicine of the Pennsylvania Germans than any other individual.

Hohman calls himself "author and original publisher of this book" and adds that he himself "could take an oath at any time upon the fact of his having successfully applied many of the prescriptions contained herein." Although the book is commonly ascribed to Hohman by those who have not studied it carefully, he was simply compiler, as he himself admits at the close of his section of "Testimonials": "This book is partly derived from a work published by a Gypsey, and partly from secret writings, and collected with much pain and trouble, from all parts of the world, at different periods, by the author, John George Hohman."

No one has yet pointed out the European sources for Hohman's book. One of its principal sources was the German-language charm book called the *Romanusbüchlein*,[14] the earliest known edition of which appeared at Glatz in Silesia in southeastern Germany (now in Poland) in 1788, only fourteen years before Hohman's emigration. In the nineteenth-century the book spread widely until it became the leading charm collection for the German-speaking countries of Europe, where it is still in print and in use.

If one takes the trouble to number Hohman's charms and lay them out comparatively—synoptically, to use the word from the textual criticism of the Bible—we find that Hohman borrowed long sections of Romanus, copying them with almost no textual change. He did not simply borrow individual charms and rescramble the Romanus order; he lifted long sections of charms and published them in the same order as Romanus. For example, Hohman 118 is identical with Romanus 1, H119 = R7, H122 = R9, H123 = R6, H127 = R5, H128-147 = R10-29, H148 = R25, H149-165 = R30-46, H166 = R48, H167-175 = R47-56, H176 = R58, H177 = R61, H179 = R62, H180 = R60, H182 = R59, H183-184 = R63-64, H186-187 = R65-66, and H189 = R2. Of Hohman's total of 189 charms, the Romanus component involves 60 charms, or approximately one-third of the total.

The additional charms have been brought together from other sources, including Albertus Magnus and several American works. Hohman's book is a kind of popular catchall with the focus on folk healing, but it extends in one direction into ritual magic—how to charm guns, catch fish, stop thieves—and in the other direction into practical household hints on such things as dyeing; how to destroy worms in beehives; how to make soap powder, curing salves, diarrhea remedies, and others. In addition there is a fourth category—long, prayerlike charms, actually benedictions, for the protection of house and individual.[15]

> The Holy Trinity guard me, and be and remain with me on the water and upon the land, in the water or in the fields, in cities or villages, in the whole world wherever I am.

The same benediction asks the Trinity to protect against enemies, imprisonment, assault, and wounds from firearms.

Although Hohman's book standardized the charm repertory for many powwowers, there preceded it in the colonial period and existed alongside it for generations an independent or related manuscript charm book tradition in which individual powwowers preserved variants of Hohman's charms or additional charms which they preferred to use instead of Hohman. This body of charm tradition, some of which has come down to the present time, was, so to speak, the "minority report" on powwowing, while *The Long Lost Friend* became the "majority report."

Occasionally the manuscript charm literature provides us with valuable insights into the Hohman collection. My favorite example is one of Hohman's cures for snakebite:

To Cure the Bite of a Snake

God has created all things and they were good;
Thou only, serpent, art damned,
Cursed be thou and thy sting.

* * *

Zing, zing, zing!

The manuscript charms provide an alternate reading for the "Zing, zing, zing":

und gott had alles erschaffen, was im himmel und auf erden ist, und alles war gud, nichts als allein die schlange hat gott verflucht, verflucht solst du bleiben, schlangen, geschwülst ich stelle dich, gift und schmerz ich döde dich, zian dein güft, zian dein güft, zian dein güft, amen X X X

REGINA SELZSER 1 8 3 7[16]

[And God created everything that was in heaven and upon earth, and everything was good, except that God cursed the serpent. Cursed shalt thou remain, O serpent. Swelling, I still thee, poison and pain, I kill thee. Draw thy poison, draw thy poison, draw thy poison! Amen, in the name of God the Father, God the Son, and God the Holy Ghost.

Regina Selzser 1837.]

The rationale here is similar to that of certain types of primitive medicine. The healer begins with a narrative statement about the Creation and the cursing of the serpent from his part in the Fall of Man in Eden.[17] Next the healer addresses the serpent directly and reinforces the curse by repeating it. Then, after addressing the symptoms and the wound which the snake has caused, the serpent is again directly addressed and ordered to draw back its poison (*zieh an dein Gift*). It is of course possible that "Zing, zing, zing" was the original form, and that "zieh an dein Gift" was an early "conjectural emendation."[18]

An analysis of the manuscript charm literature provides not only information on the texts of the Hohman charms, but also information on alternate procedures and beliefs associated with the way the powwow charm was thought to work. The ending of the charms, which frames the healing situation with powerful Christian symbolism, making the charm in a sense into a prayer, involves what Pennsylvania Germans refer to as "the three highest names"—the trinitarian formula "In the name of God the Father, God the Son, and God the Holy Ghost." Occasionally Hohman ends his charms with a direct blessing which focuses the efficacy of the charm upon the patient, whose name is then repeated as part of the charm. From my interviewing of powwow doctors of the twentieth century, I find that they use Hohman's charms and after the trinitarian formula add the phrase "help to this"; then they give the baptized name of the patient and close the charm with an amen.[19]

Among my own collection of Pennsylvania German manuscript powwow booklets are several that provide both materials parallel to Hohman's charms and, as I said above, insights into the beliefs about how powwow medicine "worked." One of these is the "Ohl Family Account Book," used to record the settling of the estate of Andrew Ohl of Northampton County, Pennsylvania, 1808-1812. In the back of the little homemade booklet are thirteen powwow charms from the same period. What makes these charms different from Hohman's is the fact that the practitioner added at the end of each charm the words "Dass zehl ich dir zur wahrer bus X X X," "This I credit unto thee as true penance—in the name of God the Father, God the Son, and God the Holy Ghost." In this case one senses echoes of the healings attributed to Christ in the New Testament where he told the person whom he healed, "Thy sins are forgiven thee."[20] And in a wider context we can see here the relation of folk medicine to the concepts of sin and guilt, confession, forgiveness, absolution, even redemption.

In a lengthy article on the relation of religion and healing,[21] Paul Tillich points out that in every one of the great traditions that lie at the base of Western civilization, healing was integrally related to salvation. Salvation, like healing, restores broken unities. This is reflected linguistically in the identity of the words for health, healing, and salvation in several European languages, for one example *Heil, heilen,* and *Heiland* in German. Our English word *health* derives from the concept of "wholeness" and is cognate with the German *Heil*. We sense touches of this earlier, almost universal identification of health, wholeness, and salvation not only in folk versions of Christianity, but even on the official levels of Christianity. Examples include the ancient references to the Eucharist as the "medicine of immortality" and the phrase in the King James Version of the Bible (1611) used in connection with the healings attributed to Christ: "Thy faith hath made thee whole."

Among the large shelf of occult literature used by the Pennsylvania Germans, the only other major volume besides Hohman that may have been indigenous to Pennsylvania German culture is the curious volume *Dr. G. F. Helfenstein's vielfältig erprobter Hausschatz der Sympathie; oder, Enthüllte Zauberkräfte und Geheimnisse der Natur.* This was published in 1853 at Harrisburg, Pennsylvania, by Scheffer and Beck in a joint edition, consecutively paged, with Hohman's *Der lang verborgene Freund.* In this relatively rare and obscure volume, which has not been analyzed before, the Hohman book takes up pages 1-74, and the Helfenstein charms, pages 75-108. Like Hohman, Helfenstein underscores the religious roots of his book. On the title page he cites Mark 11:22-24 and adds, "These are very useful writings for a Christian to have in his house," since, he points out (as Hohman did), keeping the book in one's house will provide protection from fire and sickness.

The foreword gives a brief biography of the "compiler," Georg Friedrich Helfenstein, who says that he was born of poor parents in 1730 in Rotterdam. In his ninth year his wealthy cousin, Carl August Helfenstein, took him to raise and later sent him to the university, where he studied medicine. At the age of twenty-one he returned to Rotterdam, where he took up the practice of medicine. Coming in contact with a "sympathy doctor," he learned to "heal the sick with words, as Christ the Lord had done," the healer teaching him the *Geheimnisse der Sympathie.*[22] The "doctor" recommends this method to his readers, brethren and sisters, but cautions them to "make no misuse of these formulas, but only in the name of and firm trust in the Holy Trinity." His formulas are accompanied with sympathetic gestures—stroking with the hand three times, stroking crosswise with the hand, the use of spittle, blowing three or nine times, the laying on of hands. Helfenstein also increases the power by naming the baptismal name of the patient seven times. This rubbing or stroking is prescribed for animals as well as humans.[23] Helfenstein, like Hohman, peppers his text with a few household hints—for one example: to keep flies out of the house, hang a wolf's tail on the house. For inflammation of the eyes he prescribes the juice crushed out of quince seeds and for whooping cough in children, a salve of garlic and lard.

At the end of his book, as he takes polite leave of his reader, Helfenstein again urges him to remember that this book was writ-

ten, not for profit (correcting Hohman here), but out of philan-
thropy and is intended for the good of man and beast. His reader
will find it, he predicts, "a precious treasure, a jewel, that is better
than silver and gold. . . . I am fully convinced that you will not
regret it but it will make you great joy and you will consider it as a
house friend, a savior in dangers, a refuge in pain and suffering, a
consoler of body and soul." And as he bids his "dear reader" a final
farewell, he commends him to the protection and assistance of the
Holy Trinity.

Several editions of Helfenstein also appeared printed on separate sheets of paper, one charm per page and on only one side of
the sheet. Some of these have turned up kept in homemade tin or
paper boxes for protection and special honor. In some cases these
individual sheets have been bound together into a sixty-eight-page
booklet. These are extremely rare. It is possible that some of the
individual pages were used as amulets in powwow healing, as the
book itself was.

In 1976 I will be publishing a complete translation and analysis
of the Helfenstein volume, after collating each charm with the
available charm literature. As to the identity of the compiler, I am
inclined at present to doubt the authenticity of the foreword and
treat it as fictional, although I have written to archives in both the
Netherlands and West Germany for any possible identification of a
Dr. G. F. Helfenstein and for evidence of prior publication of the
volume in Europe. There was, of course, a distinguished Helfenstein family of Reformed ministers in Pennsylvania, and a Judge
Helfenstein of Northumberland County, in which area, curiously
enough, the current English version of the Helfenstein book has
appeared.[24]

In addition to Hohman and Helfenstein, there was a whole shelf
of occult books published for the Pennsylvania German trade
which were used by powwow doctors and other occult practitioners. For example, the first American edition of the folk medical
book known as *Albertus Magnus* or *Egyptische Geheimnisse* [Egyptian
secrets] appeared in German in Pennsylvania in 1842. The title is
*Albertus Magnus bewährte und approbirte sympathetische und natürliche
egyptische Geheimnisse für Menschen und Vieh*. This volume, which
often appears under the false imprint "Braband," is divided into
four books and includes magical as well as folk medical materials.
An English edition from which the present trade editions are
derived made its appearance in Harrisburg, Pennsylvania, in
1875.[25]

The first American edition of the much-feared and mysterious volume *The Sixth and Seventh Books of Moses*[26] also appeared first in German in Pennsylvania and now, like Hohman, is available in English. It consists of Christianized cabbalistic plates and circles, which use the mystical names of God and the archangels, and a treatise on the medical uses of the Psalms.[27] This book was for the occult specialist, the witch doctor rather than the ordinary powwower, and was much feared by the common people, who warned each other against reading it lest, as they said, "one read oneself fast."

One of the most curious of the smaller powwow books to appear in Pennsylvania is *Der Freund in der Noth; oder, Geheime Sympathetische Wissenschaft, welche nie zuvor im Druck erschienen.*[28] The title page bears the legend *Aus dem Spanischen übersetzt* and bears the false imprint and date *Gedruckt in der Calender-Fabrike, zu Offenbach, am Mayn, in Deutschland, auf Ansuchung eines Tyrolers, 1790.* It is obviously a Pennsylvania imprint and after 1800. A copy which I have, much chewed by mice in a Pennsylvania attic but otherwise intact, bears the following mystifying preface on the provenance of the book:

> The following secret remedies were taken from an old Spanish manuscript, which was found at an old hermit's who for over a hundred years had lived in a cave in the dark valleys of the Graubünden land, performing in the same region many wondrous works, among others totally expelling from said regions the monstrous dragon with four young, which dwelt upon those very fearsome mountains in Unterwalden—as indeed one can read in his legend which was published at Freyburg in Ichtland by Hans von Leixner in the year 1752.

Like Hohman's book, this little twenty-four-page collection combines medical cures with magical charms. The usual range of the latter is from stopping thieves to charming guns and extinguishing fire. It includes the SATOR-formula with *S* instead of *N* in the central square and adds that these twenty-five letters represent "the song which the three men, Shadrach, Meschach and Abednego sang, whom King Nebuchadnezzar had cast into the fiery furnace." Whoever carries this "song" with him or has it in his house will avoid any harm to house or person.[29]

The European collection of blessings *Ein schöner und wohl approbirter Heil. Seegen Zu Wasser und Land, Wider Alle seine Feinde, so ihm begegnen auf allen Wegen und Stegen* frequently turns up in Pennsylvania German book collections. It is a composite of various blessings, including (1) *Eine schöne Offenbahrung, so Christus denen H.H.H. drey Frauen, Elizabeth, Brigitta und Mechtildis mündlich geoffenbahret,*[30] (2) the *Geistlicher Schild,*[31] (3) the *Geistliche Schild-Wacht,*[32] and (4) *Das*

Gebet Manasse.[33] The many copies that I have examined in Pennsylvania are all in miniature or pocket format, bear the license of the censor of the Archbishop of Trier (the edition which was popular in the Palatinate and adjoining regions), and say on the title page "Gedruckt zu Wien, in Oesterreich." This may be so, but more probably it is a false imprint, and there is a possibility that the little book was even reprinted in Pennsylvania.

There is in occult folk medicine no distinction between human and veterinary medicine. As in the case of the household medical books, occult charms appear in the Pennsylvania German veterinary manuals alongside natural cures. One example is Isaac Leib's *Wohlerfahrner Pferde-Arzt; enthaltend Mittel für die Heilung aller bekannten und verschiedenartigen Krankheiten und Seuchen der Pferde; welche nach einer fünf und zwanzigjährigen Ausübung der Ross-Heilkunst bewährt und untrüglich befunden wurden* (Lebanon, 1842). This includes several examples of word-magic, among them this one for blood stopping:

> If anyone comes and asks you to stop blood, ask him who owns the animal, then go alone to one side and say the charm:
> Three holy virgins went walking. The one is bleeding, the second is dropping, and the third is stopping. In the beginning was the Word, and the Word was with God, and the Word was God; the same was in the beginning with God, and by the same Word we command that all veins must stop which are now bleeding, i.e., with the three high holy names.

This provides evidence on the use of name-magic in healing animals. Evidently, instead of using the animal's name, the practitioner makes use of the owner's name.

What conclusions can be drawn from this brief survey of the occult literature of the Pennsylvania Germans?

1. The Pennsylvania German occult literature forms an important chapter, a transatlantic chapter, in the diffusion of the occult literature of German-speaking central Europe. Not only was it important for Pennsylvania, but through the Pennsylvania German diaspora it was diffused into the South, the Middle West, and Ontario. In addition it may have reached Louisiana; there is the possibility that it reached certain areas of the Caribbean (through contacts set up via the Moravian missions); and there is evidence that it blended with Negro conjuring traditions in the Border States, particularly Maryland.

2. When analyzed, the materials transmitted in this literature can provide us with guidelines for determining the intersection

points between religion and medicine, an area of interface which deserves much more serious study among the European cultures in the United States than it has formerly received.

3. A study of the charm literature of both Europe and America will enable us to take a diachronic view of Western folk medicine and relate the pre-Christian, the medieval Catholic, and the Protestant forms of folk healing. Particularly urgent is the necessity of studying the effects of the Protestant Reformation in breaking the medieval cultural matrix by banning religious healing from organized religion. In a sense Protestantism desacralized its world; this process happened in stages which are documentable. In the sixteenth century Protestantism weakened the sacramental under-structure of organized religion by removing the sacrament of penance, which had provided emotional security for medieval man. At the same time Protestantism expunged the saints from its world view and thus removed another source of security for everyday living, as well as the principal channel for religious heal-ing. In the eighteenth century, Pietism, with its sharp shift to individual converson, further desacralized the Protestant world by atomizing or breaking up even the old folk community and substi-tuting the sect for it. Within Protestant contexts religious healing was driven underground. Banned by the official church, it flow-ered into occult folk healing practiced by individuals who set themselves up as a kind of folk clergy existing in tension in a power triangle between the ordained clergyman, on the one hand, and, on the other, the local practitioner of black arts, the witch. For four centuries folk healing of this sort has continued to exist in Protestant contexts. In the nineteenth and twentieth centuries religious healing has begun to appear above ground, entering again into official forms of religion, first in the world of the sects (for example, Christian Science and the Pentecostal Movement) and now in the world of the older churches (for example, the Protestant Episcopal Church and the United Church of Christ). Thus, it would appear that in this ecumenical century Protestant-ism is gradually taking back some of the "Catholic" practices which it exscinded from its realm of possibilities at the time of the Reformation. The Pennsylvania German charm literature provides the fullest entrée to an understanding of the relation between these historical strands in organized and folk religion since the Reformation.

4. Finally, the charm literature in particular can demonstrate to modern-day Americans, lost in their identity crises, the vital importance of our ancestral folk cultures, where the individual was

subsumed under the community, where healing was related to faith and sympathy and community integration. Above all, this charm literature can reveal to us that unity of all things which was so often a part of the world view of European peasant cultures—a unity which brought together religion and medicine, salvation and health, "haleness" and "wholeness." Like some of the oriental and primitive religions, this folk cultural world view in its outer reaches united cosmos and individual, heaven and earth, man and environment, man and animal life, body and spirit, and the living and the dead.

NOTES

1. For a general introduction to occult folk healing in Europe and the United States, with bibliography, see Don Yoder, "Folk Medicine," in *Folklore and Folklife: An Introduction*, ed. Richard M. Dorson (Chicago: University of Chicago Press, 1972), pp. 191-215.

2. For tracing the charms to antiquity, see C. Bakker, *Volksgeneeskunde in Waterland: Een vergelijkende Studie met de Geneeskunde der Grieken en Romeinen* (Amsterdam: H. J. Paris, 1928). For transitions in the middle ages, see Wilfrid Bonser, *The Medical Background of Anglo-Saxon England: A Study in History, Psychology, and Folklore* (London: The Wellcome Historical Medical Library, 1963), and C. H. Talbot, *Medicine in Medieval England* (London: Oldbourne, 1967).

3. Germanists disagree on the origins of this usage of the common verb *brauchen*, the basic meaning of which is, of course, "to use." The once common older derivation via Yiddish from Hebrew *berakha* is now generally given up. The commonest explanation appears to be that of Fritz Heeger, who simply calls it a pseudonym or code word (*Deckname*) for secret arts (*Pfälzer Volksheilkunde: Ein Beitrag zur Volkskunde der Westmark* [Neustadt/Weinstrasse: Verlag Daniel Meininger, 1936], p. 19). For the term *brauchen* and its many synonyms in German, see the lengthy article "besprechen," in the *Handwörterbuch des Deutschen Aberglaubens*, I, cols. 1157-1172. For Pennsylvania German *Brauche, Braucherei*, and *Brauchbuch*, see Marcus Bachman Lambert, *A Dictionary of the Non-English Words of the Pennsylvania-German Dialect*, The Pennsylvania-German Society, Vol. XXX (1924) (Lancaster, Pa.: Lancaster Press, 1924.)

4. The basic history of the transfer of the Algonquin word *powwow* into English both as a noun and as a verb is given in *The Oxford English Dictionary*, VII, 1216. The transfer appears to have been made in New England, where the whites used the word first for the Indian medicine men and their practice of medicine and later for their own folk healers. The word *powwow* is the only thing Indian about the occult folk healing beliefs and practices of the Pennsylvania Germans.

5. For recent ethnographic information on powwowing in Pennsylvania, see the following articles: (1) Betty Snellenburg, "Four Interviews with Powwowers," *Pennsylvania Folklife*, 18, 4 (Summer 1969), 40-45; (2) Marcia Westkott, "Powwowing in Berks County," *Pennsylvania Folklife*, 19, 2 (Winter 1969-1970), 2-9; (3) Robert L. Dluge, Jr., "My Interview with a Powwower," *Pennsylvania Folklife*, 21, 4 (Summer 1972), 39-42.

6. Basic information on Hohman is given in Wilbur H. Oda, "John George Hohman: Man of Many Parts," *The Pennsylvania Dutchman*, 1, 16 (August 18, 1949), 1.

7. The idea of a letter from heaven, which is used as an amulet to protect house or person, dates from the apocryphal Christian literature of Hellenistic times; see *Handwörterbuch des Deutschen Aberglaubens*, IV, cols. 21-27. There are several parallel

textual traditions that have come into the Pennsylvania German culture from northern Europe; see Edwin M. Fogel, "The Himmelsbrief," *German American Annals*, n.s. 6 (1908), 286-311. For the parallel Italian tradition, the *Santa Lettera di Gesú Cristo*, which circulates in Italian American communities, see Phyllis H. Williams, *South Italian Folkways in Europe and America* (New Haven, Conn.: Yale University Press, 1938; reissue New York: Russell and Russell, 1969).

8. *Die Land- und Haus-Apotheke . . ., Enthaltend die allerbesten Mittel, sowohl für die Menschen als für das Vieh: Nebst einem grossen Anhang von der Aechten Färberey: Erste americanische Auflage* (Reading, Pa.: Carl A. Bruckman, 1818).

9. *Das Evangelium Nicodemi* (Reading, Pa.: C.A. Bruckman, 1819).

10. For one example, in which Hohman advertises his services as rhymester: *Ein schön geistig Lied von dem Nichtsseyn des menschlichen Lebens: Neu verfasset und gedruckt für Georg Hohmann, welcher seine Deinste anbietet, um Sprüche, Gebeter und Lieder aufzusetzen und um geneigte Kundschaft bittet* (n.p. [1810?]).

11. Sophia Bailer of Schuylkill County, a powwower whom I recorded on several occasions, attributed the healings to God, saying that she was only God's instrument in the healing process. She disliked the word *powwowing*, preferring to use the locution "calling a blessing on" a person.

12. Hohman's intense role-consciousness in relation to the clergy was shared by the powwowers whom I have recorded in the twentieth century. In a sense, the powwower was a type of folk clergy, whose major task was healing and who stood in a special relation to God, just as the ordained clergyman was necessary, too, with his control over the sacraments, particularly baptism. Powwowers insist on using the "baptized name of the person" for the charm to be valid. There is one exception to this. Among the "plain" sects, who refuse infant baptism, the given name of the patient is used without reference to baptism.

13. *Der Fromme zu Gott in der Andacht; oder, Merkwürdige Begebenheiten unsers Herrn Jesu . . .*(Reading, Pa.: 1846).

14. For the Romanus book, its text and comparative analysis of its charms, see Adolf Spamer, *Romanusbüchlein: Historisch-philologischer Kommentar zu einem deutschen Zauberbuch: Aus seinem Nachlass*, ed. Johanna Nickel (Berlin: Akademie-Verlag, 1958). At least one European edition of the *Romanusbüchlein* was published, by the Louis Ensslin firm of Reutlingen, with a false "Lancaster" imprint (*ibid.*, pp. 29, 408). Whether this was for export reasons or to mystify everybody further cannot be determined at this time. The Ensslin press also used "Reading" for editions of *Albertus Magnus* (*ibid.*, p. 407) and of *Der wahre Geistliche Schild* (*ibid.*, p. 38), although "Toledo," "Braband," and "Boston" were the commonest of the false imprints for German occult literature.

15. See Adolph Franz, *Die kirchlichen Benediktionen im Mittelalter*, 2 vols. (Freiburg im Breisgau: Verlag Herder, 1909; reprint ed., Graz: Akademische Druck- und Verlagsanstalt, 1960).

16. For a facsimile of this document, the original of which is in the Don Yoder Collection, see Phares H. Hertzog, "Snakelore in Pennsylvania German Folk Medicine," *Pennsylvania Folklife*, 17, 2 (Winter 1967-1968), 24-25.

17. For the best textual analysis of the charms and their ramifications into religion and magic, see Irmgard Hampp, *Beschwörung Segen Gebet: Untersuchungen zum Zauberspruch aus dem Bereich der Volksheilkunde* (Stuttgart: Silberburg-Verlag, Werner Jäckh, 1961).

18. It has been suggested also that perhaps the "zing, zing, zing" represents onomatopoetically the motion and sound of the snake's tongue darting back and forth. Dr. W. J. Hoffman recorded that each time the powwower pronounced the word *tsing*, he made the sign of the cross three times over the wound with the index finger extended (*Popular Science Monthly* [November, 1896] p. 97, cited in Carleton F. Brown, ed., "The Long Hidden Friend by John George Hohman," *The Journal of American Folk-Lore*, 17 [1904], 147).

19. Both Sophia Bailer and her niece, Sophia Eberley, of Tremont, Schuylkill County, Pennsylvania, used this formula when powwowing in English.

20. This phrase is used only once in Hohman, between each line of the Gypsy fire charm which begins "Sei willkommen, du feuriger Gast," but in this case the penance is rendered to the fire and credited to the person saying the charm. The relation of healing and penance is reflected in the word *Büsser*, a synonym for *Braucher* (*Handwörterbuch des Deutschen Aberglaubens*, I, col. 1162).

21. Paul Tillich, "The Relation of Religion and Healing," *The Review of Religion*, 10 (1946), 348-384.

22. Sympathy healing was part of academic medicine in the seventeenth century, whence it passed into folk healing, where it remained long after it was discarded on the scientific level. The once "scientific" appeal of the word *sympathy* is registered in many of the titles of the occult healing books which we cite in this article. For sympathy and folk medicine, see the *Handwörterbuch des Deutschen Aberglaubens*, VIII, cols. 619-627.

23. One of the earliest references I have located to this practice comes from the journal of William Colbert, a Methodist circuit rider in central Pennsylvania, May 2, 1797: "With my sick horse, and myself very weak, I have made out to travel about 20 miles, and lodged at one Punches a dutch mans who it is said can cure sick horses, and a strange method he fell on to cure mine—stroking him from his nose up his face, and down his mane and back to the end of his tail and lightly slap[p]ing him on the flank very gravely for three times successively. And tho' I was pensive enough I could scarcely help laughing at the way of effecting a cure." Next day he wrote: "I was used well at my strange friend Bunches, who was kind enough not to take anything for what he did for me and my horse. I rode on to Northumberland upwards of 50 miles, and was very sorry I did not git [there] to preach" (William Colbert, *Journal*, II, 145-146, Garrett Biblical Institute Library, Evanston, Ill.).

24. William Beisel, of Leck Kill, Northumberland County, Pennsylvania, a powwow doctor, in 1938 published a small pamphlet of translations from Helfenstein, appropriately entitled *Secrets of Sympathy*. In the booklet he refers to the charms as "sympathies."

25. For the European background of the book, see "Albertus Magnus," *Handwörterbuch des Deutschen Aberglaubens*, I, cols. 241-243; also "Kunst," V, cols. 817-836.

26. For the European background, see "Das sechste und siebente Buch Mosis," *Handwörterbuch des Deutschen Aberglaubens*, VI, cols. 584-593.

27. For the influence of the cabala on Christianity, see Ernst Benz, *Die christliche Kabbalah, ein Stiefkind der Theologie* (Zürich: Rhein-Verlag, 1958).

28. Tobias Hirte, an itinerant Moravian herbalist, published a volume in 1793 entitled *Der Freund in der Noth: oder, Zweyter Theil des Neuen Auserlesenen Gemeinnützigen Hand-Büchlein Für die Deutschen in America* (Germantown, Pa.: Peter Leibert, 1793). There is, however, nothing occult in it, and it is the sequel to *Ein Neues, auserlesenes gemeinnütziges Hand-Büchlein* (Chestnuthill, Pa.: Samuel Saur, 1792).

29. Recent literature on the SATOR-formula has been summarized in Charles Douglas Gunn, "The Sator-Arepo Palindrome: A New Inquiry into the Composition of an Ancient Word Square" (Ph.D. diss. in Religion, Yale University, 1969).

30. The revelation to Saints Elizabeth, Brigitta, and Mathilda appears in the Italian *Santa Lettera di Gesú Cristo* (see n. 6) and in Hohman's edition of *Das Evangelium Nicodemi* (1819).

31. For the *Geistlicher Schild*, see the *Handwörterbuch des Deutschen Aberglaubens*, III, cols. 566-567.

32. The *Geistliche Schildwacht* is a prayer course of twenty-four hours, each hour dedicated to a different Catholic saint.

33. The prayer of Manasseh is an apocryphal composition referring back to the prayer mentioned but not given in 2 Chron. 33:12-13. It appeared in the apocrypha section of Protestant German Bibles used by the Pennsylvania Germans.

Folk Medicine and Sympathy Healing among the Amish

JOHN A. HOSTETLER, *Temple University*

Every known society has developed methods for coping with threats to health and well-being. Each has created a body of therapeutic knowledge in keeping with its ongoing culture. As a member of a folk society,[1] the sick individual will act according to the norms and assumptions held by his society. Decisions about treatment and who should provide the treatment depend upon the knowledge made available to the individual from his culture. The healing arts of the folk society are frequently regarded by literate people as a queer collection of errors and superstitions. The tendency of modern medical institutions and their personnel to scorn folk concepts of illness and treatment has delayed unnecessarily long the much-needed perspective of the holistic therapeutic processes. This conference is a concrete step, a historic venture, in exploring knowledge derived from two of man's greatest sources of knowledge, the oral tradition and science. It is to be hoped that we will learn more about the integration of these methods of healing.

"Folk medicine," as Don Yoder has so effectively pointed out, "has many *gesunkenes Kulturgut* items in its repertory."[2] Modern healing practices deriving from folk medical knowledge are today in all probability very limited; and when a breakthrough is made, it is "accidental." There are practitioners, grandmothers, and sages in mass culture who as individuals perpetuate a knowledge of folk beliefs and curing. This is idiosyncratic behavior rather than a cultural phenomenon. When we come to the Old Order Amish, however, we are dealing with an enclave of humanity, a segment of interrelated people who have retained a style of living that is

credible in its "strain toward consistency."[3] The function and place
of folk medicine in the process of consistency remains yet to be
thoroughly investigated. Though the Amish are not in every
respect an ideal-typical folk society,[4] they have retained many of its
basic characteristics—distinctiveness, smallness, homogeneity, and
self-sufficiency. The Amish derive from the sixteenth-century
Anabaptist tradition and along with other Germanic-speaking
peoples migrated from Switzerland and Germany to the United
States in the eighteenth century. They have grown in population,
almost wholly from natural increase, from about eight thousand in
1905 to approximately seventy thousand in 1970. Eighty percent of
their population is located in the three states of Pennsylvania,
Ohio, and Indiana.

Aside from my personal knowledge of folk medical practices as a
product of growing up in an Old Order Amish home, I have collected data on this subject in connection with my fieldwork over the
past twenty years. The sources for this paper are personal interviews with Amish informants and with physicians who serve the
Amish people and a content analysis of the Amish newspaper, *The
Budget*. The Amish rules of discipline prevent members from
securing higher education; thus they have no physicians among
their members. In order to understand folk medicine in Amish
society, I maintain, we must observe the totality of Amish medical
practices and observe how both folk and scientific knowledge
function in a cultural system.

ATTITUDES TOWARD SICKNESS

Concern for the sick constitutes a subject of major interest in every
Amish community. *The Budget* (a weekly) reflects the attitudes,
happenings, and interests of the Amish people from scores of
communities in the United States and Canada and covers illness,
diagnosis, and treatment. An analysis of the content indicates that
the Amish are extremely health-conscious.[5] Scribes who report
illnesses frequently give lengthy and detailed reports of not only
the ailment, but also the method of treatment and the progress of
the patient. Scribes invite readers to send letters to the sick person.
It becomes the duty of members to visit, especially the chronically ill
and the aged relatives.

Modern medical terminology forms a substantial part of the
Amish medical vocabulary. The range of complaints and diseases
varies widely in Amish writings. Treatment for an ailment is
generally that prescribed by the modern medical profession,

although there are also terms used that designate home remedies, patent medicines, and traditional forms of treatment.

Modern science has penetrated the Amish culture to a far greater extent than have other aspects of "wordly" culture, such as new forms of recreation and leisure. The services of clinics, hospitals, and physicians constitute linkages with outside social systems. While the Amish have maintained boundaries against some dominant values of American culture—the automobile, radio, television, and even technological improvements—they have erected no boundaries against hospital or improved medical care. There is no need to resist health improvement, since such values are not in conflict with the values of their religion. Medical science constitutes no direct threat to the breakdown of the community. The Amish, as a culture group, find nothing in the Bible which prevents them from using hospitals, dentists, fluoridation, surgeons, or anesthetists. Yet folk beliefs and cures are still practiced for some types of illnesses.

The penetration of medical science into Amish life, the acceptance of scientific explanations of disease and treatment, suggests that medical knowledge may be one of the points most vulnerable to the inroads of change in a folk culture. Children at early ages are exposed to outside health and hygiene practices in the public school. Where health and life are at stake, new concepts of disease and treatment are not labeled "too worldly." There is, however, a selective principle which determines the method of treatment. For critical, incapacitating illnesses such as appendicitis, infections, and broken bones, scientific modes of healing are accepted. For chronic, nonincapacitating malfunctions or for treatments not responding to scientific modes of healing, folk treatments tend to play an important role.

Illnesses which are not understood or do not respond to treatment bring both scientific and folk sources of knowledge into the experience of the sick person. Much of the medical folk knowledge does not get into the columns of the Amish newspaper. The space devoted to health advertisements in *The Budget* is consistent through the years from 1890 to the present. This is a source of folk knowledge for the chronically ill reader, but it is also a form of borrowing. The advertisements are from non-Amish sources. The patent names for these remedies have varied greatly over the years, but the ailments they would cure remain about the same. Remedies for rheumatism and arthritis are most numerous, but there are also tonics, vitamins, and bitters to cure constipation and to relieve itch and other ailments. Tranquilizers and sedatives are also advertised.

Many Amish have told me, "Too many pills and strong medicine is not good for a person." For persons who believe in bone therapy and have a fear of "strong medicine," advertisements have considerable appeal. Teas and homemade formulas constitute another source of Amish medical treatment. "They use all kinds of teas for all kinds of ills and I don't interfere with it unless I know it to be detrimental," said one physician.

FOLK TREATMENTS

Amish folk medicine is composed of the two recognized branches of folk medicine: (1) natural folk medicine (use of natural phenomena, herbs, plants, minerals, and animal substances for curing), and (2) occult folk medicine (the use of charms and supernatural forms of support).[6] Both are maintained by a strong oral tradition through which, for example, knowledge of plant lore as well as charms are transmitted from generation to generation. In recent years the traditional Amish use of herbs and plants has been reinforced by the health movements in the larger American culture. I shall mention two specific linkages. One is William McGrath, a convert to the Anabaptist faith (though he did join the Old Order Amish), who has privately published a book entitled *God-Given Herbs for the Healing of Mankind* (1970), now widely circulating among the Amish people.[7] The book combines "What the Bible Says About Sickness and Health" (chapter 1) with healing methods, natural healing, herbs, and testimonials. The second illustration is the rather widespread acceptance by the Amish of the method of "reflexology," or zone therapy, attributed to Eunice D. Ingham.[8] This treatment proposes that the proper massaging of the nerves in the toes has beneficial effects on the head, neck, spine, stomach, digestive system, and other parts of the body. The Amish not only patronize non-Amish foot masseurs, but some have taken the required course to become certified as foot-massage specialists.

Occult practices in various forms, including sorcery, have been observed by those who have done fieldwork in Amish communities. The five widespread theories of disease and treatment based on magical causation as reported by Clements[9] have been observed in the Amish by Janice A. Egeland.[10] They are: (1) imitative and contagious magic; (2) intrusion of a disease-causing object; (3) soul loss, in which the victim's soul is thought to have been stolen and he is left to fall ill and die; (4) spirit intrusion, in which a person is believed to be possessed by a spirit; and (5) breach of taboo.

A common form of healing among the Amish is *Brauche* or

Braucherei, which may be translated as "sympathy healing," or "secrets of sympathy."[11] The English equivalent is usually rendered as *powwowing,* though the cultural and psychological context is very different from that of the Indian medicine man. The traditional Amish have retained this source of knowledge from the ancient past. Though it is a source of mysterious power based on the use of incantations, it is not witchcraft, as the more progressive and evangelistic affiliations of the Amish would have it. The old charms used in this connection were in the German language. Many of the charms and recipes I have found in family Bibles are in the English language.

Brauche is usually performed by one of the older Amish members in the community. Practitioners receive no remuneration for their services. The patient does not always need to be present when the actual incantations are performed, but the patient must believe in the practice to experience healing. One who desires to acquire the skill can obtain it only from an older person of the opposite sex after promising that the formula will be kept secret. The chief features of *Brauche* are the silent repeating of certain verses or charms at appropriate times. It is performed for hemorrhaging, toothache, burns or scalds, the common cold, bed-wetting, wild fire, mortification, sores in the mouth, and warts.

There are several Amish folk practitioners of varied reputation. One regularly visits Amish communities in several states in the interest of "curing." He claims to possess a special gift of healing. He asserts that his practice is neither *Brauche* nor powwowing but says he can tell what is wrong with a person by simply laying his hands on that person.

Amish persons who turn from scientific personnel to folk practitioners show little preference for Amish over non-Amish practitioners. One state inspector who investigates "quack healers" states that invariably he finds Amish patients at the offices of these healers, sometimes far from an Amish settlement.

The general tendency to rely on oral tradition and testimony, so characteristic of the whole Amish culture, is specifically manifest in the areas of the healing arts.

A mysterious ailment called "livergrown" (*a-gewachse*—literally meaning "hidebound" or "grown together") is common among Amish infants. Livergrown is thought to be caused by too sudden exposure to the outside atmosphere or by being shaken up by a buggy ride. The symptoms are similar to colic in babies. A sure diagnosis of the ailment is made by placing the child on his abdomen on a table, then bringing together, if possible, the left arm and the right foot (or vice versa) of the child. If the two do not come together with ease, the child has livergrown. The only cure for this illness is *Brauche*. This ailment and its cure is cited by Brendle and Unger in their extensive collection of folk medicine among the Pennsylvania Germans.[12] Livergrown seems to have no equivalent in modern medical terminology.

The Biblical practice of anointing with oil has never found widespread acceptance among the Amish, as it has in some of the Mennonite groups, although there are instances when it is observed. No record of the practice of anointing exists among the Amish or Mennonite groups in Europe.

Certain types of illnesses are taken to the physician and other types to the folk practitioner. Critical, incapacitating malfunctions are taken to the scientifically trained practitioner, while the chronic, nonincapacitating ailments are treated by the folk practitioner and by traditional means. For a sudden illness, broken bones, wounds, or pregnancy, the physician is consulted first. For nameless pains and long-standing disorders or for ailments which do not respond to the physician's treatment, *Brauche,* folk diagnosis, and folk treatment are prescribed. Chiropracters and naturopaths are believed to treat the "causes" of illnesses, while medical doctors tend to be regarded as specialists in treating the "effects." The former is believed to work with the slow but fundamental forces of nature; the latter gives immediate but short-range treatment by an injection of "strong" chemicals. The latter is considered necessary in emergency cases but is regarded as inferior to the slow-working "natural" cures.

The Amish have a standard practice known as "changing doctors." This is upsetting to the medical practitioner, but to the Amish it is a means of achieving social integration by acquiring all available means of healing.

PHYSICIANS AND THE AMISH

Many physicians who serve the Amish express the opinion that there is a difference in symptomatology between Amish and non-Amish patients. In an effort to discover whether the Amish have complaints and symptoms that are different from non-Amish, I conducted a survey among physicians in four states.[13] Forty-six physicians cooperated in the survey, which was conducted by the interview and direct-mail method. Eighty percent of these physicians had been in professional contact with the Amish for more than ten years, and over half estimated that they had been consulted by over one hundred Amish persons during the preceding year. On a checklist of symptoms, there was a high degree of consensus on some of the items.[14] Consensus does not prove that the physicians are right. There is, however, a somewhat greater than random chance that they might be, as indicated by applying tests of significance to the data.

The Amish are believed to have more of the following symptoms than non-Amish patients (significant at the 0.01 percent level of confidence): obesity, fats in the diet, salt in the diet, and capacity to endure pain. They are believed to have more chronic bed-wetting after the age of six and more chronic digestive disturbances but are believed to show more dependability in personal relationships than non-Amish clients. The physicians were of the opinion that there is a difference in physical and mental health between Amish and non-Amish patients (though not significant at the 0.05 level of confidence). Amish patients were judged to have less fainting, nervous tics, hysterical seizures, stuttering, chronic headaches, eczema, spastic colitis, arterial hypertension under the age of forty, coronary heart disease, complaints of menstrual disorders, aggressiveness in personal relationships, nevertheless, they were considered to have less general good mental health.

Amish patients are believed to have fewer of the following symptoms than non-Amish patients, as indicated by clinical judgments of the physicians (significant at the 0.01 percent level of confidence): chronic insomnia, chronic use of sleeping pills, drug addiction, extreme alcoholism, chronic nightmares, food allergies, and syphilis. Amish patients were also believed to have fewer of the following additional symptoms than non-Amish (significant at the 0.05 percent level of confidence): amnesia, suicide, peptic ulcers, complaints of poor appetite, coronary heart disease, malingering, fear of death, parental concern over enuresis, parental emphasis on early toilet training. They also showed less interest in birth control information.

Little or no difference between Amish and non-Amish patients is thought to exist in the frequency of the following symptoms: hypochondriacal complaints, asthma, hay fever, sleepwalking, cancer, chronic constipation, kidney malfunctions, urinary tract infections, arterial hypertension over age forty, arteriosclerosis, hypertensive complications in pregnancy, worry about illness, feeling of personal inadequacy, average life expectancy, and general good physical health.

Many of these professional clinical judgments substantiate what we would expect. As a rural people, the Amish work hard and have no difficulty sleeping at night; therefore they need no sleeping pills. Their traditional teachings have generally prevented them from alcoholic excesses. They want large families, since children are not an economic liability but rather an asset to the farm. They do not lack good appetites and apparently have less heart failure than people who work in offices and in nonfarm occupations. Once on the way to recovery, getting over an illness is not difficult, and they show little anxiety over the fear of death. The Amish infant is generally not forced into early toilet training.

Some Amish symptoms are probably associated with conditions of stress and culture change. Amish persons are believed to lack aggressiveness in personal relationships and manifest less general good mental health according to the physicians. Chronic bed-wetting after the age of six and more digestive disturbances suggest the presence of social and cultural problems. The Amish apparently complain about illness as much as other people.

Most of the physicians cooperating in the study offered comments about their Amish clients, their social relations, and their health conditions. Their observations may be summarized as follows:[15]

1. The Amish are generally regarded as being desirable patients by physicians.

2. The Amish, in the view of medical doctors, pay less attention to preventative medicine; physicians attribute this to a lack of formal education.

3. The Amish are more inclined than other patients toward using home remedies and patronizing unscientific practitioners.

4. The Amish have special health problems that are associated with social and cultural changes.

Thirty-one of the forty-six physicians believed that the incidence of possible hereditary pathologies was greater among the Amish than among non-Amish patients. Since 1965 the Amish have made a significant contribution to medical genetics by permitting medical scientists to study their hereditary problems.[16] Several recessive genetic disorders have been found to have a relatively high oc-curence: a rare type of anemia, phenylketonuria, hemophilia, six-fingered dwarfism, and a new form of dwarfism affecting the growth of cartilage and hair. Because the Amish are a well-de-fined population and have good family records, it is possible to trace many of the cases to a common ancestor. The Amish prohibit first-cousin marriages, but even though they appear not to marry close, there has been much intermarriage for generations in con-fined communities.

SUMMARY AND CONCLUSIONS

The relationship between medicine and social change is still a field which deserves much investigation. Medicine in any society, in a broad sense, is understood as we understand its relation to integration and the culture. In a changing world, medicine, as well as other social institutions, is influenced by the forces that are changing the general social order.

In Amish society changes occur selectively, by the processes of reinterpretation and syncretism. In Amish tradition there are no manifest beliefs that militate against the use of hospital or surgical methods. Nevertheless, it would appear in the case of the Amish that the practice of folk medicine persists in a culture that places a premium on isolation. Major innovations flow outward from cities to country. The sixty or more Amish settlements in the United States are agrarian communities with a preference for isolation from the general society. The Amish have preserved what the society around them has discarded long ago. In pioneer times the Amish and many rural people lived far from a physician. In case of sudden illness they were forced to use those cures at hand or to search the memory for those treatments used by their forefathers. Amish culture is slow-moving and, by tradition, slow to accept new ideas. The old ways are not only familiar ways but preferred ways in a society that ranks "practical" above "theoretical" knowledge. "Folkways" are ranked high in the scheme of things, while "new ways" are ranked lower. In a society that places a high value on face-to-face associations, the advice of a friend (especially an old person) concerning medical treatment carries more weight than the advice of a scientifically trained man. This is especially true in a society that is suspicious of higher learning in general.

Finally, the folk concepts of disease, diagnosis, and treatment are culturally consistent with the whole of Amish culture. In a mentality of slowness, of suspicion against newness, of uncertainty in general about the outside world, the old conservative ways are preferred. Another reason for the persistence of folk medicine is that the Amish are probably experiencing psychotherapeutic results which they do not find in the highly rational non-Amish world. That effective results are obtained from any number of folk treatments contributes to the persistence of folk medicine. This is a phenomenon which anthropologists and the medical sciences have yet to probe further.

NOTES

1. "Folk society" in this discussion connotes the model developed by Robert Redfield: a small, isolated, traditional, simple, homogeneous society where oral communication and conventionalized ways are important in integrating the whole of life. See "The Folk Society," *American Journal of Sociology* (January, 1947), 293-308.

2. Don Yoder, "Folk Medicine," in *Folklore and Folklife: An Introduction*, ed. Richard M. Dorson (Chicago: University of Chicago Press, 1972), p. 191.

3. The phrase is from W. G. Sumner, *Folkways* (Boston: Ginn and Co., 1906).

4. For a discussion of the Amish as a folk society see J. A. Hostetler, *Amish Society* (Baltimore: Johns Hopkins Press, 1968), pp. 3-22; and for a thorough anthropological study see G. E. Huntington, "Dove at the Window: A Study of an Old Order Amish Community in Ohio" (Ph.D. diss., Yale University, 1956).

5. For a detailed discussion of the analysis of *The Budget* on matters of health vocabulary see table I in J. A. Hostetler, "Folk and Scientific Medicine in Amish Society," *Human Organization*, 22 (Winter 1963-1964), p. 271.

6. Yoder, *op. cit.*, p. 192.

7. William R. McGrath, *God-Given Herbs for the Healing of Mankind*, 3d. ed. (n.p., 1970). 87 pp. Distributor: Dan J. B. Byler, Route 2, Seymour, Missouri.

8. Eunice D. Ingham, *Stories the Feet Can Tell* (n.p., n.d.). 109 pp. plus "Reflexology Chart." Distributor: Post Office Box 948, Rochester, N.Y.

9. Forrest E. Clements, "Primitive Concepts of Disease," *University of California Publications in American Archaeology and Ethnology*, 32 (1932), 185-252.

10. From an address at Johns Hopkins University School of Medicine, June 1, 1965. Also Janice Egeland, "Beliefs and Behavior as Related to Illness: A Community Case Study of the Old Order Amish" 2 vols. (Ph.D. diss., Department of Sociology, Yale University, 1967). For a limited study of the Iowa Amish medical practices, see Thomas McCorkle and J. von Herringen, "Culture and Medical Behavior of the Old Order Amish of Johnson County, Iowa," mimeographed, State University of Iowa, Institute of Agricultural Medicine Bulletin no. 2 (Iowa City, Iowa, 1958).

11. *Brauchen (Brauche, Braucherei)* was commonly practiced in Europe. See Fritz Heeger, *Pfälzer Volksheilkunde: Ein Beitrag zur Volkskunde der Westmark* (Neustadt/ Weinstrasse: Verlag Daniel Meininger, 1936) pp. 19-31. Sympathy healing connotes a high degree of empathy and forms of community involvement. See also G. F. Helfenstein, . . . *Hausschatz der Sympathie* (1839). *Powwow* (meaning "to council" or "confer") as applied to faith healing may be "a fundamental misapplication of meaning," says John Joseph Stoudt, in *Sunbonnets and Shoofly Pies* (New York: A. S. Barnes Co., 1973), p. 174.

12. T. R. Brendle and C. W. Unger, *Folk Medicine of the Pennsylvania Germans*, (Norristown, Pa., 1935), pp. 192-195.

13. The survey was conducted in 1961 and involved Pennsylvania, Ohio, Indiana, Iowa, and Ontario. The results were published in Hostetler, *Human Organization*.

14. The checklist was used with the permission of J. W. Eaton and R. J. Weil and appears in their book *Culture and Mental Disorders* (Glencoe, Ill.: The Free Press, 1955), pp. 233-237.

15. For quotations supporting these generalizations, refer to Hostetler, *Human Organization*.

16. Hereditary diseases have been studied by Victor A. McKusick at Johns Hopkins University School of Medicine, by his students and associates and by other medical scientists. See especially V. A. McKusick et al., "The Distribution of Certain Genes in the Old Order Amish," *Cold Spring Harbor Symposia on Quantitative Biology*, vol. 29 (1964); and Harold E. Cross, *Genetic Studies in an Amish Isolate* (Ph.D. diss., School of Medicine, Johns Hopkins University).

The Other Kind of Doctor: Conjure and Magic in Black American Folk Medicine

BRUCE JACKSON, *State University of New York, Buffalo*

There is a remarkable account of conjure work in the *Narrative of the Life Adventures of Henry Bibb: An American Slave Written by Himself*, originally published in 1849. Bibb tells of slaves who adopted various techniques to avoid whippings. "The remedy is most generally some kind of bitter root; they are directed to chew it and spit towards their masters when they are angry with the slaves. At other times they prepare certain kind of powders, to sprinkle about their master's dwellings."[1] Bibb says he got into a scrape for slipping off one time. He expected to be flogged; so he went to a conjurer who gave him both a powder to sprinkle and a root to chew, and "for some cause I was let pass without being flogged that time."[2] The next week, encouraged by his apparent power over the master, Bibb stayed away most of the weekend and on his return talked back to the master. "He became so enraged at me for saucing him, that he grasped a handful of switches and punished me severely, in spite of all my roots and powders."[3] Bibb went to another conjure doctor who told him the first doctor was a quack; the second supplied him with a sneezing powder to sprinkle about the master's bed; it would, he said, turn feelings of anger to love. The only effect was the master and his wife both suffered violent sneezing fits. Bibb "was then convinced that running away was the most effectual way by which a slave could escape cruel punishment."[4]

His interest in flight was suspended for a while when he got interested in women. Even though he'd been ill served by conjure doctors before, he once again turned to them for help. "One of these conjurers, for a small sum agreed to teach me to make any girl love me that I wished. After I had paid him, he told me to get a bull frog, and take a certain bone out of the frog, dry it, and when I got a chance I must step up to any girl whom I wished to love me, and scratch her somewhere on her naked skin with this bone, and she would be certain to love me, and would follow me in spite of herself, no matter who she might be engaged to, nor who she might be walking with."[5] One Sunday, Bibb saw a woman he liked walking with her lover. He "fetched her a tremendous rasp across her neck with this bone, which made her jump." It also made her rather angry. He went to still another conjure adviser, an old slave who told him to place a lock of his lady's hair in his shoes, an act which would "cause her to love me above all other persons." He was by that time interested in another girl, but she refused him the hair. "Believing that my success depended greatly upon this bunch of hair, I was bent on having a lock before I left that night let it cost what it might. As it was time for me to start home in order to get any sleep that night, I grasped hold of a lock of her hair, which caused her to screech, but I never let go until I had pulled it out. This of course made the girl mad with me and I accomplished nothing but gained her displeasure."[6]

To the modern reader, Bibb's experience must seem absurd on at least two major counts: how could he believe such devices would function? and after he saw they didn't help him, why didn't he learn from experience that the conjure doctor's advice was not only not helpful but sometimes downright dangerous to him?

We must change the logic a bit, shift the basic premises. What if we assume that events in this world are *causally* rather than *randomly* linked? What if we assume the world has a sense to it greater than accident and less than total divine plan? Then the only real problem is to find out how to influence the various operations. The *donnée* would be that the world *can* be influenced for good or ill, that both events and persons can be directed in significant ways. The various failures Bibb reports could then be viewed as resulting from incompetence on the part of the practitioners or some mistake on Bibb's part, but they do not themselves invalidate the theory, the process, the art.

The curious thing about the stuff so often referred to as "primitive" medicine or magic is that it is terrifically logical. It assumes the operation of the universe is causal, not gratuitous. The educated executive in New York may attribute his fall down a flight of steps to bad luck, his missing a plane to uncommon traffic congestion, but the so-called primitive would ask why he—rather than someone else—had the mass of cars in his way that afternoon and why he should have missed that top step he had always found in the past. The "logical" answer is that something caused it to happen.

A. B. Ellis, writing of Gold Coast folklore, said:

> To the uncivilized man there are no such deaths as those we term natural or accidental. All deaths are attributed directly to the actions of men or to the invisible powers. If a man be shot or his skull be fractured by another man, the cause of death appears to the uncivilized man obvious. Such and such an injury has been inflicted by So-and-so, and experience, either personal or derived, has shown him that death results from such injuries. But should a man be drowned, be crushed by a falling tree in the forest, or be killed by lightning, such an occurrence would not be considered an accident; and a man who met his death in one of these modes would be believed to have perished through the deliberate act of a malignant being. And such, to us, accidental deaths, prove to the uncivilized man both the existence and the malignancy of these beings. A man is drowned. Who has killed him? So-and-so, a local spirit of the sea or a river has dragged him down. . . .
>
> Thus far for violence and sudden deaths; but the same belief is held with regard to deaths which are really due to disease or old age. These are likewise attributed to the action of the invisible powers directly, or to witchcraft, that is to say, to the indirect action of the same powers; for it is from them that wizards and witches obtain assistance and mysterious knowledge.[7]

An extraordinary amount of folk culture is devoted to ways of dealing with what highly literate groups like to consider luck. If there are potent beings in the universe, they can do well or ill; if they exist, they can probably be influenced; if they can be influenced for good, they can be influenced for ill; if someone has caused an evil influence, perhaps someone else can cause a good one, or at least undo the evil. The world of folk magic and medicine, as many commentators have noted, assumes a total coherence in the operation of the world.

What has been assumed to be learned fatalism among lower-class American blacks in the seventeenth, eighteenth, and nineteenth centuries wasn't fatalism at all: most *knew* quite well that whatever happened was *caused*. Some things were beyond their power of influence. That didn't mean it was beyond anyone's influence— only theirs, in that place at that time.[8]

If the magic didn't work, it meant either that it was done imperfectly or that someone else was working something stronger. It is curious that a high degree of learning is directed away from the "logical" and toward the gratuitous. But the random and gratuitous are far harder to accept and live with, far more fearful exactly because one cannot cope with them.[9]

In a recent article on folk medicine, Don Yoder writes:

> Of folk medicine there are essentially two varieties, two branches: (1) natural folk medicine, and (2) magico-religious folk medicine. The first of these represents one of man's earliest reactions to his natural environment, and involves the seeking of cures for his ills in the herbs, plants, minerals, and animal substances of nature. Natural medicine, which is sometimes called "rational" folk medicine, and sometimes "herbal" folk medicine because of the predominance of herbs in its materia medica, is shared with primitive cultures, and in some cases some of is many effective cures have made their way into scientific medicine. The second branch of folk medicine is the magico-religious variety, sometimes called "occult" folk medicine, which attempts to use charms, holy words, and holy actions to cure disease. This type commonly involves a complicated, prescientific world view.[10]

The important difference between the two kinds of folk medicine is that the first assumes a direct cause and effect between application of some substance to some somatic problem while the other attempts to influence some agent other than the doctor or patient or subject. The first is quite close to what we usually consider proper medical practice; the second is closer to what we consider religious manipulation.

In Old World black culture, the two were often combined. The medicine man or voodun in Africa or Haiti would not only cure with herbs but would also act as intermediary with various divinities in the manipulation of a variety of situations. What is curious about the American situation is that the second aspect survived, but it survived without the theological framework upon which it was based. George J. McCall, for example, reports:

> "Hoodoo" represents the syncretistic blend of Christian and Nigritic religious traditions in the United States, corresponding to *vodun* ("voodoo") and *obeah* in Haiti, *shango* in Trinidad, *candomble* and *macumba* in Brazil, *santeria* in Cuba, and *cumina* in Jamaica. In twentieth century hoodoo, however, Catholic elements are less prominent than in the other variants, and Nigritic collective rituals have largely disappeared. Instead, hoodoo has been assimilated to the bewildering variety of store-front spiritualist churches in its truly religious aspect, leaving a heavy residue of sorcery and fetishism as the remaining native elements.
>
> As with sorcery among other peoples, the major foci of hoodoo sorcery lie in the realms of health, love, economic success, and interpersonal power. In all these cases, hoodoo doctors—after careful spiri-

tual "reading" of the client—prescribe courses of action (which always include some hoodoo ritual) and gladly sell him the charms, potions, and amulets the ritual requires.[11]

At its most fully developed, as in Haiti and nineteenth-century New Orleans, voodoo is a system which explains the world; it has various deities assigned a variety of tasks, deities who may be supplicated or motivated in various ways. The voodoo doctors are trained in such manipulation. But rootwork, the more common form found in the rest of the United States, is only technique; much of the work done by root doctors and conjure men has to do with common folk remedies and with good luck (or bad luck for others) charms. The voodoo doctors sometimes engaged in simple medical work, but they originally did such work through the agency of a powerful outsider, a god.

The function of the voodoo doctor in the Haitian and Louisiana traditions is close enough to the function of African medicine man that we may cite John S. Mbiti's long description of the medicine man's work:

First and foremost, medicine-men are concerned with sickness, disease and misfortune. In African societies these are generally believed to be caused by the ill-will or ill-action of one person against another, normally through the agency of witchcraft and magic. The medicine-man has therefore to discover the cause of the sickness, find out who the criminal is, diagnose the nature of the disease, apply the right treatment and supply a means of preventing the misfortune from occurring again. This is the process that medicine-men follow in dealing with illness and misfortune: it is partly psychological and partly physical. Thus, the medicine-man applies both physical and "spiritual" (or psychological) treatment, which assures the sufferer that all is and will be well. The medicine-man is in effect both doctor and pastor to the sick person. His medicines are made from plants, herbs, powders, bones, seeds, roots, juices, leaves, liquids, minerals, charcoal and the like; and in dealing with a patient, he may apply massages, needles or thorns, and he may bleed the patient; he may jump over the patient, he may use incantations and ventriloquism, and he may ask the patient to perform various things like sacrificing a chicken or goat, observing some taboos or avoiding certain foods and persons—all these are in addition to giving the patient physical medicines. In African villages, disease and misfortune are religious experiences, and it requires a religious approach to deal with them. The medicine-men are aware of this, and make attempts to meet the need in a religious (or quasi-religious) manner— whether or not that turns out to be genuine or false or a mixture of both. . . .

On the whole, the medicine-man gives much time and personal attention to the patient, which enables him to penetrate deep into the psy-

chological state of the patient. Even if it is explained to a patient that he
has malaria because a mosquito carrying malaria parasites has stung
him he will still want to know why that mosquito stung him and not
another person. The only answer which people find satisfactory to that
question is that someone has "caused" (or "sent") the mosquito to sting
a particular individual, by means of magical manipulations. Suffering,
misfortune, disease and accident, all are "caused" mystically, as far as
African peoples are concerned. To combat the misfortune or ailment
the cause must also be found, and either counteracted, uprooted or
punished. This is where the value of the traditional medicine-man
comes into the picture.[12]

The most complex and highly structured voodoo work in this
country apparently occurred in and around New Orleans because
both the black and white populations there had strong ties with
Haiti. One of the most interesting descriptions of that scene is
offered by Zora Neale Hurston. In the second half of *Mules and
Men*, she describes how, while doing research as a Columbia
graduate student, she was several times initiated as a voodoo
doctor. She offers formulas for various influences: "Concerning
Sudden Death," "To Rent a House," "For Bad Work," "Court
Scrapes," "To Kill and Harm," "Running Feet," "To Make a Man
Come Home," "To Make People Love You," "To Break Up a Love
Affair";[13] and she quotes some "Prescriptions of Root Doctors."[14]

The tradition she describes is essentially Caribbean and African;
it operates with the claimed mediation of deities and through the
application of chemicals, and some of the practitioners claim
temporary apotheosis as the source of their power. Luke Turner,
descendant of famed voudooienne Marie Leveau, gives Hurston a
long description of Leveau's work and says, "Marie Leveau is not a
woman when she answer one who ask. She is a god, yes. What
ever she say, it will come so."[15]

Turner described in some detail Leveau's method of affixing a
curse:

> She set the altar for the curse with black candles that have been dressed
> in vinegar. She would write the name of the person to be cursed on the
> candle with a needle. Then she place fifteen cents in the lap of Death
> upon the altar to pay the spirit to obey her orders. Then she place her
> hands flat upon the table and say the curse-prayer.
>
> "To the Man God: O great One, I have been sorely tried by my
> enemies and have been blasphemed and lied against. My good
> thoughts and my honest actions have been turned to bad actions and
> dishonest ideas. My home has been disrespected, my children have
> been cursed and ill-treated. My dear ones have been backbitten and

their virtue questioned. O Man God, I beg this that I ask for my enemies shall come to pass:

"That the South wind shall scorch their bodies and make them wither and shall not be tempered to them. That the North Wind shall freeze their blood and numb their muscles and that it shall not be tempered to them."

There follows a catalog of bodily afflictions and diseases and infirmities that make the plagues of Exodus seem a mild sentence in comparison.[16]

It is difficult to estimate the actual spread of voodoo worship in Louisiana in the nineteenth century, but the practice was extensive enough to get wide contemporary coverage in popular magazines in other parts of the country. George Washington Cable, for example, told the urban readers of *Century Magazine* in April 1886 of the potency of voodoo worship:

> Whatever the quantity of Voodoo *worship* left in Louisiana, its superstitions are many and are everywhere. Its charms are resorted to by the malicious, the jealous, the revengeful, or the avaricious, or held in terror, not by the timorous only, but by the strong, the courageous, the desperate. To find under his mattress an acorn hollowed out, stuffed with the hair of some dead person, pierced with four holes on four sides, and two small chicken feathers drawn through them so as to cross inside the acorn; or to discover on his door-sill at daybreak a little box containing a dough or waxen heart stuck full of pins; or to hear that his avowed foe or rival has been pouring cheap champagne in the four corners of Congo Square at midnight, when there was no moon, will strike more abject fear into the heart of many a stalwart negro or melancholy quadroon than to face a leveled revolver. And it is not only the colored man that holds to these practices and fears. Many a white Creole gives them full credence."[17]

But outside of the curious situation in southern Louisiana, black folk medicine on the mainland United States has in general lacked an overarching theory or any coherent oganization of deities. Much of what Hurston's doctors do is simply the uttering of folk superstitions, many of which are common to European traditions. ("If you kill and step backwards over the body, they will never catch you. . . . If you are murdered or commit suicide, you are dead before your time comes. God is not ready for you, and so your soul must prowl about until your time comes. . . .Bury the victim with his hat on and the murderer will never get away. . .")[18] Her root doctor prescriptions cover common diseases—bladder trouble, rheumatism, swelling, blindness, lockjaw, upset stomach, loss of mind, poisons. Though some of the salves for swelling might work well enough, it is hard to see how some of the treatments for gonorrhea ("parch egg shells and drink the tea" or "fifty cents iodide potash to one quart sarsaparilla; take three teaspoons three times a day in water") or for syphilis ("ashes of one good cigar, fifteen cents worth of blue ointment; mix and put on the sores" or "get the heart of a rotten log and powder it fine; tie it up in a muslin cloth; wash the sores with good castile soap and powder them with the wood dust")[19] would help sufferers much. (Of course, the techniques of medical doctors at the time weren't any better for treating those diseases.)

Although there was—and still is in some rural areas—much belief in the efficacy of various magical practices and the potency of folk doctors and the existence of certain supernatural beings, that body of belief does not form a system so much as a great mass of techniques varying widely from place to place; and just about everywhere in this country, it is the technological, rather than the theological, aspect which is operative.

The most spectacular collection of black folk medicine is Dr. Harry M. Hyatt's *Hoodoo—Conjuration—Witchcraft—Rootwork*.[20] The first four volumes of this projected five-volume work consist of almost thirty-eight hundred pages of interviews with hoodoo doctors and thousands of samples of techniques for various situations and afflictions. The fifth volume, an index being done under the direction of Wayland D. Hand, should make this enormous mass of rare data more easily accessible and approachable. At present, it is pretty much like wandering in a cataloged but unindexed archive, where we have the names and titles of performers but can only sense the holding by experiencing the entire collection. Dr. Hyatt is quite aware of his collection's value and limitations. "Though *Hoodoo* is full of magic rites and cures," he wrote me recently,

> always I sought the professional operator, the *doctor*, his appearance, personal mannerisms, origin of his power, possible descent from a predecessor, activities, beliefs, methods and the atmosphere surrounding him. The latter also means a study of his clients. As you can see, *Hoodoo* is an archive, not a logical presentation of material or a *Golden Bough* trying to prove a theory; but a picture of living people, talking, demonstrating rites in front of you, 1600 of us, asking study by the scholar.

The literature on black folk medicine and magic, on conjure and such, is quite extensive.[21] In the nineteenth century, long before F. J. Child began his monumental library work at Harvard, gifted amateurs were already hard at work in the field collecting Negro folk tales (Joel Chandler Harris's first Remus book was published in 1880)[22] and folk song (Thomas Wentworth Higginson's influential article "Negro Spirituals" was published in *The Atlantic Monthly* in June 1867, and the first book-length collection of black American songs, *Slave Songs of the United States*, was published in the same year).[23] There were numerous articles about black superstition, magic, and medicine in the third quarter of the nineteenth century,[24] and when the American Folklore Society was organized in the late 1880s, its founders set forth as one of its areas of special concern the folklore of the Negro.

But there is another reason why there is so much material on black folk medical and magical practices and customs: there was in fact a great deal of such material around. There were few other sources of power available to the slaves and ex-slaves; there was no justice in the courts for them and no regular source of financially reasonable medical aid from the white doctors in town. Because of custom and the policy of the controlling class, those practices among the folk survived long after they had become moribund in other groups. It is still difficult to know how much of that nineteenth-century material was African survival and how much was European material translated into black idiom and style. Just as with spirituals, there remains something of both. But those things remained because they were necessary, because more sophisticated devices of control were absent. I think John Dollard expresses this as well as anyone else:

> There is another means of accomodating to life when it is not arranged according to one's wishes. This is the use of magic. Of course, one can think of magical practices among the Negroes as lagging culture patterns, which they are, but one can also think of them as forms of action in reference to current social life. Magic accepts the *status quo*; it takes the place of political activity, agitation, organization, solidarity, or any real moves to change status. It is interesting and harmless from the standpoint of the caste system and it probably has great private value for those who practice it. . . . Magic, in brief, is a control gesture, a comfort to the individual, an accomodation attitude to helplessness. There is no doubt that magic is actively believed in and practiced in Southerntown and county.[25]

I think it is clear that one of the reasons many of these practices have become rarer in the past three decades is that those lacks Dollard notes have become realities: there has been considerable "political activity, agitation, organization, solidarity, [and other] real moves to change status." But the remembrance of such times is

still with us. Mrs. Janie Hunter told Guy and Candie Carawan in
the early 1960s:

> We didn't go to no doctor. My daddy used to cook medicine—herbs
> medicine: seamuckle, pine top, lison molasses, shoemaker root, ground
> moss, peachtree leave, big-root, bloodroot, red oak bark, terrywuk.
> And you hear about children have worm? We get something call
> jimsey weed. You put it in a cloth and beat it. And when you done beat
> it, you squeeze the juice out of it, and you put four, five drop of
> turpentine in it, give children that to drink. You give a dose of castor oil
> behind 'em. You don't have to take 'em to no doctor. . . .
> All this from old people time when they hardly been any doctor.
> People couldn't afford doctor, so they have to have and guess. Those
> old people dead out now, but they worked their own remedy and
> their own remedy come out good.[26]

But it wasn't just for medical problems that people visited the
folk doctors. Social affairs were just as much in their domain.
There are many reports similar to the story told by Henry Bibb
about people visiting hoodoo or conjure doctors to try to get help
in managing the difficulties of simply getting on in the world. John
Dollard wasn't the first observer to understand how such belief
compensated for a sense of impotence or for a lack of other kinds
of organization. Leonora Herron and Alice M. Bacon, writing in
the *Southern Workman* in 1895, said:

> Overt and natural means of obtaining justice being forbidden the
> Negro, was it surprising that, brought up in ignorance, and trained in
> superstition, he should invoke secret and supernatural powers to
> redress his wrongs and afford him vengeance on those of his fellows
> whom envy, jealousy or anger prompt him to injure?
> The agent of this vengeance was usually the Conjure Doctor. This
> individual might be a man or a woman, white or colored, but was found
> in every large Negro community, where though held in fear and hor-
> ror, his supernatural powers were still implicitly believed in. The source
> of these powers is but ill defined.[27]

As the source of power some of their informants cite the devil;
some God; some, education. Basically, they say, "The conjure
doctor's business was of two kinds: to conjure, or 'trick,' a person,
and to cure persons already 'conjured.'"[28]

The conjure doctor is simply a library of folk beliefs and techniques in the areas of contagious and homeopathic magic. Many
people know of these matters and can cite a limited number of
cures or techniques, but he is the man (or woman) one goes to for
the best technique for a specific situation. He is known by various
names, but his functions are relatively constant. Richard Dorson

describes categories of such operators when he discusses the term
two-head: "Although 'two-head' designates any person with esoteric gifts, the Southern Negro speaks of three separate kinds. The
hoodoo doctor diagnoses and treats diseases caused by hoodoo evil.
The fortuneteller, like renowned Aunt Caroline Dye of Newport,
Arkansas, prophesies the future, and locates lost persons and
property. The healer cures natural ailments that baffle doctors
through his secret arts. Some of the most graphic stories told by
Negroes involve these two-header practitioners."[29]

Dorson is no doubt correct that there are three separate kinds of
practitioners in this area, but the boundaries dividing them are
sometimes rather amorphous. Most of the reports in this century
suggest that the practitioners assume a variety of functions which
seem to depend as much on neighborhood needs as on professional divisions of labor.

Carl Carmer, for example, describes an Alabama conjure woman
whose name is Seven Sisters. "It's a spirit in me that tells," she told
Carmer, "a spirit from the Lord Jesus Christ. Used to be old
voodoo woman lived next to my mammy's cabin. She tol' me how to
trick. She say her mammy in Africa teached her. But she was a bad
ol' woman—a voodoo conjure woman. I tricks in the name o' the
Lord."[30] She offers recipes and techniques for various conjure acts.
One will "keep your wife from flirting around; take a persimmon
sprout about six inches long and bury it under the doorstep while
her flirting spell is on." Other cures have to do with getting good
crops, inflicting revenge on an enemy, knowing when you've been
tricked by another conjurer, or curing warts. You can get a girl to
sleep with you if you "steal something dirty from being next to her
skin—a string from her drawers, moisture from under her right
arm, best of all a menstruation cloth—stick nine pins in it and bury
it under the eaves of the house" or "take hair from her head, make
it into a ball, sew it up, and wear it under your right arm."[31]
Norman Whitten, reporting on such practices in North Carolina,
found a similar combination of activity. The conjurer, he said, "is
the professional diviner, curer, agent finder, and general control-
ler of the occult arts. Local synonyms for the conjurer are "root
doctor,' 'herb doctor,' 'herb man,' 'underworld man,' 'conjure
man,' and 'goofuhdus man.' [This last is probably *gooferdust man*,
referring to the graveyard dust such doctors sometimes use.] The
principal function and role of the conjurer is to deal with and
control the occult. This he does for a fee."[32] And Loudell F. Snow,
reporting on a voodoo practitioner in Tucson, Arizona, says her
informant will treat any sort of disorder: "I don't turn down

nothin'," the practitioner said to Snow, "I don't care what's wrong with 'em, I just have confidence. I tell you what. I believe in God. I believe God can do anything and everything. That is a high power, faith and the belief. I never lose faith, I never doubt myself. I know there's nothin' I can do *without* him, and I feel like He's with me at all times."[33]

This last is in many ways close to the white fundamentalist preacher who sometimes also assumes the power of healing; she is clearly a long way from the complex theological framework of the African slaves and New Orleans devotees of Haitian voodoo of the last century. It would be difficult to separate which of her techniques derive from European and white American tradition and which derive from African and black American tradition. Clearly some significant melding has occurred, and many old contexts have disappeared. I don't think this informant is anomalous: although there are remnants of those older traditions still around, one would now be hard put to duplicate the monumental fieldwork of Hyatt or the important collection of Puckett.

But it isn't completely dead. Although these practices are not much in evidence in modern American cities (and the majority of America's population—white and black—lives in urban centers now), there are occasional reports that suggest some of the old power is still there, that it still influences behavior in significant ways. Though fewer people may be involved in the various levels of practice than in previous years (as is the case with most rural folk traditions brought to the city), many still take them with as much seriousness as ever, with deadly seriousness. Both the folk remedies and the techniques for control still surface as significant elements in certain communities. Consider the following item, an Associated Press dispatch datelined Miami, February 12, 1974:

COURT REFUSES TO APPOINT VOODOO DOCTOR

The court was bedeviled when a defense lawyer asked to have the defendant examined by a voodoo doctor or an exorcist.

"What's a voodoo doctor?" Circuit Court Judge Dan Satin asked at a hearing Monday.

"One who by training has learned about the powers of voodoo," replied defense lawyer David Cerf.

Mr. Cerf pointed out that the defendant, Harvey Lee Outler, has been determined competent for the murder of his common law wife but the evaluating doctor said Outler believed he was under a curse.

Mr. Cerf said Outler, 36, believed that Mable Young, 31, had put a curse on him. Police say Outler shot Mrs. Young with a pistol April 13.

"Your honor, a voodoo curse is just as deadly as a threat with a gun," Mr. Cerf said.

Judge Satin said: "I respect any man's rights. But if you think I'm going to appoint a voodoo doctor, you've got another think coming." Mr. Cerf's motion was denied.

NOTES

1. In Gilbert Osofsky, ed., *Puttin' On Ole Massa: The Slave Narratives of Henry Bibb, William Wells Brown, and Solomon Northup* (New York: Harper and Row, 1969), p. 70.

2. *Ibid.*, p. 70.

3. *Ibid.*, p. 71.

4. *Ibid.*

5. *Ibid.*, p. 73.

6. *Ibid.*

7. A. B. Ellis, *The Tshi-Speaking Peoples of the Gold Coasts of West Africa: Their Religion, Manners, Customs, Laws, Languages, Etc.* (London: Chapman and Hall, 1887), p. 13.

8. See, for example, Norman E. Whitten, Jr., "Contemporary Patterns of Malign Occultism Among Negroes in North Carolina," *Journal of American Folklore*, 75 (1962), 311-325; reprinted in Alan Dundes, ed., *Mother Wit from the Laughing Barrel* (Englewood Cliffs, N.J.: Prentice-Hall, 1973), pp. 402-418. Whitten notes: "Everything has its antithesis. For instance, for every disease there is an antidote if man can only find it" (p. 413). See also Ruth Bass, "Mojo, " in *Scribner's Magazine*, 87 (1930), 83-90, reprinted in Dundes, *op. cit.*, pp. 380-387. Bass writes: "So far as I have been able to discover, there seems to be a trick for every kind of occupation and desire in life. To the swamp Negroes nothing is inanimate, incapable of being tricked. I have heard a swamp Negress talking about to her pot because it was slow about boiling. She begged it to boil, pointed out the advantages of boiling over not boiling, and when it remained obstinate she resorted to a trick which consisted of rubbing her belly. The pot promptly cooked faster" (p. 383).

9. The story of Job, which is one of the most popular stories in the Old Testament, is of course an attempt to deal with exactly this problem: it suggests the Lord acts in ways which are not for man to question. The problematic nature of the solution put forth in Job is attested to by the fact that it is the most frequently analyzed book of the Old Testament.

10. Don Yoder, "Folk Medicine," in *Folklore and Folklife: An Introduction*, ed. Richard M. Dorson (Chicago: University of Chicago Press, 1972), p. 192.

11. George J. McCall, "Symbiosis: The Case of Hoodoo and the Numbers Racket," in Dundes, *op cit.*, p. 420.

12. John S. Mbiti, *African Religions and Philosophy* (Garden City, N.Y.: Doubleday Anchor, 1970), pp. 221-222.

13. Zora Neal Hurston, *Mules and Men* (New York and Evanston, Ill.: Perennial Library, 1970), pp. 332-335.

14. *Ibid.*, pp. 340-343.

15. *Ibid.*, p. 243.

16. *Ibid.*, pp. 245-246.

17. George Washington Cable, "Creole Slave Songs," *Century Magazine*, 11 (April, 1886); reprinted in *The Negro and His Folklore in Nineteenth Century Periodicals*, ed. Bruce Jackson (Austin: University of Texas Press and the American Folklore Society, 1967), pp. 237-238.

18. Hurston, *op. cit.*, p. 332.

19. *Ibid.*, pp. 340-341.

20. Harry M. Hyatt, *Hoodoo—Conjuration—Witchcraft—Rootwork*, 4 vols. (Hannibal, Mo.: Memoirs of the Alma Egan Hyatt Foundation, 1970-1975).

21. See, for example, quoted material and reference in Dundes, *op. cit.*; Jackson, *op. cit.*; Richard M. Dorson, *American Negro Folktales* (New York: Fawcett, 1967); Newbell Niles Puckett, *Folk Beliefs of the Southern Negro* (Chapel Hill: University of North Carolina Press, 1926); Georgia Writer's project of the Works Project Administration, *Drums and Shadows* (Athens: University of Georgia Press, 1940); Robert Tallant, *Voodoo in New Orleans* (New York: Macmillan, 1946).

22. Joel Chandler Harris, *Uncle Remus: His Songs and His Sayings* (New York: D. Appleton, 1880).

23. *Slave Songs of the United States*, ed. William Francis Allen, Charles Pickard Ware, Lucy McKim Garrison (New York, 1867; reprint ed., New York: Peter Smith, 1951).

24. See Jackson, *op. cit.*, p. 134 ff.

25. John Dollard, *Caste and Class in a Southern Town* (Garden City, N.Y.: Doubleday Anchor, 1957), p. 265.

26. Guy and Candie Carawan, *Ain't You Got a Right to the Tree of Life?* (New York: Simon and Schuster, 1966), p. 45. The photograph on the opposite page (p. 44) shows an old woman (who may not be Mrs. Hunter, since the photos and interviews were arranged separately) sitting in a wooden chair before an old iron stove. The walls beyond her are papered with pages of newspapers. It may be that the newspapers serve because nothing else is at hand—but anyone from that area knows full well that *hants* (spirits, ghosts, demons), who sometimes possess people at night, are compulsive counters, and grains of salt or pages of a newspaper will serve as adequate protection because it takes so long to count the grains or letters that dawn comes before the hants can do any harm. I am reminded of a visit to the Massachusetts Hospital for the Criminally Insane at Bridgewater about ten years ago. A guard tried to prove to me how batty one particular old black inmate was. He called the man over and asked him about the devils in his room at night. The man said there weren't any devils in his room; "The devil's in your army, not mine." That seemed rational enough a position. The guard urged the man to tell me how he kept the devils out, and the man said it wasn't devils he kept out.

"Is it hants?" I asked.

He said it was hants and looked at the guard, who at that point was starting to look oddly at me.

"Tell him what you do," the guard said, "about the newspapers."

"You put newspapers on the floor to keep them out?" I asked.

"That's right."

"Where are you from? South Carolina? Georgia?"

He named a coastal town in northern Florida.

I asked the guard just what it was about the man that was supposed to be so batty. He scowled and asked, "How'd you know where he was from?"

"Because of the hants." I pointed out that no southern doctor would consider that sort of superstition adequate grounds for incarceration. "Lots of the old people there used to do that." The guard, obviously no student of folklore, looked at me as if I were as batty as the inmate and walked way, shaking his head.

27. Leonora Herron and Alice M. Bacon, "Conjuring and Conjure Dotors," in Dundes, *op. cit.*, p. 360. (Originally in *Southern Workman*, 24)

28. *Ibid.*

29. Dorson, *op. cit.*, p. 187.

30. Carl Carmer, *Stars Fell on Alabama* (1934; reprint ed., New York: Hill and Wang, 1961), p. 218.

31. *Ibid.*

32. Whitten, *op. cit.*, p. 409.

33. Loudell F. Snow, "'I was Born Just Exactly With the Gift': An Interview with a Voodoo Practitioner," *Journal of American Folklore*, 86 (1973), 277-278.

Birthmarks and Psychic Imprinting of Babies in Utah Folk Medicine

AUSTIN E. FIFE, *Utah State University*

Notions that there are supernatural bonds between mother and fetus must be universal and of prehistoric origin. The fetus is of the mother's flesh and blood, always there to share whatever sensations she might be subjected to and, magnetlike, to attract certain of these sensations and to record them as "marks" upon its skin, as deformities, or in extraordinary behavior patterns. Nor could it be otherwise: so long as there have been or are to be born babies with discernible abnormalities—physical or behavioral, visible or hidden—speculation about their causes will occur; and explanations will be based upon the mother's experience during her pregnancy.

Mrs. Fife and I took our first steps as field collectors of Mormon and western lore thirty-five years ago. We were persistent though untrained collectors, using the "vacuum cleaner" technique, which is to say that we took almost everything that came our way, including folk medicine when we encountered it. As for data on prenatal influence, we made our richest finds in interviews at Moab, Utah, during the summer of 1953 and from students in folklore classes at Utah State University since 1970. We have not interviewed a sufficient number of informants nor visited a sufficient number of communities to reach final conclusions about the nature and distribution of this belief, but some tentative conclusions are still indicated.

The central idea is that if a woman's emotions get sufficiently stirred up during pregnancy, then the fetus itself may feel and register the shock as a blemish on the body, as a deformity, or as a pattern of behavior. The mark frequently resembles the object or circumstance which produced the mother's emotional state.

FRIGHT

A sudden fright, of undetermined cause or by a wide variety of objects, animals, or events, is frequently cited.

> It was a common belief then that if the pregnant mother saw something frightful it would cause the child to be deformed or marked (Vernal, 1970 [FAC I 703]).[1] (Also, in 1970, from Tooele; Fairview, Wyoming; and Red Deer, Alberta, Canada.)

Note that one report comes from western Wyoming and one from Canada. Both of these communities were settled by Mormon groups, and the data have been reported from their descendants. Many of the western Wyoming and southern Idaho towns are both tangential to and part of the Mormon colonizing experience.

Often the mother's fright is caused by an animal: a mouse, rat, snake, bear, or—in one case—a two-headed monster.

> He has a gray spot on his body which he claims is the result of his mother being frightened by a mouse during her pregnancy (Fairview, Wyoming, 1970).

> If you're pregnant and you see a rat, your baby will be marked (Ogden, 1972).

> If an expectant mother is frightened by a snake, her baby will have a birthmark on it shaped like a snake (Vernal, 1970).

> If she is bit by a snake it will have snake marks on it; whatever scares her will be marked there (Moab, 1953 [FMC I 874]).

> Margaret said she knew a woman who was scared by a snake when she was pregnant, and when the baby was born the outline of the snake went all the way around its head and face, and the snake's head was right between its eyes (Moab, 1953 [FMC I 882]).

> A pregnant woman went to a circus sideshow and saw a crocodile. When her baby was born, it had the skin of a crocodile (Manitowac, Wisconsin, 1970).

> If a two-headed animal is born don't look at him while you are pregnant or it will mark the baby (Murtah, Idaho, 1972).

> A pregnant woman got scared by a bear. When her baby was born it had bear fur all over it (Manitowac, Wisconsin, 1970).

> We really have some big bears up here. They're rarely seen by the people though. Once a couple of years ago some lady was out hiking with her husband, she was pregnant, and they saw a bear. The bear came up and mauled them but they were saved by the Rangers. They

weren't hurt, but when the baby was born it had the signs of the bear there. It was born with bare feet (Logan, 1973). (First heard at Watertown Lakes, Canada, 1973.)

This is, of course, a spoof on belief in prenatal influence for the benefit of a sophisticated audience.

The mother's fright may be the result of seeing a fire, witnessing a crime of violence, or receiving news of disaster by word of mouth or by telephone. Seeing a corpse is to be avoided.

When you're pregnant don't look on the dead or it will mark the baby (Murtah, Idaho, 1972).

If a pregnant mother views a fire, then her baby will be born with a birthmark resembling red burns on its face (Salt Lake City, 1973). (This was first heard by the informant in Oslo, Norway, in 1920, prior to her migration to Utah.)

"There used to be a person here that one side of her face looked like it had been burned."
"The Dalton girl."
"Yes, the Dalton girl . . ." (Moab, 1953 [FMC I 904]).

There is a spot on my forehead—Dad had been in town and had been hit on his head and it was all bloody, and he came in and Mama looked up and seen this, and when I was born I had this red streak on my head. It shows up most when I am not well (Moab, 1953 [FMC I 866]).

Often the mark is difficult to detect or even invisible except when the person bearing it is himself under stress. It may take a bit of imagination to see the mark even when it is pointed out. One is almost led to conclude that the informant is forcing the issue in order to establish evidence to corroborate the belief.

In cases where the pregnant woman has been subjected to a fright, the added effect of actual physical contact is often present, thus assuring the flow of magical energy to the fetus through both sight and touch. In some cases there is no mention of a fright, though its presence is implicit because of the nature of the experience.

Don't rest fingers on face or around the neck during pregnancy or your unborn child will have a birthmark (Orem, 1970).

Pug Stocks has finger marks where Aunt Rose grabbed hold of somebody (Moab, 1953 [FMC I 882]).

Before Nicholas was born Mama was standing on the ground and Tom was up in a tree and threw a cherry down and hit her on the leg. When he was born he had a big cherry on his leg (Moab, 1953 [FMC I 866]).

If a pregnant woman works with warm meat—like if they've just killed a pig or something—if she touches the warm meat, she's supposed to lose her baby (Moab, 1953 [FMC I 878]).

Pregnant women should not pick raspberries or strawberries or their child will be marked with a birthmark that appears like unto the fruit (Orem, 1970).

The informant told me of a person who rode on a street car and felt something on her hip. She reached for it and found a mouse. She held the mouse there until she was off the street car and in her father's store. After the baby was born, her baby had a perfect shape of a mouse on the hip. It was even fuzzy (Preston, Idaho, 1970).

A young Hurricane wife who was eight months pregnant was hanging out clothes when she felt something around her ankle. It was a snake coiling around her leg. She flung it off. When her baby was born it had snake skin, and its tongue flicked in and out constantly like a snake's. The doctor said it would live 12 hours, 12 days, or 12 years. It lived 12 days (Lancaster, Wisconsin, 1970).

ACTS OF VIOLENCE

I have an uncle in Los Angeles that's got a blood tumor on one whole side of his face. Well, they claim that was caused from my grandmother watching a man hit his wife in the face with a hatchet—the blunt end of it, I mean (Moab, 1957 [FMC I 975]).

Mrs. R. told me her brother got killed and her mother was expecting a baby at that time. When they came and told her mother she put her hands up on her head and fainted, and the baby was born with its head crushed (Moab, 1953 [FMC I 882])

My brother-in-law's brother was the sheriff—this is a fact—in Price, and they had a jail break and the fellows got an old shotgun and shot his hand clear off, and shot him in the arm and in the stomach and killed him. They told his sister about it and she was expecting a baby. When the baby was born—I've seen it a thousand times . . . when the child was born it didn't have a hand, and it had shot marks on its arm just as plain as day.

"Now I'll tell you a story opposite to that. I knew I was pregnant and that was all. My husband's brother-in-law's sister committed suicide and killed her three children all at the same time. There was nobody in town to do anything except me and [named two women], and we went up there about seven in the morning, and nobody knew anything about me being pregnant, but they thought Ida was pregnant, and she didn't go into the room where this mess was, but I went in, and somebody said, 'Ida's pregnant and she can't come in.' But I went in and laid all four of them out and handled their dead bodies all day, but it didn't have any effect on me." (Moab, 1953 [FMC I 882]).

TOUCH

Where deformity is involved, magical and psychic factors of a somewhat more complex nature come into play. Parents, and even grandparents, may carry a deep sense of guilt because of a feeling that the deformity is hereditary. Or they may see it as divine retribution for moral lapses, especially premarital or extramarital sex relations. Hence they are predisposed to cite beliefs about marking as an "out." Thus a family etiological tale may come into being.

Mr. H.: My brother that was older than me, when he was born he had a crooked foot. He walked on the side of his foot—his foot was just turned right around and they had to cut the cord. You can see my foot—my foot was crooked the same way. My mother—I can remember well when she used to take my foot and straighten it up—I run barefoot a lot, and she would set me on her lap and hold my foot straight, and when she let me down she would make me promise I'd walk on my foot straight so my foot would grow straight. My brother had to wear a brace but I never did wear one.

Mrs. H.: She told me—she said that fooling with Len's foot every day, trying to straighten it up and working with it and rubbing it before they put the brace on, she knew that she marked Will . . .

Fife: She was doing that while she was carrying him?

Mrs. H.: Yes.

Fife: Have you heard of any other cases?

Mrs. H.: . . . She had a baby and . . . she said she was looking at Len's foot, and he was showing it to her, showing her the ankle and she was looking at his ankle, and when Leonard was born he was the same way. (conversation in Moab, 1953 [FMC I 904]).

CRAVING—REVULSION

The fetus may also be marked by the pregnant woman's craving for a particular kind of food. When such a craving occurs, every effort is made to find the desired item so that the mother may satisfy her appetite and thus reduce or suppress the craving before the fetus is damaged. Less often the marking takes place because the mother has eaten too much of a certain food and has thereby developed a revulsion for it.

Jim had a mark on him, a strawberry on him. It was caused because Mother wanted strawberries (Moab, 1953 [FMC 913]). (Also from Preston, Idaho, 1970.)

Do not eat strawberries when pregnant because the child will be born with the mark of the strawberry (Salt Lake City, 1973).

I've got a piece of bacon somewhere on my neck because my mother wanted bacon (Moab, 1953 [FMC I 881]).

I have a niece who marked her baby with a strawberry: it's just as natural as could be. When strawberries get ripe it gets red and has dots in it (Moab, 1953 [FMC I 910]).

If an expectant mother eats too many strawberries before delivery, the baby will have a birthmark shaped like a strawberry (Vernal, 1970).

They say you can't mark a child, but I know better because my mother, when they first came here, didn't have much to eat . . . and they went fishing lots. She got so sick of fish she said she thought she couldn't stand it when she was pregnant, and I have a fish this long [measuring on her index finger and hand for about four or five inches] on my leg. She just had a horror of fish (Moab, 1953 [FMC I 910]).

Rae Thompson told me that her brother was marked with a chicken, a roast chicken, and she said it was just as plain a roast chicken as you ever saw. Right on his thigh here, right there [pointing]. She said her mother, before he was born, went into a neighbor's house and just as she went in there this neighbor had opened the oven and pulled this chicken out to baste it, and she said it just looked so good she just went home and all day she wanted some of that chicken . . . and just kept it on her mind so much, and when Steve was born he had that chicken on him, and she said the leg stuck up just like a chicken will. And she said it was just as plain and just as brown as any roast chicken you ever saw (Moab, 1953 [FMC I 904]).

If, while pregnant, you crave something very bad and cannot obtain it, the child will be marked. . . . When she was pregnant with her third child, one day at around three or four she saw a boy walk down the street with a string of trout he had just caught. Late in the night, twelve or one o'clock, she had a very strong craving for those fish and sent her husband to the home of the boy to buy some. The mother of the boy understood what was going on but could not help for they had eaten all the fish that night. For fear of marking the baby Mrs. West sent her husband out in the middle of the night to knock on their neighbor's doors and wake them up till he found some fish (Smithfield, 1973).

Mrs. F.: Oh, well, I claim that a woman can get a craving for some particular kind of food and can mark the baby.

Fife: You mean, by marking the baby, some design on the skin, or something?

Mrs. F.: Yeah. Of course they claim now days that you can't do that, but I claim that they used to, anyway.

Fife: Do you know of any cases?

Mrs. F.: Yes. Especially my own. When first I discovered that I was in the family way with my boy, I thought I could smell cheese in the middle of the night. I waked up, and oh, I wanted some cheese. I didn't have any, and I went up to my neighbor's that I knew had some, and I never tasted such good cheese in my life as that was. I ate what I wanted, and that craving was all gone, that's all there was to it. When the child was born, he always did like cheese. [Laughter.]

But I really marked him with fresh meat. Mr. F. was on the mountain, riding for cattle, and I was in the valley, and he came down, and he brought some fresh beef. And I said, "Well, I'd better go and start supper." And he said, "I'll cut some of that meat." And he cut some of that fresh meat, and I made up my mind that I knew just how I wanted it cooked, so I put the skillet on the stove, and put quite a bit of grease in it and got it just good and smoky hot, and took that meat, the slices on my hand, and laid it in that grease, and it just all quivered, and the blood came to the top, and oh, it smelled good.

And I went on and put all the meat in there, and the water was in my mouth, the saliva, and I stood there looking at it, and I turned around and scratched my buttocks. And they say, "Wherever you touch yourself, there's where the mark will be." And when that child was born he had the prettiest bite of raw meat on him you ever saw. It lasted there all his life.

Fife: Is that right? Just a kind of a raw place?

Mrs. F.: It wasn't raw. It was smooth, just as smooth, but it was just the color of red, and it had the dark red veins like it was in the meat all across that bite. . . .

Our little girl, before she was born, of course—I was young and didn't know much of anything, and I had a picture of huckleberries hanging on the wall above our bed. And I waked up one morning and looked at that and I said, "Oh, I would like to have some of those. I wonder if they have any of those in the West." During the day, I think I talked to my mother about it. She says, "Well, if there's any huckleberries in town we'll get them." So they went downtown and got some canned huckleberries, but they didn't taste good. They didn't taste like I imagined the ones back east did. And, it went on, and when she was born there was huckleberries right across the bottom of her lower jaw. They were blue, and kind of raised up a little, and they looked just like huckleberries that I imagined I seen. But we were afraid at the time that as she grew they'd grow out and bother her teeth. But they didn't. As she grew, the huckleberries grew down in her mouth. They didn't hurt her teeth none, but they were always there" (conversation in Moab, 1953 [FMC I 896]).

FOOD TABOO

In a few cases the mark or deformity may result simply from the pregnant woman's having eaten a food which is taboo or which has some special virtue. The food itself, not the mother's craving for the food, appears to be the agent.

If you're pregnant and you eat a potato with a spoiled spot, even if the spot has been removed, the baby will be born deformed (Logan, 1973).

Eat carrots while pregnant and the child will have good eyesight (Orem, 1970).

If a pregnant woman eats a large amount of tomatoes, the child will be born with rosy cheeks (Venice Beach, California, 1973).

REACHING

Pregnant women are admonished not to reach high above their heads lest they entangle the navel cord and strangle the child. No magical phenomenon is involved, just the mechanical fact of the displacement of the cord itself.

Her daughter was pregnant and was reaching above her head to get something on a high shelf. She told her not to do that because the cord would get wrapped around the baby's neck and strangle when it was born (Iona, Idaho, 1973).

When you are pregnant, never raise your hands above your head or you will cause the cord to wrap around the baby's neck and possibly choke the baby (Ogden, 1970). (Also from Murtah, Idaho, 1972.)

PSYCHIC IMPRINTING

Psychic imprinting is akin to marking in that certain experiences of the mother during pregnancy influence the fetus in remarkable ways. But there are important differences: the mother need not be subjected to any sudden and overpowering sensation. Quite the contrary; her sustained mental condition, good or bad, is transferred to the fetus. Indeed, the mother may voluntarily subject herself to a regimen throughout the period of pregnancy in the belief that the benefits thereof will be transmitted to the child. Or she may unwittingly endow the child with undesirable behavior patterns deriving from her own unwise behavior.

Well, everybody has heard that. In olden times, they thought if you wanted an artist you admired artists' work and all; if you wanted a beautiful child, you admired a beautiful person; and if you wanted a talented child—well, it was all the same. That was the superstition, of course (Moab, 1957 [FMC I 975]).

The disposition of a pregnant woman will be the same in the child (Charleston, 1972).

The amount of sleep a woman gets while she is pregnant determines what her baby will be like. If a lot of sleep, then baby will be congenial—if little sleep, then the baby will be cranky (Logan, 1971).

In order to have a happy child an expectant mother must be cheerful at all times (Orem, 1970).

If you go swimming when you are pregnant your baby will not be afraid of water or swimming (Logan, 1973).

The informant said she had heard that a pregnant woman can make her child talented by playing the piano a great deal while the mother is pregnant (Preston, Idaho, 1970).

If the mother reads late at night or in bad light, the child will be born with weak eyes and need glasses (Logan, 1973).

One interesting superstition of her mother [in Sweden] was concerning the marking of an unborn child. She always ate with a very small spoon so that her child would have a small mouth (Thornton, Idaho, 1970).

If an expectant mother sees three crows flying in the same direction in the same day, the child will tend to grow up to be a vagabond (Salt Lake City, 1973).

Well, there is a man . . . he's a very prominent man here in town, but he's just insanely jealous of his wife. And he has no reason in the world to be. Absolutely no reason to be. And his mother told me that she marked him that way. Because when she carried him, his father was just stepping out with everybody and anybody, and they had a girl working for them, and he would sit with this girl on his lap right in front of her, to torment her. And any time that he was gone, she just watched at the windows for him, and walked the floor. And she said, "I know I marked this boy." You'd be shocked if I told you who it was (Moab, 1953 [FMC I 895]).

That's what I say I did with my last child. I don't know that it was possible, or anything. She probably would have been born a tomboy anyway. But she's twenty-three years old now, and she's lots more boy than girl, and she's married and got two little boys. And she's just a little boy right with them, and she's been a boy all her life. Well, she was my sixth child, and I wanted another boy. That would make me three of each, and I just knew she was going to be a boy, and I didn't even have a girl's name picked for her, or nothing. She was just born like a boy. . . . She's definitely been more boy all her life. And when she went to school out on the dry farm, she never wore a dress, she always wore overalls. And one day an airplane flew over, just awful close—it just grazed the tops of the cedar trees near my house. And the schoolhouse was right close, and she come home and she said, "Mama, did you see the airplane today?" And I said, "Yes, I saw it, and it was just above the big old cedar tree, it was so low." And she said, "Well, just us boys saw it. The girls were in the house and didn't see it. . . ." She was just a first grader. . . . She was always the one to get the buckskin [that is, shoot a deer] and come home. She was the best shot. She went to the Christian Camp out to Musselman's Ranch several years ago, after we moved down here—went out with the Baptist kids, and she beat all the boys at rifle practice, and they were just burned up with her. And she just hates to wear a dress, even today. She's married. She made the cutest bride you ever saw, in her long dress and her veil (Moab, 1953 [FMC I 895]).

Basic in the lore of many cultures is the concept that man must avoid the usurpation of prerogatives belonging to God or to nature. Wishing too strongly for a child of either sex is often seen as such a transgression and is punished in one way or another.

TABOOS FOR PREGNANT WOMEN

There are taboos that circumscribe the behavior of pregnant women in order to shield offspring from marks, deformities, or undesirable psychic imprints. Some of these apply specifically to the period of pregnancy; others, to the behavior of married women throughout the fertile years of their life.

> While a mother is pregnant she shouldn't open an umbrella in the house or the newborn child will have a birthmark on the top of the head (Salt Lake City, 1973).

> Moles on a baby are caused by the pregnant mother having intercourse, the number of moles being the number of times she participated (Lava Hot Springs, Idaho, 1971).

> The wife should not indulge her husband while he is under the influence of alcohol, for idiocy and other serious maladies are liable to be passed on to the child (Hyde Park, 1973).

> My mother's sister married a distant cousin, and the family always feared that their child would have crooked noses [sic], because if you married your cousin your children would have crooked noses (Knoxville, Tennessee, 1973).

> Don't get your teeth filled while you're pregnant or they will fall out (Logan, 1971).

> If a mother has a bad complexion during her pregnancy, the baby is a girl, because she is taking beauty from her mother (Salt Lake City, 1973).

These last two items suggest that there also may be a reverse effect in prenatal influence: the fetus imposes certain conditions upon the mother.

CONCLUSIONS

Beliefs and superstitions concerning the marking and psychic imprinting of babies are encountered quite generally in Utah. The topic, naturally, interests and preoccupies women more than it does men. Women at all levels of the society seem to be aware of these beliefs, though they find a more ready acceptance among the least educated. Whether believed or rejected, they are live topics for conversation. Moreover, they seem to be about as well known now as they were twenty years ago. Nothing has been found to indicate that any aspects concerning prenatal influences have been shaped by or adapted to Mormon beliefs or social experience: Mormon women seem to share them with other English-speaking women of the United States and Canada.

NOTE

1. Sources of materials used in this paper are identified as follows:

FMC I = Fife Mormon Collection (bound volumes of field interviews between 1939 and 1958).

FAC I = Fife American Collection (also bound volumes, similar to FMC I, collected since 1958).

All items not identified by FMC or FAC were collected by students in folklore classes at Utah State University since 1970.

If an item was collected in Utah, the town name only is given; items from other locations are so identified.

Healing in a Balmyard: The Practice of Folk Healing in Jamaica, W.I.

LEONARD E. BARRETT, *Temple University*

It is estimated that between 60 and 70 percent of all man's illnesses are psychosomatic—literally of body and mind. Such illness starts in the mind and affects the body, and vice versa. Those individuals who have excessive worries, tensions, and insecurities may develop various kinds of somatic illnesses which, in turn, may cause discomfort to the mind. These psychic infections can even cause death. Folk healers have always dealt with illness, real and imagined; and if we are not blind or prejudiced, we must agree that they seemed to have done a good job in curing because the population of developing countries, which have been backward in the fields of science, seems to grow rather than decline over the centuries. We now know that thousands of people the world over have been treated for curable and incurable diseases by herbs, prayers or just the "healers' touch." In our day, the process continues unabated. This paper deals with herbal curing in the Caribbean, one area where folk curing is still influential. I begin with a personal experience.

· INTRODUCTION

My interest in folk medicine stems from my contact with it at about the age of eleven. For a period of two years, I had suffered periodically from malarial fever which grew worse each year. At the age of eleven, I suffered an attack which was rather serious. My mother would go to the druggist during these periods for the regular allotment of quinine, but in time this medication became ineffective because my physical condition grew progressively weaker. I was aware that my condition was becoming grave because of the weakness of my body from excessive ague and vomiting. During one such attack, the last I remember, very early one morning I was awakened, dressed, and taken out of the house to an awaiting donkey which was to take me on a journey. Because of the weakness of my body, I was able to ride by myself for only one-fourth of the way. I finished the rest of the journey riding on the backs of my mother and my uncle. It was not long before it occurred to me that we were not on our way to the medical specialist, the only physician in the community. Our journey took us on strange country roads which finally led us into a healing center with banners flying on tall poles, drumming, singing, and a lot of other strange activities. Soon after our arrival, I was made ready for what seemed to be a bathing experience. I was taken to a booth and given a vigorous sponging from head to foot with a herbal mixture, then dressed again and ushered into the presence of a large woman with a most compassionate face. A period of discussion went on between my mother and the healer about my illness. I received from the healer a glass of medicine, which was taken in her presence; my mother took a bottle of medicine for me with instructions on the kinds of bushes to boil after the bottle was finished; and we were on our way home soon thereafter.

The thing I remembered most vividly was that on my journey to the healer I had to be carried, but on my return home I walked. It was this experience that led me to know, and later to develop an interest in, Jamaican folk healers and their medicines. This paper is an introduction to this Jamaican healing center, which has been in continuous operation for over one hundred years under the leadership of two women, Mother Rozanne Forbes, the healer who treated me, and her daughter, Mother Rita Adams, the present healer.

THE BLAKE'S PEN HEALING CENTER

In the interest of time I shall concentrate on the setting of the center, the personality of the present healer, her methods of operation, and an analysis of the syncretism of primitive medicine and modern faith-healing techniques as they now exist in the island. But the study also depicts the situation that is prevalent in most of the islands of the Caribbean and the Antilles.

The Location and Origin

Driving on the main highway south from Kingston, the capital city of Jamaica, through May Pen and Mandeville, one will arrive before long at the great mountain divide (Don Figuerero Mountain), which separates the hill country from the savannahs to the south. At the foot of the mountain there is a road to the left which leads southward through that wedge of savannah which is bordered to the right (west) by Burnt Savannah Mountain, on the left (east) by Plowden Mountain, and on the south by the sea. The area is flat and dry and without rainfall six months of the year. Until a few years ago this was considered one of the disaster zones of the island, but a rich vein of bauxite was discovered in the area, and it now has one of the largest bauxite-processing factories in the island. But despite this seeming bonanza, very few people of this area can find work because the factory needs special skills; consequently, most of the work is done by foreigners and skilled workers from other parts of the island.

In spite of the austerity of this region and long before the bauxite bonanza was discovered, this area has been known to thousands of Jamaicans as a center of herbal curing for over one hundred years. It all began in 1871, when a young woman by the name of Rozanne Forbes received the vision to "rise up and heal the people."

Rozanne Forbes was the daughter of an African slave mother who was herself an expert in herbs. At her call, Rozanne Forbes was a member of the local Anglican Church (Episcopal). But it seems that she had become affected by the 1860 revival which swept the island in that period. This revival brought into being the new syncretistic cults known today as Revival Zion and Pukumina.

In response to the call, Rozanne is said to have been led by an angel near the mouth of a remote cave at the foot of Plowden Mountain, where she remained for fourteen days in fasting, eating only bread and water provided daily by her husband. For the first seven days she was instructed by the angel in seventy-seven different weeds and leaves, which were to be medicine for balming. The following seven days she was instructed in the properties and uses of herbs to be taken internally. She was also instructed in the ritual forms to be used—for example, the size of her tabernacle; the ritual colors; the time of day for healing, fasting, and worship; and the fee for her service. Among other things, she was told to dig in the center of the camp a hole ten feet square and five deep, from which a healing fountain would rise. This fountain was to be dug by the hands of women only and without metal instruments. One hundred years have past, but to this day the fountain has not emerged. The present healer told me that the water has never appeared because of the breaking of a taboo by her mother; she did not elaborate, but she expects the water to appear at any time.[1]

Rozanne Forbes continued her work from 1871 to 1929, when she died, leaving her daughter, Rita, to carry on her work. During her lifetime she served an area of fifty square miles, with auxiliary centers in Brompton, where I was taken to her in my childhood, and at Lacovia, where Martha Beckwith of Vassar College studied her in 1920.[2]

The Balmyard, or Healing Center

The Blake's Pen healing center is located on a seventeen-acre plot of ground in the parish of Manchester and is partially obscured from the view of passersby by the homes of the Forbes' relatives. To enter the center one climbs a steep incline, at the top of which is the "yard." At the entrance is a four-cornered concrete floor with flags at each corner and a cross in the center. This is called the "four-pole square" and symbolizes the four corners of the earth. All believers or patients coming to the center must circle this square counterclockwise before entering the consecrated grounds. Fifty yards from the square, one passes through what looks like a Japanese torii gate in front of which is a tall pole called the "Dial," which must also be circled. A few yards away from this pole is the healer's house, with living quarters and consulting rooms. There is also a chapel where service is held; a kitchen where medicine is prepared; two bathrooms, one for women and the other for men; and the fountain in which there is no water. The chapel is furnished with benches, a platform and a preaching stand, two tables with numerous glass tumblers, and an enamel basin with water. Among the other ritual equipment are three drums and several banners of the colors red, white, and blue with scriptural passages printed on them; there are also many flags all over the center, but because of the vigorous breeze coming off the sea, they are always ragged.

The center as described above remains essentially in the same pattern as it was laid out by the founder. Services are held each morning from 5 to 6 A.M., from 12 to 1 P.M., and from 6 to 7 P.M. Monday is set aside for fasting. The service begins at 9 A.M. to 12 noon with a break of one hour, and then resumes from 1 to 6 P.M. There is no Sunday service, which is quite unlike the ritual patterns of other centers and the religious tradition of Jamaica. No reason was given to me for this deviation.

The Passing of the Mantle: The Present Healer

At the death of Mother Forbes, the traditional role passed to her daughter, Rita. But Rita was not a stranger to her mother's work. As a child, she was her mother's medium. During her early childhood, she received dreams and visions which she related to her

mother, who acted on them. Recalling her childhood experiences
in elementary school, she relates that many times she experienced
spirit possession and had to be sent home; she returned to school,
as she puts it, "only when the spirit was through with me." It was
during her childhood that she received the vision of the exact year
her mother was to die and the exact place where she should be
buried. Her mother is said to have accepted the vision calmly, and
she gave orders that the spot be marked. Mother Forbes is today
buried at the very spot.

The present healer is seventy-eight years old, of medium height
and size, light in complexion, with an intelligent face, bright,
piercing eyes and a warm, compassionate smile. Even at age
seventy-eight, she displays a charming personality; she enjoys a
good laugh and in her free moments recalls humorous stories for
the enjoyment of her guests. Although she would be classed with
illiterates according to Jamaican standards, she is blessed with a
strong memory and will often recall incidents surrounding a
patient whom she has not seen in a year. She is in full control of the
varied activities around her—from the boiling of herbs to the
domestic care of her grandchild and her animals in the field to the
orders for a special lunch for the researchers who may be present.

Each person in the balmyard may share in the numerous
presents of food and fruits which are brought to her daily by her
patients; no one leaves the premises without a gift even if it is cold
water. The name "Mother" is both a religious title and a feeling of
affection by all who come to her. She is to them a mother, a healer,
and an adviser. She ministers not only to human illness, but to
animals also.

At the age of seventy-eight, she still visits the parish capital,
Mandeville, six miles away. This she does twice weekly in order to
buy her needed medical supplies. She also goes out each month on
missions, sometimes as far as Montego Bay, a hundred miles away.
Although physical and mental weakness is slowly setting in, she still
displays remarkable agility of body and mind.

A Day at the Balmyard

The major service at the center is on Monday, the day of fasting.
The followers arrive in buses, trucks, or private cars, on donkeys,
bicycles, or foot from distances up to seventy miles away; as many
as fifty patients may arrive in one day.

The colors for this service are white and blue: white for initiated
members and blue for new converts. The order of service is flexi-
ble; the major portion of the first part is given over to choruses in
which the drums are employed. It is a time of dancing, clapping of

hands, and testimonials—this may be designated as a praise service. The second part is marked by a more serious atmosphere, in which the songs of the Church of England are used. In this section the ritual for the Lord's Supper, according to the Book of Common Prayer, is used word for word. (Incidentally, the members know the ritual and the gestures accompanying it from memory.) This section of the service is closed with the breaking of bread and the drinking of water! Following this, there is a short sermon by Mother and then the benedictions. I say "benedictions" because there seems to be a never-ending recitation of various benedictions. The morning service now ends, and a period of feasting begins. This may last for an hour, after which the service of "travailing" begins. This period generally coincides with the balming of the sick in herbal baths and spiritual reading and prescriptions by Mother Rita in her consulting room.

The service of travailing is a kind peculiar to the Revival cult throughout Jamaica. It is conducted by a leader known as the "warrior shepherd." The members form in a circle in the chapel or outside of it on what is known as the "dial seal." Accompanied by chants, the members dance in counterclockwise movement, bending forward and backward from head to waist, chopping the air with both hands while emitting a hissing or grunting sound. The sound is the result of inhaling air and letting out the compressed air through the lips.

This exercise may continue for hours or sometimes days, depending on the dimension of evil revealed. During the ritual, members are said to be "at war" with the evil spirits that are present. The more vigorous the travailing, the greater will be the success in healing the sick. During this ritual many of the evils affecting the sick are revealed. Some members will fall under spirit possession and in this state will prophesy of impending dangers, like hurricanes, earthquakes, sudden death by poison, and witchcraft. Some will receive elaborate messages which they write on the ground in cabalistic signs similar to the *vever* of vodun in Haiti. Others pour libations on the ground. The ritual of travailing develops an atmosphere of tension among the insecure and is only abated in the process of consultation and balming as a means of protection.

Methods of Healing

As we shall see, the method of healing in the center is both ritual and herbal. The herb is used externally as a bath or taken internally in liquid decoction as medicine. Every patient visiting the center from the time of the founder to the present day receives a bath. Time will not permit me to detail the method of the founder as told to me by the present healer. I therefore will concentrate on the method of the present healer, the bathing procedure, her consulting techniques, and various samples of her herbal prescriptions.

The bath.—To acquaint myself better with the experience of my youth, I decided to take a herbal bath. When my turn came, I entered the roofless enclosure of corrugated zinc sheets. An enamel tub filled with herbal mixture was in the center of the enclosure, and nearby was a stone slab on which the patient stands. The attendant entered and asked that fifty cents in coin be thrown in the tub. This done, I was asked to assume a squatting position. With towel in hand, the balmer applied the mixture to my head and sponged down my back while he recited Psalm 23. He continued this operation from my waist to my heels and, reciting a new psalm, followed the same procedure from my face to my toes. Much attention was paid to the small of my back and my thighs, where the balmer administered vigorous blows with the sodden towel. After all the parts of the body had been thoroughly sponged, he made the sign of the cross from the nape of my neck to my waist, crossing at the shoulders. The sign was repeated in front, but this time he made the cross from the right shoulder to the toes of the left foot and from the left shoulder to the right foot as he recited the benediction: "In the name of the Father, Son, and Holy Ghost, as it was in the beginning now and ever shall be world without end, amen." The incantation was timed to conclude at the toes with the words "world without end." I was then asked to dress myself and refrain from taking a bath for twelve hours to allow the medical properties of the herbs to be absorbed into the pores.

Since I was the last to bathe and there were several people ahead of me awaiting consultation and prescription, I encouraged the balmer to divulge the names of the weeds used in the bath. Such disclosures were not allowed, but with the gentle bribe of a Parliament cigarette, he gave me the names of those of the seventy-seven weeds he could remember. He soon ran out of names and apologized that some of the names of these weeds are not known. Here are the few he remembered: yellow saunders bush, casha-marrior, sweetsop bush, sowersop bush, willow bush, Rosemarie weed, lakka bush, candle wood bush, leaf-of-life. High-John-The-Conqueror weed, soap bush, ballad weed, rickkie-rocher bush, wild cinnamon, semen-contra, strong-back, dead-and-wake; and here he ran out of the bushes.

Consulting techniques and prescriptions.—In the consulting room

there are three impotant chairs. The first is the chair of the
founder, which is always empty. Beside it is the chair in which the
present healer sits, and in front of the healer is the patient's chair.
The diagnostic techniques of the present healer differ from those
of her mother. During the days of the founder, when a patient
appeared before her for healing, she requested a basin with the
herbal decoction in which the person was later to bathe. The
patient was asked to dip both hands in the basin. Mother Forbes
then wet the palms of her hands with the water, struck both her
hands together, and read the patient's sickness from the palms of
her hands. The water was then sent back to the balming tent and
became part of the water with which the patient was later treated.
This method was clearly a process of divination, in which the water
was the medium. The present healer does her work in a different
way. First, the patient is bathed in the mixture and then appears
before the healer. The first few minutes of the consultation are
informal. The healer may open with a statement such as "I was
looking forward to seeing you," or "You have finally decided to
come," or "What took you so long?" Or she may recall some
incident that took place on the patient's journey. Then she requests
the patient to show his/her tongue. She now relates to the patient,
without asking the symptoms of the sickness, when the sickness
began and how it came about. I will give only four examples from
the large number of taped consultations I observed over two
summers.

1. A woman fifty years old. The healer looked steadily at her
face, glancing now and then at her legs. Then she asked: "How
long have you had the pain in your head? Pain in your joints? Pain
on the left side of your womb? Dizziness in the morning? Nausea
after eating?" Note that she did not ask whether the patient was
experiencing these conditions; she was relating the kinds of things
the patient was experiencing. I have yet to hear a patient deny her
statements.

Prescription: Summoning her secretary, she called out the following remedy: button-weed, sweet-cup weed, half-leaf of aloes,
juba bush. Boil in five pints of water to five half-pints. Mix this
with Gilby's Wine and take a half-glass daily.

2. A woman on behalf of her mother. She brought her mother's
handkerchief. The healer took it in her hands, concentrated a
moment, and then said: "Your mother suffers with pain in the legs.
It is because of an infected kidney. She has pain in her sinuses; pain

in her womb; she has a disposition of confusion and cancer in the womb. I cannot cure her but I can make her to feel better."

Prescription: A bottle of High-John-The-Conqueror's oil. Anoint the hands daily, making the sign of the cross. Sprinkle a little around the room while repeating Psalm 23.

3. A girl about seven years of age suffering with pains which prevented her sleeping at night. Mother Rita looked at her tongue and felt her stomach. The healer told the child's mother that the child had recently fallen from a tree and dislocated her womb but had concealed it. After much prompting the child admitted that she had fallen from a tree three weeks before coming. This was not known to the child's parents. Mother gave her some words of admonition.

Prescription: Womb weed, garden bitters bush, bladder weed, horse bath, button-weed, strong-back weed, leaf-of-life. Boil seven half-pints to three half-pints. Take also a bottle of Indian-root pills.

4. A man who suffered from insomnia. The healer questioned him about a recent court case in which he was involved. She informed him that evil powers generated in that case were still affecting him.

Prescription: Buy some black-puss incense and burn it in the bedroom; this will clear up the destruction that is following. No bush.

Before I leave this section, let me list a few ailments and the remedies for them as dictated to me on tape by the healer.

Gonorrhea: Kwaku bush, juba bush, one-leaf aloes, horse bath, Bahama grass, dead-and-wake, sweet-cup bush, bladder weed, vervine.

Boil in nine pints of water to nine half-pints; take with Gilby's Wine.

Mental disorders: Wet the head with oil of nutmeg or lavender water. Several doses of brain tonic until patient begins to "come around." After this period, put him on the bushes. Seatime, nine coconut leaves, hard-shell sweet-cup bush, mauve water grass, one leaf of aloes, white sage, hug-me-close, dead-and-wake.

Boil in nine pints of water to nine half-pints. Add to this Wincarnis Wine. Take a glass a day.

Gastric troubles: Camphor weed, black joint, one leaf of aloes, nine cotton leaves, dead-and-wake, three chips of birchwood bark, hug-me-close, and horse bath.

Kidney troubles: Cucumber bush, hug-me-close, baby-gripe, garden bitters, nine cotton leaves, black joint, leaf-of-life, sweet-cup that runs on the ground.

Heart trouble: Search-me-heart, horse bath, three leaves of cow foot, mauve water grass, Bahama grass, nine cotton leaves, ten sprigs of balsam, and a sprig of sea-time.

SOME ANALYSES

It is clear that Jamaican healers of the type under consideration are an integral part of the folkways of the island. They serve a large community and are always in great demand. It is not unusual for one of them to see and serve eighty people a day. Healers like Mother Rita are so influential that the government seeks to encourage them rather than obstruct them. This is not the case with the other class of native specialists, the obeah-men or sorcerers, who also use weeds and heal but hurt by magical means as well. The class to which Mother Rita belongs always performs work within the context of the native religion, but the sorcerer is a private person with a client-professional relationship. The difference between these two classes of specialists will become clearer in my concluding statement.

The work of Mother Rita combines healing and divination. She is believed to have a "spiritual eye" through which she can "see" the patient's complaint, whether this be physical illness or supernormal interference. She explained to me that sometimes she is able to see "ghosts" or spirits accompanying the patients as they approach her residence. In such cases she would first send the patients to the chapel for spiritual "decontamination" before allowing them to sit in the chair. She also related that while she is working with a patient, a "weed" will be revealed to her unconsciously, and she then sets its name down. Here again her mediumship reveals itself.

There are many features of her center which are similar to those of other folk healing centers the world over. For example the ritual numbers—seventy-seven weeds and seven days and nights for the learning of herbs—are reminiscent of a similar center in Ghana which deals with ninety-nine weeds. The flags and banners are typical of Revival groups all over the Caribbean. The fountain of water is also an important feature in Jamaican healing lore. Several centers, some of which I have studied, specialize in healing with water. In Mother Rita's center, water is used in the fasting ritual and the pouring of libation. One healer told me that the spirit of prophesy comes over him only when it rains. A comparative study of these centers must be made before we can get a picture of their main features.

Most of Rita's patients are people close to the soil who grew up in the cultural milieu of herbal lore. Many of them are acquainted with the names of these "medicines" and know exactly where to find them. What they lack is the knowledge of their combinations. As in Africa, so it is in Jamaica: the majority of rural people often cultivate a small garden of herbs and use the well-known ones for common ailments. So the average person who is sick will first medicate himself before seeking the aid of any physician, native or trained. The native healer is far more sought after than the European-trained doctors. In the urban centers of the island, there are about two thousand patients to a doctor, but in some rural areas there are as many as twenty thousand. Most doctors reside in the town and visit the rural communities infrequently; thus the native healer is closer in every respect to the village community. A visit to the European-trained specialist is in many cases indulged in only for his scientific advice. Most rural people come to him to have him put his stethoscope on them. This the Jamaican calls "sounding." Then they will take his diagnosis to the healer and take the healer's prescription and ignore that of the doctor. There are two reasons for this: first, the doctor's medicine is usually too expensive, and, second, the rural Jamaicans have little faith in it. The one thing the average Jamaican will take from a medical doctor is an injection; this is considered to have a special effect even if the doctor uses only water or vitamins. One of the reasons for the high respect and confidence for the native healer is his combination of religious ritual with healing. Sickness of any kind to Jamaican folk is a visitation from God or the devil. In either case it is considered of supernatural origin, and there is nothing that touches the Jamaican's emotion more deeply than the folk religion. In the hands of the religious healer he feels safe. Therefore the healing centers, with their drumming, singing, and healing, are natural settings for the restoration of body and mind.

As to the effectiveness of these healers' medicine, no scientific study has yet been done on this subject. The only evidence we have is the testimonies of people who have had experiences with them. If one is to go by these testimonies, the evidence is heavily in favor of the healers. As in most magico-religious healing, those who have had no cures are reluctant to speak because there is always the fear that the prescription was not followed correctly or that they themselves were the causes of failure.

There seems to be no question that the weeds are high in

medicinal properties. The use of these weeds is pervasive, whether they are given English names, as in Jamaica; French, as in Haiti; or Spanish, as in Santo Domingo. It is surprising how the uses of them are uniform in all the Caribbean islands.

This leads me to a point which has never been made before: most of the herbs, barks, and roots originally bore African names, and that fact suggests the handing down of the tradition from one generation to the next. Some seem to bear the names of the original healers who made them famous, such as Kwaku bush, Cudjoe weed, or Packy bush, myal weed, pimpe, mapimpe, pem-pem, and various others of African origin. Most names of weeds and bushes are now Jamaicanized; examples of these are hug-me-close, dead-and-wake, heal-and-draw, seed-under-leaf, and cure-for-all. Although the first groups of Africans brought to Jamaica met and socialized with the Arawak Indians, their medical lore seems to have had little or no influence on the African community. Almost all of the names of plants and herbs still keep their Ashanti names, and those translated in English are words referring only to their properties.

SOME CONCLUSIONS

It is impossible for anyone to understand Caribbean folk medicine without taking into account the provenance of the people who inhabit the area and their methods of healing before and after they arrived in the islands. Eighty percent of all Caribbean peoples are of African descent; in Jamaica it is 90 percent. The African medicine man is not a Johnny-come-lately. He belongs to a healing fraternity that goes back to antiquity. In his book *African Religions and Philosophy* John S. Mbiti has this to say of them:

> To African societies the medicine-men are the greatest gift, and the most useful sources of help. Other names for them are "herbalists," "traditional doctors," "Wanganga" (to use a Swahili word). These are the specialists who have suffered most from European-American writers and speakers, who so often and wrongly call them "witch-doctors"—a term which should be buried and forgotten forever. Every village in Africa has a medicine man within reach, and he is the friend of the community. He is accessible to everybody and at almost all times, and comes into the picture at many points in individual and community life.[3]

About their calling and behavior he says:

> There is no fixed rule governing the "calling" of someone to become a medicine-man. This may come when he is still young and unmarried, or

in his middle or later life. In other cases, a medicine-man passes on the
profession to his son or other relatives. . . . There are both men and
women in this profession. Their personal qualities vary, but medicine-
men are expected to be trustworthy, upright morally, friendly, willing
and ready to serve, able to discern peoples' needs and not be exorbitant
in their charges.[4]

Speaking of their knowledge of the craft Mbiti states:

Candidates acquire knowledge in matters pertaining to: the medical
value, quality and use of different herbs, leaves, roots, fruits, barks,
grasses and various objects like minerals, dead insects, bones, feathers,
powders; . . . the causes, cures and prevention of diseases and other
forms of suffering; . . . magic, witchcraft and sorcery and how to combat them, the nature and handling of spirits and the living dead; and
various other secrets some of which may not be divulged to outsiders.[5]

Mbiti, as we have seen, discusses folk medicine and the medicine
man within the religious context of African peoples. This is most
important because sickness and diseases in African traditional
thought fall within the realm of the supernatural, and both the
medicine man and his archenemy, the sorcerer, are men who deal
with supernatural forces. During the period of slave trade, many of
these spiritual functionaries were brought to the islands, and we
are fortunate that early scholars were keen enough to observe their
works and to leave in writing a few details on them. One such
writer is the Jamaican historian Herbert G. DeLisser, who was well
acquainted with the African influence in the island. He writes:

Both witches and wizards, priests and priestesses, were brought to
Jamaica in the days of the slave trade, and the slaves recognized the distinction between the former and the latter. Even the masters saw that
the two classes were not identical, and so they (the masters) called the
latter 'myal-men' and 'myal-women'—the people who cured those that
the obeah-men had injured.[6]

Time will not permit me to go into a detailed discussion of the two
words that DeLisser uses in this quotation. But let me quickly differentiate them in the Jamaican context. The words *obeah* and
obeah-man are known throughout the Caribbean. The word comes
from the Akan language of Ghana, West Africa, where the word
Obayi means witchcraft.[7] Thus, an obeah-man is one who casts
spells and sells deadly charms. His work is antisocial, and to this day
his influence in Jamaica is sinister. The words *myal* and *myal-man*
refer to that class of African specialists who under spirit possession
(myal) can detect the evil influence of the obeah-man, and they are

the ones who prescribe the herbal cures for the healing of those who are bewitched. The myalmen are descendants of the "priests and priestesses" referred to by DeLisser.

During the years of slavery, the legitimate priest and priestess, unable to function in the slave setting, joined hands with the obeahman to fight the witchcraft of the masters. They functioned as a secret society, offering bullet-liquifying potions to the slaves, performing ceremonial oaths, and administering herbal poisons to the enemy. These secret societies became strong institutions among the slaves, and they were never challenged until the late nineteenth-century, when missionary work began in earnest.

One of the important factors that aided the medicine man in the islands was the availability of the weeds and bushes with which he had been familiar in Africa. Sir Spencer St. John, the nineteenth-century British ambassador to Haiti, related how the slaves used herbs to cause the death and derangement of many Haitian masters and concluded:

> And if it be doubted, that the individuals without even common sense, can understand so thoroughly the properties of herbs and their combinations . . . I can say that tradition is a great book, and that they receive these instructions as a sacred deposit from one generation to another, with the further advantage that in the hills and mountains of this island grow in abundance similar herbs to those which in Africa they employ in their incantations.[8]

For a period of nearly two hundred years, the preaching of the Christian gospel was forbidden to the slaves in Jamaica; and although some kinds of religious instructions were allowed, it was not the rule. It was not until 1815 that the Church of England grudgingly began to instruct the slaves in Christianity in order to oppose the Nonconformists. But it was mainly through the work of the Baptists and Methodists and Moravians that Christianity became island-wide. In 1860 a great religious awakening, similar to that which occurred in the United States, began. The slaves were stirred by this phenomenon, but since they had no knowledge of the new teaching, a period of syncretistic formation followed. The slaves merged the Biblical teachings and the Christian rituals of the various denominations with their African beliefs, and thus began the Afro-Christian cults which now flourish in the islands. It is in this context that we observe in the Blake's Pen healing center the high syncretism of Anglican rituals neatly wedded with African healing lore. It is under the guise of these cults that the wider dimension of African retentions, which are the main cultural and emotional foundations of Caribbean peoples, is found today. Even the Jamaican elite, who emulate the English way of life sometimes even beyond the standards of the Englishman, are not quite able to rid themselves of their early cultural upbringing. I vividly recall a medical doctor, a graduate of a prestigious British university, who, on learning of my plans to study Mother Rozanne, cautioned me to be discreet in my reporting because, as he put it, "That woman saved my life." He then related in detail how as a young boy he had come down with the vomiting sickness that had already caused the death of his sister. His parents, who were Moravians, finally decided to visit the founder of the center, and it was her medicine that saved him. On my second visit, I found out why he cautioned me: he suffered with diabetes and the present healer had been treating him for over a year. I was rather amused when just before I left his house for my second summer at the center, the doctor took me aside, presented me with a large bottle, and asked that I have Mother Rita send him a supply of the usual medicine. The story of the doctor is only one example of the confidence still shown in the medicine man in the island.

I do not have time to discuss the strong beliefs in some other aspects of Jamaican folk medicine. It would take another paper of some length to relate the uses of incenses, oils, and talismans, which seem to be a big business for the drugstores. One healer who works mostly with these items told me that since January of 1973, he had spent at one store about four hundred pounds, or $1,120, for oils, roots, and incenses.

As a final documentation, I quote Professor Katumi Kiteme of Kenya, presently teaching at the City University of New York, who recently wrote about his father, a medicine man in Africa, and his own experience in the Caribbean:

> From my father's medicine collections, he has (or can prepare) medicine for snakebites, abdominal disorders, venereal diseases, . . . birth control and abortions for women who are too weak and ill to give birth; malaria, migraine headache; colds, pneumonia, fresh or infected open wounds; poor sight and blindness; toothaches, diarrhea; stomach ulcers and all other illnesses which strike the Africans in our area. It is significant to note that the use of herbs for medicines is still found among African descendants in the West Indies, Brazil and Southern United States. My visit to a Haitian "leaves doctor" revealed very similar medical practices.[9]

As recently as June 1973, news came out of Nigeria that the government had decided to set up an institute for the study of native herbs and roots to preserve the age-old tradition of the medicine man.

With the rising cost of synthetic medicine and the scarcity of trained medical practitioners in the developing Caribbean and the Third World, Nigeria has hit upon a sound plan. It is my belief that folk traditions, despite their placebos, have much to offer; and until such time science as is able to serve the rich and the poor, a large section of the world population will still be in the bush.

NOTES

1. The content of this paper is based on taped interviews between the author and Mother Margarite Adams (Rita) in the summers of 1970-1973.

2. See Martha Beckwith, *Black Roadways: A Study of Jamaican Folk Life* (Chapel Hill: University of North Carolina Press, 1929), pp. 171-173.

3. John S. Mbiti, *African Religions and Philosophy* (New York: Frederick A. Praeger, 1969), p. 166.

4. *Ibid.*, pp. 166-167.

5. *Ibid.*

6. Herbert G. DeLisser, *Twentieth Century Jamaica* (Kingston, 1913), p. 108.

7. See J. G. Christaller, *Dictionary of the Asante and Fante Language*, 2d ed. (Basel, 1933), p. 11.

8. Sir Spencer St. John, *Haiti; or, The Black Republic* (London: Smith, Elder and Co., 1884) p. 215; emphasis mine.

9. *Ebony*, 27, 7 (May 1973), pp. 114-122.

Doing What, with Which, and to Whom? The Relationship of Case History Accounts to Curing

MICHAEL OWEN JONES,
University of California, Los Angeles

The best-known case that "Uncle" Jim treated concerned young Joey Martin, who had warts on his vocal cords. "There was nothing the doctors could do," exclaimed Jim's daughter Gladys; "he was dying! He would eventually have choked."

Many of the people in the village where Jim was raised commented on the events to me. So did Jim Gallagher,[1] the eighty-five-year-old man who had been divinely bestowed with the gift of healing because he had been born a seventh son.[2] Gallagher's daughter and her husband also mentioned aspects of this illness frequently in our conversations, noting the striking nature of the malady. "It was never encountered here before,"[3] remarked Gladys, who described the events three or four times. When she communicated information about the incident to me, Gladys tended to emphasize the futility of professional treatment and to focus attention on the boy's suffering.

"He was choking," declared Gladys. "They had a tube in his throat, here, and that's what he was breathing through—it was like a silver, a little silver tube about as big as a half dollar, and it had to be taken out—the mucus," she said. "He'd choke up this tube, and they'd have to take it out ever so often, and clean it, and put it back in. Just keeping Joey alive," she told me. "And he was so bad that the bishop prayed for Joey, had special prayers for Joey Martin."

Gladys's husband, who worked with Joey's father, had told Jim about Joey's problem, and Jim Gallagher went to the hospital on the condition that nobody but the parents would be with the boy.

"And so when he went in," explained Gladys, "Father saw that Joey couldn't breathe through this hole—right here it was in his throat. And Father said, 'Well, I'll see.' And he warned them of what he was scared of," that the dislodged warts would choke the boy. "And he put his hand on him, and when he put his hand on him, the hand was shaking mad and Mr. and Mrs. Martin never saw anything like it before. And Mother was scared stiff that Joey would choke—the warts would come off and choke him."

Gladys paused for a moment. "And then Father rubbed Joey's throat," she continued, "and he rubbed his chest. And he said, 'Yes, I'll cure that young fella,' he said. 'I'll cure him.'"

By the third night of treatment, however, something else was wrong. Jim Gallagher told the parents that he found something amiss, not in the throat, but with the lungs, for his quivering left hand, used in both diagnosis and therapy, shook more intensely as it neared the boy's chest. Because of Jim's insistence, the parents agreed to have the doctor x-ray Joey.

When Jim saw the boy the next night, according to Gladys, "he said, 'They had X rays, and Joey's lung damned near collapsed.' That's the report from the doctor. And it was caused," claimed Gladys, "through the tube being inserted into his throat. That caused it. They attributed it to inserting the tube in too far; it punctured a vein leading into the lung."

That problem attended to, Jim then predicted that within a few days the warts would be gone because his hand had been quivering with decreased intensity.

"And the fifth or sixth day, I'm not too sure," continued Gladys, "Father went down, and they were after taking X rays, and Dr. Malone and the nurse came, and the doctor said, 'The warts on his vocal cords,' he said, 'were flattened out like the head of a nail.' And they couldn't understand why."

"Father warned the parents not to tell anyone he was there," explained Gladys, when I raised my eyebrows in question. "If they did, he wouldn't go again. He didn't want any publicity, see. He wanted to cure Joey—he knew definitely he could cure Joey—but he didn't want any publicity. And within a week Joey Martin was sitting up in bed. And they took more X rays, and the warts were gone. They didn't know what happened, and they still did not."

At this point Gladys changed to a somewhat disparaging tone as she told me that the doctor was about to leave on his vacation, and despite evidence that the warts were nearly gone, he predicted the imminent demise of the boy.

"'Anyhow, I'm going; nothing else I can do for you,'" he told the parents according to Gladys's account of the event. "'Joey Martin won't be alive when I come back.' He said, 'There's no way for him to live that length of time.' And he want away and Joey Martin kept getting better," said Gladys, "and they let him off the bed and me father went out and said, 'I'm going out on the bay; the young fella's all right.'"

"And Dr. Malone was back from his vacation within a month," Gladys continued, "and they kept Joey in the hospital because they couldn't discharge him until the doctor came, or gave orders to discharge him, you see. And the nurse said, 'When Dr. Malone comes we're gonna make sure Joey Martin is at the top of the stairs, gonna make sure.'"

"And Dr. Malone was due in the hospital that morning," said Gladys. "Course Joey Martin was going around everywhere—he was just grand. He still had the tube in his throat—'twas a little silver tube (I can see it now)—just what he was breathing through. And when Dr. Malone came and stopped at the stairs to the hospital, and looked up to come up those stairs," said Gladys; "when he looked up and saw Joey Martin coming to meet him, he said, 'My God!' he said, 'What kind of a miracle happened here?'"

"They never told Dr. Malone," Gladys hastened to add. "Father told them not to tell. And in a couple of days they had him out of the hospital. And Dr. Malone at the hospital, the nurses at the hospital, and doctors and all of them said Joey Martin'd never talk."

Gladys did not explain this allegation more fully, but her father emphasized the erroneousness of the prediction when he communicated the incident to me later.

"He was six years old then. And that was June 1953. And that young fella's twenty-one now," said Gladys in July 1968. "And he graduated from school and's working, and all—a great big young fella," she noted, apparently satisfied with the outcome of her father's therapy.

"And when he got out of the hospital that summer," Gladys said about young Joey, "he went to see my father who was out fishing. And he hasn't had a wart since," she said, which is what Joey and his parents also told me when I talked with them later and saw for myself the evidence of Joey's having had a tracheotomy. "And that's as true, my son, as the light is shining," said Gladys. "And you know that fella, I dare say to this day, he says his prayers, he prays for Mr. Gallagher," Gladys contended, although the Martins indicated to me only that they send a five-dollar bill to Jim each Christmas. "'Thank God for Mr. Gallagher!' he used to say in his prayers," said Gladys. "His mother and his grandparents (they've died since then) said, 'Every night Joey said his prayers, he'd thank God for Mr. Gallagher.' And that's as true as the light," concluded Gladys.

What, then, is the relationship of this and similar descriptions to curing? To be considered are the following possibilities: as a source of information for historical studies of curing, as a form of therapy, as the data base for describing a tradition of healing and for determining the motivations of healers and their patients, and as a source of insights for understanding more fully the nature of human thought processes and behavior. When I was conducting research in an eastern province of Canada, I asked myself initially if descriptions of cases could be used as a data base for diachronic studies. Oral communications of specific cases might have provided some useful information about medical practices in the past if more of them had been recorded, but the paucity of such data was a problem needing attention. Consider that for more than six decades, Jim Gallagher had treated patients from many parts of the United States and Canada, as well as from his immediate vicinity. Although he had staunched bleeding wounds, banished warts, stopped the pain in aching teeth, attended to instances of gout, arthritis, and even goiter, and, especially, treated eczema for many hundreds or perhaps thousands of individuals, few actual case histories were communicated by the healer or his family, by former patients, or by friends and acquaintances of the healer and patients. The same situation obtained for other healers, too, though I focused most of my attention on Uncle Jim at this time and later in 1969, when I eventually presented myself to him as a patient. In what manner could I account for the failure of individuals to recall as many cases of treatment as I had expected, and how could I explain the number and nature of the cases communicated to me? Of the thousands of experiences that Jim had had, nineteen events were described by him, his daughter, and those acquaintances of his whom I interviewed, and many of these nineteen cases were known to the majority of people with whom I spoke.

The most likely explanation of both forgetting and remembering, in addition to other factors pertaining to one or the other but not both,[4] is that only a few incidents can be recalled under ordinary circumstances owing to the vast number of experiences that we have; and those events of the past that are remembered and described are the unusual ones. This explanation was suggested by the healer's daughter Gladys. Her father had just told me that after diagnosing or treating a patient, the left side of his body, where his healing power is manifested, sometimes broke out in crosses that formed a red, "treadlike" pattern. I asked Gladys about this phenomenon, which I found rather odd and difficult to comprehend (although later Jim pointed it out to me after he had treated me). Gladys said, "I don't know of severe cases; I have seen it, but I can't recollect of severe cases. But I have seen it. The way we grew up, we grew up with this. And it's not peculiar to us, whereas it could be peculiar to you. We grew up with it." A few minutes later I asked her about the report that earthworms died if they came in contact with Jim's left side, one of the signs that a seventh son or daughter is different from ordinary people. Again she said, "I never questioned him too much about it. Because we grew up with it."

This quality of the striking or unusual has important implications for folklore studies in many ways, and the topic of forgetting and remembering is of considerable significance.[5] All I wish to point out now, however, is that a review of the cases noted by interviewees suggests that the incidents of curing communicated to me were unusual in regard to the healer and his behavior; or the patient who had striking physical or personality traits, or responded in an unusual manner, or was the informant or a member of his family; or the illness, which was rare or of marked severity; or the treatment, which was atypical for the particular disease or the healer or was undertaken in unusual circumstances.[6] One can appreciate, then, why the people I talked to who knew Jim Gallagher or had heard about him were aware of the case of the boy with warts on his vocal cords.

Communications of specific cases might have been useful for purposes of historical reconstruction, too, were it not for the fact that the events of the past which are described relate to the present interests of those who communicate this information and to the future needs of those to whom the incidents are described.[7] This raises a question regarding the purposes served by descriptions of medical cases. Given the circumstances attending the communication of healing incidents to me as researcher, curiosity-seeker, and patient, it would appear that there were at least five reasons for the communication of these case histories, although an intent common to all seemed to be to explain and to verify. Depending on the situation, individuals described particular cases in order to explain the etiology of disease, to illustrate specific kinds of diseases and their manifestations, to indicate more fully the nature of therapeutic measures, to verify the soundness of the therapy employed, and to demonstrate the power and effectiveness of the healer (or, in some cases, to discredit the therapy and healer or to support one healer and denounce another).

For example (and by way of verification), immediately after Gladys said that she did not know of "severe cases" of her father's breaking out in crosses, she described to me an incident involving two infant sisters with a severe case of eczema who "were so bad that after Father had finished with them the scalp came right offen their head, here, and the whole works, and their head was as clean as the palm of me hand." Shortly afterward, when remarking upon the seven different kinds of eczema, she mentioned a specific case of "dry eczema" involving "this poor old gentleman from Pigeon's Cove—Henry Franklin Green." Green, as was the custom, had been invited to stay the night and was to sleep in the bed of the parents, who would spend the night in the room of the children, who would have to sleep on the floor. But Green insisted on using the daybed in the kitchen. After Jim rubbed Henry Green, said Gladys, "he had his first night's sleep, he said, in years—stopped itching. And up over our couch was the queen and the royal family. . . . And he, when he was gonna go away that day, he said, 'You see her up there?' he said. He said, 'If I was in her palace I'd have to scratch. But,' he said, 'I'm walkin' home today.' And he said, 'I'm going down,' he said, 'I'm going down and I won't have to scratch all the way.' But it was the dry eczema that could do that," said Gladys, " and dust would fall on the floor—dry eczema. Henry Franklin Green: How I can remember him, cause we were tickled to death cause we didn't have to give up our bed," she laughed. "Now that must be *forty-one years ago*."[8]

I could continue illustrating these several uses of other peoples' communications of case histories, especially those incidents described essentially for demonstrative purposes and reinforcement, by citing further examples of unusual behavior that I remember from my own experiences with other people, but I would rather proceed to the next question. Is the communication of particular cases an act that itself may be part of the therapy and directly related to the illness and recovery from it? Probably not, but perhaps so; at least this is the relationship I was considering when I was asked to contribute a paper to this conference, and it partly accounts for the title, the implication of which is that the parameters of curing may not be as easily distinguished as is usually supposed. In some situations, especially when I was a patient (but also when I inferred that others inferred that I might be doubtful of what they said), it seemed to me that specific cases were communicated to me not only to inform me in greater detail about a procedure or the nature of an illness or the causes of some afflictions, but also to *persuade* me of the veracity of what had been proposed. I noticed that Uncle Jim and his daughter referred to other cases, even described some in detail, that were far worse than mine, and I felt relief at the knowledge that I would soon recover.[9] When I complain of some minor affliction now to my wife, she will remind me of how well I really am compared with some other people we know who have broken bones, ulcers, or terminal illnesses; and if I persist in glorying in my agony, in exasperation she will describe some of these conditions to me. Close friends tend to be more sympathetic, I feel, perhaps because unlike my wife, they are not registered nurses. *They* seem to perceive my apprehensiveness about what I conceive to be a serious disorder, such as headache or perhaps a cold or allergies, and appear to recognize my need for sympathy, particularly when they allude to other instances of greater severity, which serve to distract my attention from my frail condition.

It was my belief, then, that the relationship of the communication of case histories to curing is that these communicative acts are means of expressing concern, care, even love and understanding to another individual and that as a technique of persuasion, these messages attend to the emotional dimension of pain, illness, and injury and help the patient to recover from his sickness. Furthermore, I thought that traditional procedures and faith healing are utilized because of the degree to which they are successful—and the licensed physician and the nurse and their techniques perhaps unsuccessful—in treating illness through suggestion therapy. After all, many of our health problems, I believed (though I could not *prove* beyond doubt a single instance of this) are emotional in origin or aggravated by an adverse mental state; quite a few traditional therapies learned and utilized in situations of firsthand interaction do not involve the administration of herbal or chemical substances and yet seem to be effective (well, at least the patient reportedly recovers); and faith does seem to be involved in promoting and defending certain propositions and procedures.[10] There is, of course, evidence of the use of "persuasion" or suggestion in healing which is convincing enough to help reinforce my own belief that orally communicated metaphorizations of cases of healing are aids in the curing process. Unfortunately, however, such a proposition is not conclusive for me,[11] although I wish that I could defend my belief because it has some important ramifications for certain questions: who is the healer, in what circumstances, using what techniques of therapy? (For example, anyone expressing sympathy to another person is a "healer," the curing process may occur any where and any time even though a designated "healer" is not present, and so on.)

A third relationship between descriptions of past cases and curing might be their use as a source of information regarding the healing tradition and the factors that motivate healers to assume this identify and patients to utilize the services of these healers. I did in fact attempt to use some of these metaphorizations as a data base to discover the ways in which certain individuals perceived themselves and their relations to the environment. A report of this research appeared recently as a brief monograph entitled *Why Faith Healing?*; so I will not repeat the findings here. But reference to this use of orally communicated information about particular incidents of healing suggests a fourth and even more fundamental point.

To repeat the question: what is the relationship of case history accounts to curing? Change the phrasing from "case history accounts" to "communications of case histories" and insert "understanding" before "curing," and the answer follows. The relationship of communications of case histories to understanding curing is to be found in the extent to which we are enabled to comprehend more fully, by means of a detailed examination of specific instances described to us, the mental processes of individuals who perceive themselves to be sick and who conceive as appropriate many different techniques for attending to their illnesses.

Several investigators suppose, of course, that, in the words of one researcher, "a convenient metaphor would be to view the actual cures as entities embedded in a traditional body of belief to which they owe their existence." Further, it is common to speak of a "belief network," "system," or "complex," of the "retention of cures" or their "replacements," of people who have "abandoned some cures" or who "cling to the past," and of "persisting beliefs," "the tenacity of tradition," and the "modernization of the older belief[s]."[12] In other words, just as I originally considered it convenient to speak of case history "accounts" as if these communications were "texts" with physical qualities, it is often deemed appropriate to concretize the abstract, to make static that which is dynamic, and to systematize what is actually elusive, diffuse, and disjointed. Introspection with regard to our own cognition and behavior or analysis of our interactions with other people who are attempting to communicate ideas to us, however, suggests that "beliefs" or therapeutic techniques are not simply accepted without question and that they are not things which are inherited from the past as an assemblage of objects, united by some form of regular interaction or interdependence, which may be physically substituted or discarded or clung to. Other people, and we, can tell us this, but we have to listen.

Permit me to describe one more case which seems unusual in regard to the healer and his behavior, the patient and his response, the severity of the affliction, and the circumstances of treatment, although—and this is what is really striking—the case is not atypical or peculiar with respect to the conception of therapy appropriate to the perception of illness. This case will illustrate and give support to my contention that the use of certain metaphors is actually inconvenient for purposes of understanding human behavior, and perhaps it will persuade others of the need to reconsider some of the approaches to the study of "folk medicine."[13] This case demonstrates that the kinds of treatment used depend upon the way the patient perceives the malady and the manner in which he conceives of the relationship between therapy and illness, both of which are never fixed in his mind but change constantly as he continues to experience the illness.

The case involves a young man at UCLA who recently had what he called "a relatively absurd complaint"—the hiccups—that lasted for three days, during which time, he said, "it metamorphosed into something mysterious and primary." The first day the hiccups were intermittent; they were conceived of as simply a "mild annoyance" to be treated with familiar techniques thought by this individual to have "some biological reason" for their purported effectiveness. They did not work. "I finally gave up," he said, "and the hiccups ceased some half hour after I discontinued holding my breath and drinking water," but by then he saw no correlation between the remedies and the cessation of the hiccups. Later he experienced an intense attack for two hours. "Attempts at standing on my head failed (I felt this had biological validity as a cure)," so "I began trying remedies that I felt had no correlation to scientific medical knowledge." His hiccups stopped about an hour after he put a ten-franc coin in his pocket. "I've always regarded it as being 'lucky,' that is, possibly it could effect change," he observed. "At this point I was just as skeptical about direct causal correlation as in the case of the more plausible biological cures. However, I felt that both types could effect change, but that they simply hadn't in these cases," although he did not know why they had not proved effective.

Four hours later the hiccups returned with great intensity. "My first reaction was anger," he reported. "I tried several 'head dips' (swallowing water with head between knees while standing bent at the waist), but I held on to my lucky ten-franc piece as well. Both commanded equal respect in my mind, yet neither seemed powerful enough to cure the hiccups." The question was still, why had no therapy proved successful? Shortly after midnight the hiccups ceased. "My reaction," he observed, "was one of exhaustion and I felt the absurd humor of it all. Also, I felt that I knew considerably less about hiccups, but considerably more about one's reactions to hiccups."

On the second day he used some procedures he had employed the first day, hoping for success this time but expecting failure because of his earlier experience, and "I also tried several cures not previously employed: hopping on one foot while holding breath, sugar on tongue, push-ups, sit-ups, put lucky coin in pocket, handled several other lucky objects (pinecones and personal items of old friends), reproduced several designs of pentagrams and placed them in my pocket or hand."

"At this point," he noted (and his statement is important for understanding his use of certain therapies) "I was beginning to think of the hiccups as being more mysterious than I had ever imagined. I realized that I would try any remedy without regard to its biologically plausible merit and this realization bothered me for some unknown reason."

Although the hiccups continued for another five hours, he refrained from all therapy. Instead, he focused attention on trying to understand the nature of this malady and examined medical texts which recommended the surgical procedure of crushing the glottis; this treatment was conceived by the patient as not attending, however, to what he thought was the essence of the problem itself. No, he reported, "It was as if the hiccups began to take on a very mystical character worthy of respect. I began to wonder if they indicated something: good or bad?"

He met with friends who tried to be helpful by suggesting cures to him and illustrating and supporting these remedies by reference to other cases; but most of the techniques he had already tried, though he used some again to appease his friends. He still felt that his hiccups were esoteric, and by this time he was experiencing "a growing feeling about the importance of my hiccups." Indeed, by the third day he was beginning to feel that his experience might in some way be beneficial to him, although he was uncertain how.

Still more acquaintances consoled him, suggesting remedies none of which was new to him and therefore none of which was seriously considered by him. By now the attention of other people was disturbing. "I felt that I knew so much more about the hiccups than they that I didn't even want to continue the discussion." A close friend and he agreed that the hiccups had to be met on their own ground; but what was that? Examining medical texts again simply generated further bafflement, so "the only cures I attempted at this point," he observed, "were magic drawings and forms, lucky pieces, verbal commands."

Consultation with a physician left him disappointed because the doctor could offer no treatments he had not already tried except pills that the physician said were sometimes effective but often not. So he went home and drank a pint of Jack Daniel's, and shortly afterward the hiccups stopped. Why the hiccups ceased he did not know; what the hiccups were and why he had had them were also unclear, although "I had a decided opinion of what they were *not*," he said. "I had an equally decided preference for certain cures which seemed more compatible with the mysterious nature of the experience."

The patient perceived the illness, at different times but never at a fixed moment, as a mild annoyance, an absurd complaint, a nagging muscle spasm, and something mysterious in nature; at particular moments he found the situation exhausting, humorous, or frightening; once in a while he was angered by the hiccups, which he also occasionally felt might be a meaningful experience for him; sometimes he thought he knew what his hiccups were, but on other occasions he was unsure because the remedies that were employed in relationship to changing conceptions of the malady did not seem effective, although they presumably should have been. As the sense of urgency and mystery increased and as the conception of the nature of illness varied, the individual experimented with many kinds of treatments learned from others or invented by himself; he consulted medical texts and a physician in seeking an explanation of the illness and a cure for it. The concern for reasons why a therapy might or might not have been effective, although always important in the search for a proper remedy, paled in significance as the illness continued and the patient's desire increased for a dramatic solution to a significant and distressing problem. Entities? Belief system? Retention of cures?

NOTES

1. In contrast to his daughter Gladys, Jim Gallagher stressed the parents' difficulty in reaching a decision to permit him to lay his quivering left hand on Joey's chest and throat, and he emphasized the boy's problems in speaking or regaining his speech. These concerns are especially apparent in the interview of July 9, 1968, at

2:15 P.M., which I recorded, but they were expressed in Gallagher's other references to the case of the boy with warts on his vocal cords. I interviewed Joey Martin and his parents on November 27, 1969. The father did most of the talking, emphasizing the expense of Joey's illness (the family had to sell their home and many of their belongings because they had no insurance). After reviewing the circumstances of the case, the father said, "I never did believe these things, even though my father said them; but we were so desperate, you know. You'll try anything." He did not know how Jim's healing works, he said, only that it does. He alluded again to his desperation over Joey's illness and his acceptance but lack of understanding of Jim Gallagher's healing ability. Mrs. Martin concluded the interview, "We'll always believe it now."

2. There is uncertainty on this point. Some people told me simply that Gallagher was a seventh son; others said he was the seventh of a seventh; and on one occasion he himself said he was the seventh of a seventh of a seventh, which "gives me more power." One of several skeptics and detractors, however, insisted that Gallagher had no power at all because he was really the eighth son, since there had been a miscarriage before he was conceived.

3. Although rare, the malady is not unique. The Martin father said that the specialist who had treated Joey knew of two other cases, and the same affliction was reported recently in the *Los Angeles Times*, October 6, 1973: "Throat Tumors Reappear: Boy, 2, Kept Alive by Surgery Every Month" (stressed in the article are viral tumors the size of small warts, breathing difficulties, lack of speech, removal of warts thirteen times, frequent operations, and silver trachea that needs cleaning by the mother four times daily).

4. One might argue, in regard to the apparent failure to recall specific cases, that my expectations were unrealistic, for one can remember only so many incidents; that people were reticent about discussing such things with me; that individuals have no interest in the past; and that the people with whom I talked simply had poor memories or were inarticulate. As a way of accounting for the recall of only a few cases, one might suggest that the incidents communicated to me involved the individual himself as healer or patient or as family member, which is certainly correct in many but not all instances; and to explain the second question in this fashion leaves the first question unanswered.

5. To realize the significance of the striking or unusual in folklore research, one need only examine some remarks in Stith Thompson's *The Folktale* (New York: Holt, Rinehart, and Winston, 1946), especially definitions of "motif," p. 415, and "legend," pp. 8-9. See also W. H. R. Rivers, "The Sociological Significance of Myth," in *Studies on Mythology*, ed. Robert A. Georges (Homewood, Ill.: Dorsey Press, 1968), pp. 27-49. I want to thank Professor Georges for calling my attention to Rivers' article and for his invaluable insights into the study of human behavior (the discussion of perception and conception in this paper, for example, probably would not have been emphasized had it not been for comments made to me by Professor Georges). I wish to express my gratitude also to the National Museums of Canada for supporting my research on which the present essay is based and to Bruce Giuliano and Kenneth L. Ketner, with whom I had discussions about this paper. The topics of both legend and the striking or unusual qualities in experiences deserve much greater attention than I am permitted to give them in this note. All I can say, therefore, is that while several researchers have been fortunate enough to have discovered some previously unrecognized genres of folklore or new kinds of especially interesting data that others have missed, particularly what they call legends, little attention, strangely, has been given to these descriptions of case histories. Using the categories of legends established by Jan Harold Brunvand in *The Study of American Folklore: An Introduction* (New York: W. W. Norton & Company, 1968), pp. 87-99, as a point of departure, we might ask, are these descriptions of seemingly miraculous healing incidents by extraordinary individuals in particular areas of the country supernatural legends, personal legends, local legends (specifically, historical

legends), or religious legends? Attempts by the genre specialist to define these communications of case histories and distinguish them from other examples of communicative acts would benefit from the warnings, advice, and admonitions of Robert A. Georges in "The General Concept of Legend: Some Assumptions to be Reexamined and Reassessed," in *American Folk Legend: A Symposium*, ed. Wayland D. Hand (Berkeley, Los Angeles, London: University of California Press, 1971), pp. 1-19, and Wayland D. Hand in "Status of European and American Legend Study," *Current Anthropology*, 6 (1965), 439-446.

6. I am drawing on notes used for the preparation of a paper for presentation at the American Folklore Society meeting, Atlanta, Georgia, November 1969 (which was not actually read owing to my inability to attend the meeting), entitled "Forgotten and Remembered Cases of Folk Medical Treatment," and on discussion in an unpublished report submitted to the National Museums of Canada, February 1969. More information on the healing tradition may be found in my monograph *Why Faith Healing?*, National Museum of Man, National Museums of Canada, Canadian Center for Folk Culture Studies, Mercury Series, Paper no. 3 (Ottawa, 1972). This study is concerned primarily with the motivations of health personnel, about which little is known, to judge by the published literature; see also, however, Wayland D. Hand, "The Folk Healer: Calling and Endowment," which was read at the annual meeting of the American Folklore Society, Los Angeles, November 1970. Little is known about the seventh son tradition as well, and I am indebted to Professor Hand for permitting me to examine the cards that he has accumulated on this subject archived in the Folk Medical Collection of the Center for the Study of Comparative Folklore and Mythology, University of California, Los Angeles.

7. There are many problems in the study of oral history, but this may well be the most fundamental one. For a recent example of an attempt to reconstruct the past on the basis of communications in the present, see William Lynwood Montell, *The Saga of Coe Ridge: A Study in Oral History* (Knoxville: University of Tennessee Press, 1970); the descriptions of the curing of young Joey Martin communicated to me by Jim Gallagher, his daughter Gladys, the father Peter Martin, and other people might be examined in a similar way to establish the exact events that occurred. Perhaps a more interesting study, however, would be the meaning of the event for these people twenty-five years later as it relates to the interview situation, for, after all, what these individuals tell others depends on the social situation and other aspects of the specific occasions at different times.

8. There was a brief lull in the conversation, so I said, "I didn't know there's seven different kinds of eczema."

"There's seven different kinds," repeated Gladys. "Some is called psoriasis—medical, different names for it. Father says seven kinds. I know for sure there's three kinds," she said. "There's a wet eczema, dry eczema, and then there's something that itches. Now Bob Mullen had psoriasis. It's a big sore, what Bob Mullen had is a big sore, that's spread all over him," she explained and then told me of the many unpleasant details of this case. My point is, however, that these descriptions of instances of healing occurred throughout the continuum of conversation, although I have singled them out for purposes of illustration. I also wish to note that all the names used in this report are pseudonyms.

9. Some information about my reactions is given in *Why Faith Healing?*, pp. 23-27.

10. Speaking of faith, "I'll tell you what it all boils down to, mostly," one of the villagers told me in regard to some of these medical practices with which he was familiar, "regardless of what denomination, regardless of what church you are, what it all boils down to, if you have faith in what you're doing, faith that you'll get ahead with it, then you'll do that." His son added, "See, around here we're all Catholic and I s'pose believes in these things, using prayers to cure infections, with a faith. . . . Well, maybe we can't explain how it works, and you've got to have faith. A gold ring, see, for curing," he concluded, referring to curing a sty by passing a gold wedding ring over the eye three times. But faith is obviously important in many ways in our

lives, not only for accepting certain religious tenets but also for using some propositions in scholarship as assumptions for analytical purposes or accepting the outcome of such research.

11. The literature on suggestion therapy is becoming prolific, because many investigators have begun to treat folk medicine as psychotherapy; there is much to recommend this point of view. Consider, for example, the discussion of suggestion therapy in Jerome D. Frank's *Persuasion and Healing* (Baltimore, Md.: The John Hopkins Press, 1961; reprint ed., New York: Schocken Books, 1967); Ari Kiev's "The Psychotherapeutic Aspects of Primitive Medicine," *Human Organization*, 21 (1962), 25-29; or Lauri Honko's "On the Effectivity of Folk-Medicine," *Arv*, 18-19 (1962-1963), 290-300. Worth mentioning in the present context is "A Dermatologist Talks About Warts," *Today's Health* (March 19, 1963), pp. 40-41, 52-54, and 57-58, in which William R. Vath reveals, through conversations with doctors like E. William Rosenberg of Memphis, the kinds of suggestion therapy employed by dermatologists specializing in wart cures.

12. One finds "folk belief" and "folk medicine" characterized in this manner so often that it hardly seems necessary to single out particular works other than to admit that I am quoting from Ellen J. Stekert's article "Focus for Conflict: Southern Mountain Medical Beliefs in Detroit," *Journal of American Folklore*, 83 (1970), 115-156. I refer to this article only by way of exemplification and not for purposes of criticism, for there are many useful and significant points made by the author.

13. There obviously needs to be a reexamination of concepts and perspectives in the study of "belief" and medicine. I made a minor, and limited, attempt at broadening the scope of medicine study in "Toward an Understanding of Folk Medicine in North Carolina," *North Carolina Folklore*, 15 (1967), 23-27, and the scope of belief study in "Superstition: The Virtuous Weed," a paper presented at the California Folklore Society meeting, Dominguez Hills, May 1973. Some of the meanings of the terms *belief, superstition,* and *folk medicine* and some surveys of scholarship on the subject of belief and medicine may be found in Kenneth L. Ketner, "Superstitious Pigeons, Hydrophobia, and Conventional Wisdom," *Western Folklore*, 30 (1971), 1-17 (Ketner also attempts to deal with curing processually); Wayland D. Hand, "'The Fear of the Gods': Superstition and Popular Belief," in *American Folklore: Voice of America Forum Lectures*, ed. Tristram Potter Coffin (Washington, D.C.: United States Information Service, 1968), 215-227; and Wayland D. Hand, "Introduction," in *The Frank C. Brown Collection of North Carolina Folklore*, ed. Wayland D. Hand, vol. 6, *Popular Beliefs and Superstitions from North Carolina* (Durham, N.C.: Duke University Press, 1961), pp. xix-xlvii.

Texas and Southwest Medical Lore in the Anderson Collection, University of Houston

JOHN Q. ANDERSON, *University of Houston*

Items in the John Q. Anderson Folklore Archives at the University of Houston number 27,049. Contributions to this collection were made by about five hundred students in folklore courses that I taught over a period of five years, each semester and each summer term.

Each student is given a set of the instructions (included in the Appendix) and told to accumulate thirty to forty of the slips, to be turned in a month or more later. When the slips are returned, they are categorized according to the format used by Wayland D. Hand's edition of volumes 6 and 7 of the *Brown Collection of North Carolina Folklore*.[1] At the end of each term, the thirty to thirty-five students turn in about 950 slips, all of which are readily filed according to semesters. Included in the 27,049 general items of folklore in the archives are 13,622 entries dealing with folk medicine, of which 1,333 were published as *Texas Folk Medicine* which I edited and which was published as one of the Paisano Books of the Texas Folklore Society).[2]

What is unique about the Anderson Collection is that so many of the items come from Texas and the Southwest. A survey of one semester's compilation shows that of the 735 items collected in Texas, 35 were also collected in Louisiana and 25 in Arkansas (with some 50 others collected in other states and foreign countries). Although student-collectors were not advised in advance to solicit only from informants in the Southwest, it happened that the great part of the students at the University of Houston are from that region. Among southwestern students who took the course were Mexican Americans whose cures and remedies turned out to be the most exotic of the whole collection. I found their cures and remedies and beliefs to be the kind that would have been within the province of a *curandero* among their own people. Here is an example:

> Treatment for *susto*: The person suffering from fright [*susto*] is laid on the bed, a white cloth is placed over the face, the arms stretched out to make the sign of the cross. The healer takes a sip of water and holds it in his mouth while he "sweeps" the afflicted person with a branch of *pirul* [a small tree similar to mimosa]. The branch is thrown away. Recently, the palm frond, blessed on Sunday, has been substituted for the branch and is kept for further use. [Mexico; 1971].

Second to these Mexican American cures in exoticism are the remedies and beliefs obviously still held by black Americans who grew up in the cottonlands of Central and South Texas in such valleys as the Brazos and the Colorado. Some few of these beliefs reflect misunderstanding of white words, such as "come-a-Christian" for *palma christian*, or other types of language confusion. These black Americans achieved adulthood in time to reflect the speech of their elders and therefore to imitate what sociologists once thought was the difference between blacks and whites. Although there is a certain number of voodoo traditions and practices in the speech of these black Americans, belief in their efficacy begins to fade after 1960.[3] Even the voodoo dolls, so-called, may be bought at most novelty counters. Another example of black lore is the death knot, shown in the preface to Hyatt's second edition *Folk-Lore from Adams County, Illinois.*[4]

A third element in the southwestern content of the Anderson Collection is the lore on medicinal plants and herbs—such as prickly pear, creosote, and mesquite—that appear in some remedies. A mesquite bean is used to separate toes and fingers when these members have grown together. A fourth element is the southwestern birds and animals that appear in treatments, such as curing a boil by eating all or parts of a roadrunner.

The Anderson Collection has concentrated so far on the survival of European folk cures and remedies in the United States; for example, there are 925 wart cures in the collection. Some are in the category of the magical transference of disease (nailing, notching, plugging), which must reflect the most ancient of all wart removal cures: steal a dishrag, rub it on the wart, bury the rag underneath the back doorstep; when it rots, the wart will be gone. Of more interest to me all along has been those magical transference methods which presume to move the disease from the human patient to sticks, stones, trees, and objects.

Most of the 27,049 items in the Anderson Collection concern subjects that appear in the major collections already in print in North Carolina, Illinois, and Alabama. Most of these deal with everyday diseases, such as the common cold, mumps, measles, flu, and warts. Table 1 below shows how carefully these common diseases have been worked out in the Anderson Collection. It also shows medical items in the folklore archives all the way from "Arthritis & rheumatism" to "Warts."

Table 1

ITEMS IN THE JOHN Q. ANDERSON FOLKLORE ARCHIVES UNIVERSITY OF HOUSTON

Aches ... 52	Cuts ... 244	Insomnia ... 24	Stings, from plants ... 34
Acne ... 71	Dandruff ... 32	Itch ... 120	Stomach disorder ... 225
Appendicitis ... 8	Diabetes ... 15	Jaundice ... 9	Stuttering ... 4
Arthritis & rheumatism .. 462	Diphtheria ... 14	Kidney trouble ... 88	Stys ... 233
Asthma ... 119	Diarrhea & dysentery ... 157	Labor pains ... 80	Sunburn ... 137
Athlete's foot ... 35	Earache ... 347	Lice ... 45	Swelling ... 54
Bed-wetting ... 23	Eye ... 166	Measles ... 76	Teething ... 122
Bleeding ... 212	Fever ... 239	Mumps ... 93	Thrash ... 71
Blood ... 162	Fingernails ... 25	Nervousness ... 9	Tetanus ... 110
Boils ... 406	Flu ... 40	Night sweats ... 53	Thumb sucking ... 42
Bone felon ... 4	Freckles ... 74	Nosebleeds ... 265	Tonics ... 445
Bronchitis ... 11	Frostbite ... 30	Pain ... 12	Toothache ... 207
Bruises ... 98	Hair ... 145	Pneumonia ... 104	Ulcers ... 35
Burns ... 316	Hangover ... 90	Poison ivy ... 112	Warts ... 925
Chicken pox ... 58	Hay fever ... 31	Rabies ... 15	Whooping cough ... 89
Chills ... 53	Headache ... 191	Rash ... 100	Worms ... 152
Colds ... 845	Heart trouble ... 22	Ringworm ... 103	Wounds ... 150
Colic ... 110	Hiccup ... 431	Shingles ... 13	Animal cures ... 225
Complexion ... 90	Hives ... 69	Shock ... 19	Miscellaneous ... 851
Constipation ... 142	Ingrown toenail ... 38	Smallpox ... 8	
Convulsions ... 24	Indigestion ... 73	Snakebite ... 207	
Corns ... 62	Infection ... 98	Sores ... 93	
Coughs ... 331	Insect bites & stings ... 661	Sore throat ... 426	
Cramps ... 141		Splinters & thorns ... 81	
Crick ... 4		Sprains ... 124	Total ... 13,622
Croup ... 161			

The John Q. Anderson Folklore Archives at the University of Houston show that folk medicine and beliefs may well be the simplest of all examples of folklore for beginning students to collect. A simple assignment, simply made, can bring in hundreds of items each term. These items can be turned in, filed, and analyzed. The result is a rapidly growing accumulation of bound folders in which it is possible to check back on any one item.

The Anderson Collection shows, among other things, how quickly Texas and the Southwest are becoming urbanized. Only a generation ago most farmers in the region worried that if they sent their sons off to war or to work in Houston, they would not come back; now it is certain that they will not return. Furthermore, within Houston, neighborhoods are made up of enclaves of Mexican Americans, blacks, Cajuns, Greeks, and others who now by choice wish to remain separate. These ethnic groups will not, it seems, be as readily absorbed into the mainstream of the city as optimistic sociologists thought a few years back. If our experience at the University of Houston is indicative, collecting folk cures and remedies and beliefs in these neighborhoods will remain the easiest way to study the basic nature of American beliefs and will continue to be one of the best ways to collect folklore in the nation.

APPENDIX

English 433. Collecting Folk Medicine (cures and remedies).

Folk medicine may be classified in four groups: cures, treatments, removals, and preventives and health practices. Most ailments are *cured*; warts, blemishes, freckles are *removed*; burns, cuts, rashes are *treated*; some remedies *prevent* sickness or promote good health.

Diseases that appear in folk medicine include:

aches	colds	diabetes	headache
acne	colic	diphtheria	heart trouble
arthritis	constipation	dysentery	hiccups
(rheumatism)	convulsions	earache	hives
blood disorders	coughs	eye disorders	indigestion
boils	corns	fever	infection
bruises	cramps	flu	ingrown toenail
burns	croup	frostbite	insect bites
chicken pox	cuts	hangover	itch
chills	dandruff	hayfever	kidney trouble

labor pains	smallpox	stings	thumb sucking
lice	snakebite	stomach disorder	thrash
measles	sores	styes	toothache
mumps	sore throat	sunburn	ulcers
night sweats	splinters and	swelling	warts
nosebleeds	thorns	teething	whooping cough
poison ivy	sprains	tetanus	worms

Cures and remedies are also applied to domestic animals: cats, dogs, and farm animals.

Obtain full and precise information from the informant: whether the medication is used externally or internally; measurements and dosage; names of medicines or medicinal plants. Some removal remedies (i.e. warts) employ "supernatural" means, that is, rubbing with the hand, reciting Bible verses or other formulae and tabus; obtain details. Folk healers obtain and impart their special curative powers by traditional means, some parts of which are "secret." The informant may or may not know details; inquire.

Each cure, remedy, belief is recorded on a separate 3 × 5 slip, as shown below. These slips are permanently filed in the Archives; fill them out carefully and legibly. Each entry should be as complete as possible.

NOTES

1. Wayland D. Hand, ed., *The Frank C. Brown Collection of North Carolina Folklore*, vols. 6 and 7, *Popular Beliefs and Superstitions from North Carolina* (Durham, N.C.: Duke University Press, 1961-1964).

2. John Q. Anderson, *Texas Folk Medicine* (Austin, Tex.: The Encino Press, 1970).

3. See my article, "Popular Beliefs in Texas, Louisiana, and Arkansas," *Southern Folklore Quarterly*, 32 (1968), 304-319.

4. Harry Middleton Hyatt, *Folk-Lore from Adams County, Illinois* (New York: Memoirs of the Alma Egan Hyatt Foundation, 1935); Harry Middleton Hyatt, *Folk-Lore from Adams County, Illinois*, 2d ed. (New York, 1965)

Index

"Nothing like this valuable collection has been brought together before . . . A collection like this deserves wide reading; it raises many intriguing questions for historians and for all those in the health fields." —*American Scientist*

"This intriguing and informative volume contains twenty-six papers presented before a Conference on American Folk Medicine held in 1973 . . . The papers range in time from the dawn of consciousness to the present, most treating recent and contemporary practices; in geography from Canada to South America, most centering within the United States; in cultural group from Amish to Cajun to Jamaican to Mexican American, the largest single category focusing on American Indian medicine; in theme from the madstone to the mole, from the birthmark to the balmyard, the variety too rich to credit properly here."
—*Journal of the History of Medicine*

"Until the publication of this book, no attempt had been made to provide the student of folk medicine with a collection of diverse approaches to topics in the discipline. . . . [this is] a seminal work within the realm of this major genre of folklore, and might well be understood as being a useful mirror of contemporary folkloristics."
—*Kentucky Folklore*

"The authors represent a number of fields and the articles cover a very wide variety of topics. Each is a scholarly contribution with excellent documentation, and the book as a whole is a repository of information, a function it will retain for some time. . . . Because of the multidisciplinary nature of its contents it will be consulted by a large number of individuals." —*Medical History*

University of California Press
Berkeley 94720

Cover design by Laurie Anderson

ISBN 0-520-04093-2